MINIINVASIVE FACE AND BODY LIFTS – CLOSED SUTURE LIFTS OR BARBED THREAD LIFTS

Edited by **Nikolay Serdev**

Miniinvasive Face and Body Lifts – Closed Suture Lifts or Barbed Thread Lifts
http://dx.doi.org/10.5772/2654
Edited by Nikolay Serdev

Contributors

Nikolay Serdev, M. B. Des Fernandes, Meity Hidayani, Syarief Hidayat, Dali Amiruddin, Roberto Tulli, Ronald Feiner, Chedly Bouzouaya, M.A. Sulamanidze, G.M. Sulamanidze, C.M. Sulamanidze, K. Sulamanidze, A.A. Adamyan, N.D. Skuba, Z.R. Khusnutdinova, I.S. Vozdvizhenskiy, K.M. Sulamanidze, E.G. Azizyan, M. Sulamanidze, G. Sulamanidze, I. Vozdvizhenskiy, K. Sulamanidze, A. Kadzhaya, Peter Prendergast, Pier Antonio Bacci, O. Gaziullina, O. Zhukova, S. Shostak, Vilma L. Padín

Published by InTech

Janeza Trdine 9, 51000 Rijeka, Croatia

Copyright © 2013 InTech

Notice

Publishing Process Manager Ana
Pantar **Technical Editor** InTech DTP team
Cover InTech Design team

Additional hard copies can be obtained from orders@intechopen.com

Miniinvasive Face and Body Lifts – Closed Suture Lifts or Barbed Thread Lifts,
Edited by Nikolay Serdev
p. cm.
ISBN 978-953-51-1196-2

Meet the editor

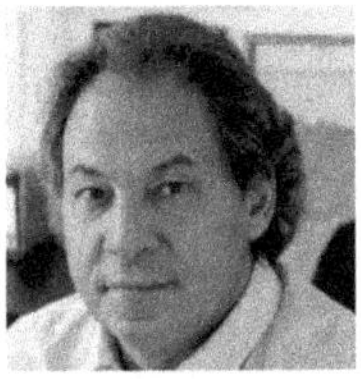

Prof. Dr. Nikolay Serdev, MD, PhD is a renowned cosmetic doctor and surgeon. He has trained hundreds of doctors globally, in minimally invasive aesthetic surgery and medical procedures. He is a founding member of the European Society of Aesthetic Surgery and the International Board of Cosmetic Surgery. He is a Honorary President of the Bulgarian Society of Aesthetic Surgery and Aesthetic Medicine, Honorary Professor of the New Bulgarian University, the International College of Cosmetic Surgery, the South East Asia College of Cosmetic Surgery, Honorary member of the Australian College of Cosmetic Surgery, South American Academy of Cosmetic Surgery, French Society of Aesthetic Surgery and numerous other international societies. Dr. Serdev is the author of "Scarless Serdev Suture® lifts" of face and body and pioneer in many mini-invasive cosmetic surgery techniques: ultrasound liposculpture of face, body; leg elongation and beautification; T-excision and columella sliding in rhinoplasty; non-surgical body contouring; and combination approaches to facial volumising and rejuvenation. He is also a world authority in ultrasound-assisted (VASER) body contouring and has trained doctors from around the world in its basic and advanced techniques. Dr. Serdev divides his time between his clinic, the New Bulgarian University in Sofia and short travels for hands-on courses in countries of all continents. He is editor of the most comprehensive textbook in Liposuction and has authored many chapters in aesthetic surgery and medicine, as well as original papers in leading medical journals.

Contents

Preface XI

Section 1 Transcutaneous Suture Lifts and Suspensions 1

Chapter 1 **Serdev Sutures® in Upper Face: Brow and Temporal Lift; Glabella Muscle Ligation 3**
Nikolay Serdev

Chapter 2 **Serdev Sutures® in Middle Face 43**
Nikolay Serdev

Chapter 3 **Serdev Sutures® in Lower Face and Neck 95**
Nikolay Serdev

Chapter 4 **Serdev Sutures® Lifts in Body Areas 127**
Nikolay Serdev

Chapter 5 **Percutaneous Suspension Sutures to Change the Nasal Tip 153**
M. B. Des Fernandes

Chapter 6 **Chin Enhancement Using Serdev Suture: Five Case Reports 163**
Meity Hidayani, Syarief Hidayat and Dali Amiruddin

Chapter 7 **Serdev Technique for Cervicoal Flaccidity and Mandibular Definition Utilizing "Serdev Sutures" 173**
Roberto Tulli

Chapter 8 **Suture Lifting and Liposculpture Integration in the Creation of Facial Esthetic Harmony 185** Ronald Feiner and Chedly Bouzouaya

Chapter 9 **The Holistic Scarless Rejuvenation of the Face 195**
M. B. Des Fernandes

Chapter 10 **Midface Thread Lifting: Method of Internal Suturing 213**
M.A. Sulamanidze, G.M. Sulamanidze and C.M. Sulamanidze

Chapter 11 **Mastopexy – How to Reach Consistent Results – New Methods 231**
M. Sulamanidze, G. Sulamanidze and K. Sulamanidze

Section 2 Barbed Thread Lifts 249

Chapter 12 **Morphological Foundations of Facelift Using APTOS Filaments 251**
A.A. Adamyan, M.A. Sulamanidze, N.D. Skuba and Z.R. Khusnutdinova

Chapter 13 **Experience in Preventive Measures and Treatment of Complications at Face and Neck Thread Rejuvenation 263**
M.A. Sulamanidze, I.S. Vozdvizhenskiy, G.M. Sulamanidze, K.M. Sulamanidze and E.G. Azizyan

Chapter 14 **New Method of Face Elastic Thread Lift 277**
M. Sulamanidze, G. Sulamanidze, I. Vozdvizhenskiy, K. Sulamanidze and A. Kadzhaya

Section 3 Barbed Threads Sutured One Side 287

Chapter 15 **Minimally Invasive Face and Neck Lift Using Silhouette Coned Sutures 289**
Peter Prendergast

Section 4 Combined Techniques - Sutures and Barbed Threads 307

Chapter 16 **T3 - Soft Face Lift by Suspension Surgery 309**
Pier Antonio Bacci

Chapter 17 **Correction of Face Involutional Changes by Method of Light Lift Elegance Thread Reinforcement 323**
O. Gaziullina, O. Zhukova and S. Shostak

Chapter 18 **Experience in the Use of Barbed Threads and Non-Barbed Serdev Sutures in Face and Body Lift – Comparison and Combination 333**
Vilma L. Padín

Preface

Both Suture lifts and Thread lifts present closed scarless techniques of tissue suspension, but they fix different tissue and use different type of fixation. These are totally dissimilar techniques and should be differentiated.

The number of such techniques is growing without precise understanding and formulation. Presently, there is no clear description and definition of the differences, results, and longevity of these two mini-invasive techniques. They use different instruments and materials in different areas and layers, and give different results.

Both suture and threads are scarless, the downtime is shortened. In some countries they are called "coffee break" or "lunch procedures".

This will be the first scientific book that could clear the false public beliefs that both suture and thread lifts are one and the same method:

- Suture liftings present a closed method to fix mobile SMAS and fascias to immobile stable tissue like periosteum, fascias, or tendons, using only skin perforations. Sutures could be used for liftings, suspension, and tissue enhancement (volumising) at the same time.
- Thread lifts are a different technique that uses barbed threads, which are not sutured, but placed in the subdermal fat. They fix subdermal tissue between barbs.

The growing public interest in mini-invasive interventions in cosmetic surgery requires clear description and differentiation of these two techniques and their results, as well as scientific information about the different instruments and materials used. This clarification will be hugely beneficial both for patients and doctors, having in mind the increasing number of such interventions.

Prof. Dr. Nikolay Serdev
National Consultant of the Ministry of Health in the Specialty of "Cosmetic (Aesthetic) Surgery" 2006-2008,
Director of University Program in Cosmetic Surgery at New Bulgarian University,
Head, Medical Center "Aesthetic Surgery, Aesthetic Medicine",
Bulgaria

Section 1

Transcutaneous Suture Lifts and Suspensions

Chapter 1

Serdev Sutures® in Upper Face: Brow and Temporal Lift; Glabella Muscle Ligation

Nikolay Serdev

Additional information is available at the end of the chapter

http://dx.doi.org/10.5772/55673

1. Introduction

Closed approach transcutaneous Serdev Suture® lifts encompass the principale concept of stable suturing and fixation of mobile fascias to immobile periosteum, tendons and fascias, resulting in suture suspension and/or volume augmentation and/or repositioning.

21 techniques and individual modifications are used on face and in body areas, even where open surgical techniques cannot be directly applied. Serdev Sutures® are scarless and uncomplicated in the post-operative period. These techniques use curved semi-blunt semi-elastic needles and smooth surgical sutures to elevate and fixate mobile fascial tissue. Polycon surgical sutures are preferred for these techniques. They are characterized by short elasticity to prevent mobilized tissue from rupture and are characterized by delayed resorption (in 2-3 years, after the fibrosis is finalized). This enables stable fibrotic fixation before suture degradation.

Fixed mobile facial tissue using Serdev Sutures® is SMAS in all face areas: upper facial SMAS (galea aponeurotica), zygomatic SMAS extension, cheek SMAS, platysma and others. It is fixed by suture to stable, immobile tissues, such as periosteum, temporal fascia, zygoma, coli fascia, mastoid, occipital bone etc.

In addition to the possibility of lifting, Serdev Sutures® follow aesthetic principles of beautification: adaptation of aesthetic proportions, volumes and angles. In art and theatre, face masks called "mask of tragedy" and "mask of comedy" are well known and used to express age, status and emotions. The concept of scarless suture lift in face is to convert the "mask of tragedy" into a "mask of comedy", i.e. to uplift the subcutaneous facial mask – the SMAS. As soft tissue and skin are attached to the SMAS by a trabecular system, an intrinsic consequence of SMAS lifting is reflected in the lifting of the face and its most important elements in the same direction.

The structuring and positioning of different face elements is not limited to facial ptosis and elderly cases. Unaesthetic face angles, volumes and proportions are responsible for lack of beauty in young patients as well. Beautification is most important in youth and rejuvenation incl. beautification in elderly. Changing SMAS position by sutures can restore aesthetic angles, shape, volume and proportions as a basis for beautification and rejuvenation, imparting a happy, youthful appearance and a smiling expression.

1.1. History

Scarless closed approach Serdev Suture® lifts present skeletal fixation using skin punctures, without incisions and excisions, as a first alternative to classic excision lifts. Sutures are the same as in open surgery, but with much more variations and even in areas not reachable in open surgery. The anatomy study, instrument creation and surgical suture selection commenced in 1990 and the entire understanding of local topographic anatomy, instrumentarium and technique of this new method was ready in 1993. Needle preparation and selection of surgical sutures was experimental. For sutures stretch, elasticity and cut through tests were performed. The long term absorption of the sutures is crucial in the author's method. In 1994, at the Second annual meeting of the National Bulgarian Society of Aesthetic Surgery and Aesthetic Medicine, most of the scarless suture techniques for correction of early ptosis and flabbiness in areas of face and body were presented, as well as the initial results with 54 patients, operated during the period from 1993 to 1994. The author's contribution is that the transcutaneous closed approach suture techniques lift the SMAS and the facial skin attached to it, without traditional incisions. Operations were ambulatory with excellent results, reported by the patients. The trauma is minimal and the follow-up period is no longer than 3 days with fast and mostly immediate return to work and social life. There are no visible scars and the needle perforations on the skin are no longer visible after days.

1.2. Technique and anatomical fixations

Operations are ambulatory, without hospital stay. Trauma is minimal. The techniques consist of passing closed sutures, by needle perforations only, to lift mobile fascias supporting the skin and fix them to immobile skeletal structures (such as periosteum) in several facial and body areas.

The author has invented and performs the following scarless transcutaneous closed approach **suture lifts**:

1. **In face areas**: **Temporal lift** (upper SMAS to upper temporal line and temporal fascia) and **supra-temporal lifting** (upper SMAS to upper temporal line), **Brow lift** (orbito-cutaneous brow fascia, discovered by the author, to upper temporal line periosteum 1.5 cm above the upper orbital rim or at the hair line), **Lateral canthus lift** (to orbital rim or to upper temporal line and temporal fascia), **Mid-face lift** (SMAS zygomatic extension to temporo-parietal tendon and to upper temporal line periosteum), **Cheekbone lift** (fascial tube of Bichat fat pad, SMAS and zygomatic SMAS extension to zygoma

periosteum, to upper temporal line and temporal fascia, to temporo-parietal tendon etc.) **as well as Augmentation** using patient's own tissue, **Smiling dimple formation, Lower SMAS-platysma face and neck lift** (platysma fixation to mastoid), **Chin enhancement, form and position correction** with or without fixation to the menton periosteum, **Chin dimple formation, Sutures in rhinoplasty** for **tip rotation** (medial crura of greater alar cartilages to nasal bone periosteum), **tip refinement** (suturing together all 4 crura of both greater alar cartilages at the dom), **alar base narrowing** (suturing the alar base incl. accessory alar cartilages), **Otoplasty** (perihondrium suture to obtain the antihelix fold) etc.

2. **In body areas: Breast lift** (fixation of breast fascia and upper glandular tissue to clavicle and/or to pectoralis major tendon), **suture technique for Simmastia, or implant position correction, Buttocks lift** (fixation of the fibrous soft tissue to the sacro-cutaneous fascia, found by the author), **Abdominal flaccidity tightening** (linea alba shortening, superficial fascia to costal line, spina iliaca superior anterior), **Inner thigh lift** etc.

1.3. Results

The suture methods became possible after creating specific curved, semi-elastic, semi-blunt needles. Best results were obtained with the Bulgarian polycaproamide sutures Polycon, which ensure semi-elastic fixation of mobile to immobile tissue (unlike other available non elastic and non-absorbable surgical sutures). The author has experimentally evaluated that they do not cut through the tissues.

Preferred **surgical suture** qualities are – short elasticity, absorbable within two-three years - after final fibrosis formation, and anti-microbial action. The author's tests have shown that only Polycon surgical sutures ensure these qualities. - http://medicaldevices-bg.com/MDI/Threads.html.

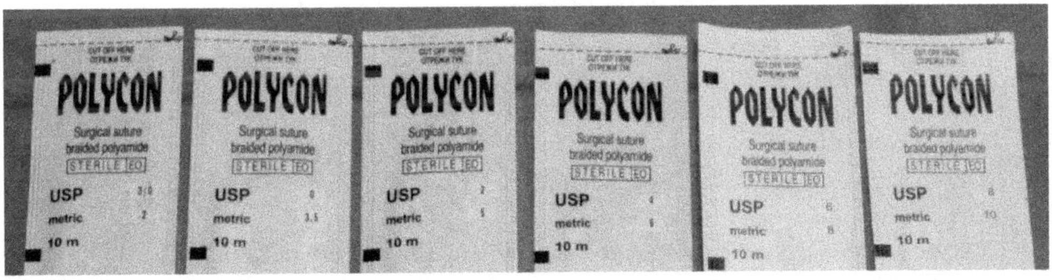

Figure 1. Polycon surgical sutures (3/0, 0, 2, 4, 6, 8) are semi-elastic (short elasticity), braided polycaproamide sutures of different thickness and have anti-microbial qualities.

USP depends on application. **6 different USPs** are suitable for different procedures and body areas:

- **USP 3/0** - for ear and nose: tip & base
- **USP 0** - for chin & brow lift
- **USP 2** - for facial, inner thigh, abdomen lifts

- **USP 4** - for temporal, mid-face lifts, buttocks & breast lifts
- **USP 6** - for bigger buttocks & large breast lifts
- **USP 8** - for bigger buttocks lifts (mostly used in Latin America)

Polycon surgical sutures are absorbed in the human body within 2-3 years, i.e. after the final fibrosis. According to the author, these are the best surgical sutures for lifting methods, because they permit semi-elastic movement of the sutured tissues.

1.4. Contributions

Serdev Suture® lifts, suspensions and volumizing present the first lifting method to replace scarring classic excision lifts as a complete method for scarless transcutaneous closed approach in total face and body lifts, where mobile fascias (holding skin by trabecular system) can be lifted and fixed to immobile periosteum, tendons and fascias.

1.4.1. Author suture techniques present

- A new method for closed approach face and body liftings – a new alternative to classic excision lifts;
- Scarless lifting, using skin punctures only (no incisions or excisions);
- Mini-invasive, no downtime procedures;
- Beautification and rejuvenation methods;
- Volumizing method without implants and transplants. When needed, tissue augmentation is performed using patient's own tissue – a new alternative without implants;
- Can be used in cosmetic, aesthetic and plastic-reconstructive surgery;
- Downtime is shortened from weeks into some days;
- No danger of hematoma formation, no nerve damage, no scars.

Serdev® Needles are specially designed and developed for best use and have the following qualities:

- Elastic curve (the curve cannot be deformed when applying pressure in patients tissue);
- Smooth surface (does not cut periosteum);
- Conical semi-blunt tip (trauma is minimized);
- Thickness depends on length (from 50 mm to 250 mm) and application - http://medicaldevices-bg.com/MDI/Serdev_Needles.html.

11 different needle lengths were developed specifically for one or more face & body lifting techniques:

- Mini Mini 50 - for ear and nose: tip and alar base
- Mini Mini 50 (bended) - for fine chin subperiosteal fixations
- Mini 60 - for brow, chin, temporal, mid-face, cheekbone etc. lifts
- Mini 60 (bended) - for fine mid-face subperiosteal fixations

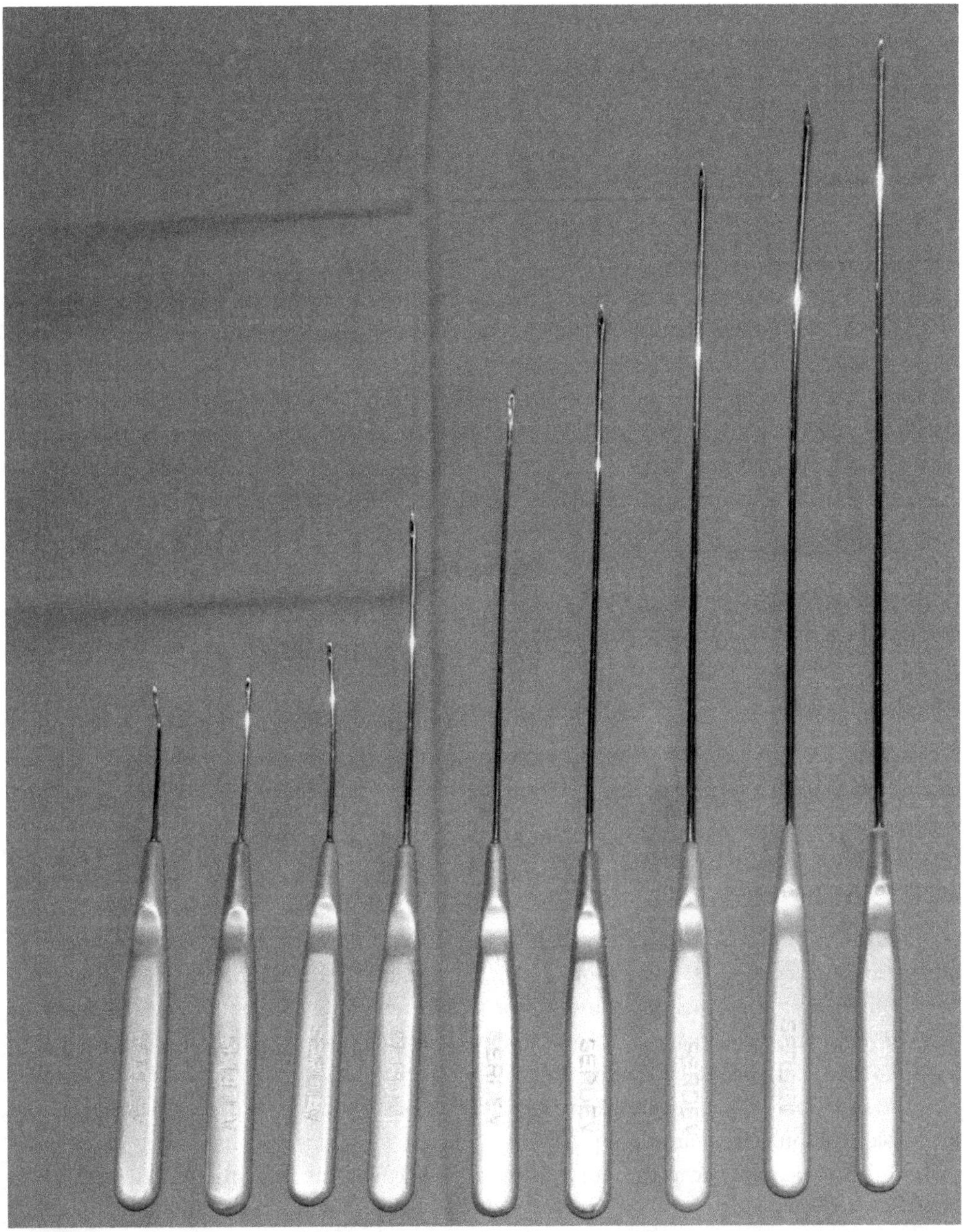

Figure 2. Serdev® needles (from left to right): Mini Mini 50 mm (bended), Mini Mini 50 mm, Mini 60 mm, Small 100 mm, Medium 140 mm, Long 170 mm, Super Long 210 & 230, and Super Super Long 250 mm (mostly used in Latin America).

- Small 80 - for neck lifts
- Small 100 - for facial, inner thigh, abdomen lifts
- Medium 140 - for mid-face, breast, abdomen lifts
- Long 170 - for buttock and breast lifts
- Super Long 210 - for buttock lifts *
- Super Long 230 - for buttock lifts *
- Super Super Long 250 - for buttock lifts *

*The choice of length depends on patient's physical characteristics

The needles are similar in shape to the currently used surgical needles with a handle to ease manipulation, with an eye at the needle tip (example Reverdin needles). However, Serdev® Needles are different in surface, elasticity, shape, size, thickness and have a curved elastic section (that retains structural curve memory regardless of the applied pressure). The elasticity and smooth polished surface allows the needles to safeguard bone-periosteal structures against cutting, regardless of the length and change of direction of the moving needle. The semi-blunt tip and elastic needle characteristics combine to avoid tissue trauma. The needle curve is specifically designed to provide ease of skin ingress, fluid movement through different soft tissue levels and periosteum, and the capture of fascial tissue. The semi-blunt tip exhibits variable penetrative qualities adapting to the application of the respective methods. The handle is flat and has a concavity mark for secure handling and display of needle tip position in the tissue.

1.5. Discussion

Scarless Serdev Suture® liftings use closed approach fixation of specific mobile fascial tissue to immobile skeleton periosteum without incisions. In Brazil they are known as "fio elastico" or "fio bulgaro". The Serdev Suture® techniques are used to correct early ptosis and flaccidity in areas of face and body, without traditional incisions. They are used also for tissue augmentation.

Observing Dr. Serdev's videos without proper training and understanding of anatomy led to "modified" techniques using non-original or straight needles, performing superficial barbed threads that are neither sutured, nor fixed, free floating in subdermal fat tissue or fixed only superiorly. Superficial threads and sutures fixed solely to the trabecular system in the subdermal fat cannot guarantee outcome longevity. Using straight needles is an over simplification that fails to secure deep fixation of mobile to immobile tissues that is essential for stable fixation. These are easy procedures for non-surgeons and this is the reason that this oversimplification became popular. However, outcomes are insecure. As little as a 1 or 2 mm change is enough to miss the topography of the important anatomical fixations such as bony rim, level of fascias and tendons. Therefore it is essential that doctors have a critical perception about the differences between suture lifts of mobile to immobile stable tissues and superficial thread lifts in subdermal fat.

2. Brow lift

Multiple invasive techniques have been described for fixation of the scalp and upper face. However, these methods do not allow the direct positioning of the brow as in the suture method described by the author. Within the past decade the demand for minimally invasive surgery, fast recovery and immediate beautification outcomes have revised the trend toward extensive surgical procedures and radically changed surgery in face-forehead beautification and rejuvenation. Even minimal incision approaches to brow lifting, using endoscopic methods or excisions of supra-brow skin, are associated with longer down time and have become undesirable options for beautification in younger patients. Improved understanding of eyebrow anatomy, pathophysiology of the aging face and advances in small - and non-incision surgery, have contributed to the new approach in correction of the eyebrow position for beautification and rejuvenation. The Serdev Suture® method with needle skin perforations between the eyebrow hairs has been reported and introduced internationally since 1994. The concept is to capture mobile but stable tissue (the orbito-supercilliar fascia, discovered by the author) and attach it to firm, immobile upper temporal line bone and periosteum.

The eye-eyebrow is the most influential region in determining facial expressions. There is only a narrow range of eyebrow positions that are perceived as attractive. Artistic location of the eyebrow is a guide line for eyebrow repositioning. The author has reviewed the young position of the eyebrow in models and also the artistic experience and aesthetic criteria for ideal female eyebrow height and shape in both international fashion models and movie stars. The preferred distance from the upper orbital rim to the eyebrow tail is on average 1.5 cm. Eyebrow shape should have a lateral apex slant. In male patients a lesser rise of the eyebrow tail has to be considered. The importance of aesthetic anatomy, aesthetic assessment and treatment planning in evaluation of the face must take into account considerations of patient selection, indications, and contraindications.

The author performs brow lift by suture in cases of ptosis, asymmetry, or in patients who desire a non-scarring and non-invasive procedure. Indications are beautification, rejuvenation, correction of proportions and angles.

2.1. Procedure

The brow lift suture is done by needle punctures only between the eyebrow hairs to prevent scaring. It presents a stable fixation of the orbito-supercilliar fascia to the periosteum of the rim of the upper temporal line, 1.5 cm above the orbital rim or at the hair line. The subperiosteal bite line (1.5 cm above the orbital rim) defines the eybrow design. An important instrument that facilitates performing this technique is the curved, semielastic, semiblunt mini-mini Serdev® needle with length of 50 mm that can be turned down and up in order to enter through the skin, capture periosteum or fascias and exit through another skin perforation point (Fig. 5). It is most important that we have at our disposal the 0 polycaproamide surgical sutures with marked elasticity that are biodegradable in the longer term (in 2-3 years), antimicrobial and braided (Fig. 1, 4). The semielastic, braided, USP 0 suture permits movements of face and muscles, fixation under elastic tension and does not traumatise or cut the sutured tissue. The extended period of resorption quality allows time for a stable fibrosis formation and does not leave foreign bodies in the tissue after the fibrotic fixation formation process and suture absorption is complete.

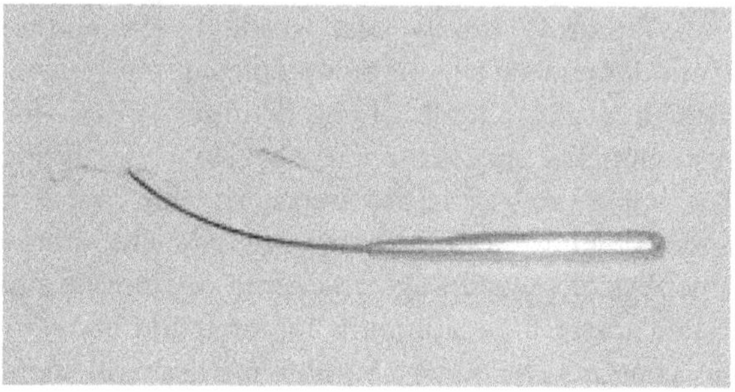

Figure 3. Curved, elastic, semi-blunt 50 mm or 60 mm Serdev® needle.

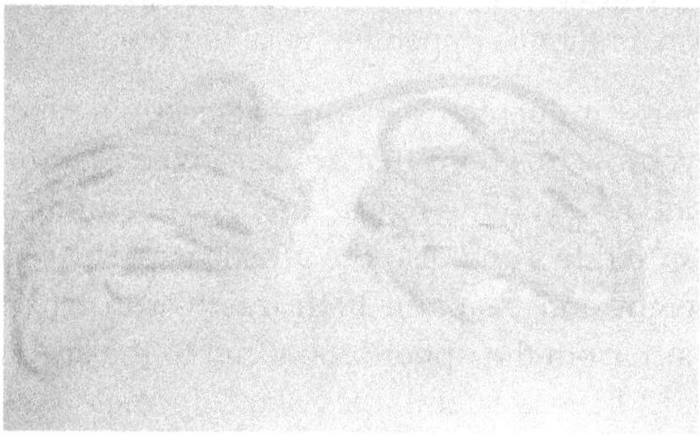

Figure 4. Semi-elastic, absorbable, braided, anti-microbial, polycaprocamide surgical sutures USP 0 are preferable and give best results.

2.2. Method for scarless brow lift by suture

1. Fixation of the orbito-supercilliar fascia to the periosteum of the upper temporal line, 1.5 cm above the orbital rim

To perform and accomplish the brow lift suture, the author uses 2 perforation points between the hairs of the brow, using the tip of a No. 11 scalpel blade. The perforation points are located on both sides of the intersection of the lateral canthus line and the eyebrow (Fig. 5A, B). The lateral canthus line is very important as the upper temporal line rim is located along this line, above the upper orbital rim. To position the eyebrow for artistic fixation, the forehead skin is pulled with a thumb placed 1 cm higher than the eyebrow, at the lateral canthus line. The maximum pull positions the eyebrow tail at the desired level of 1.5 cm over the upper orbital rim, without exeption. **NB!** Do not pull the eyebrow itself, which is looser and more mobile - it will result in a wrong brow tail position. After local anesthesia, while holding the eyebrow lifted, a 50 mm Serdev® needle is introduced through the lateral skin perforation point A with the tip pointing down, slides down on the rough surface of the upper temporal line rim, taking its periosteum, and becomes fixed. **NB!** If the needle is not

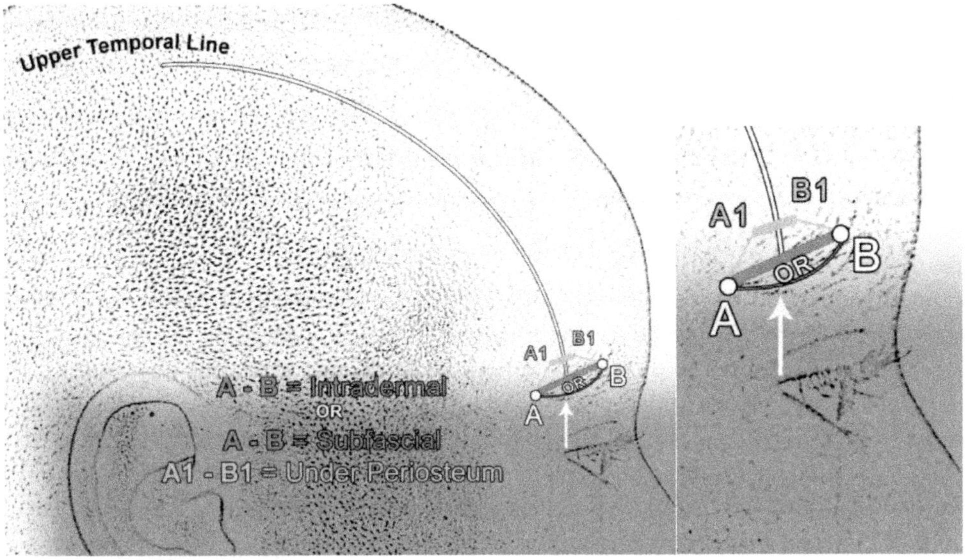

A.

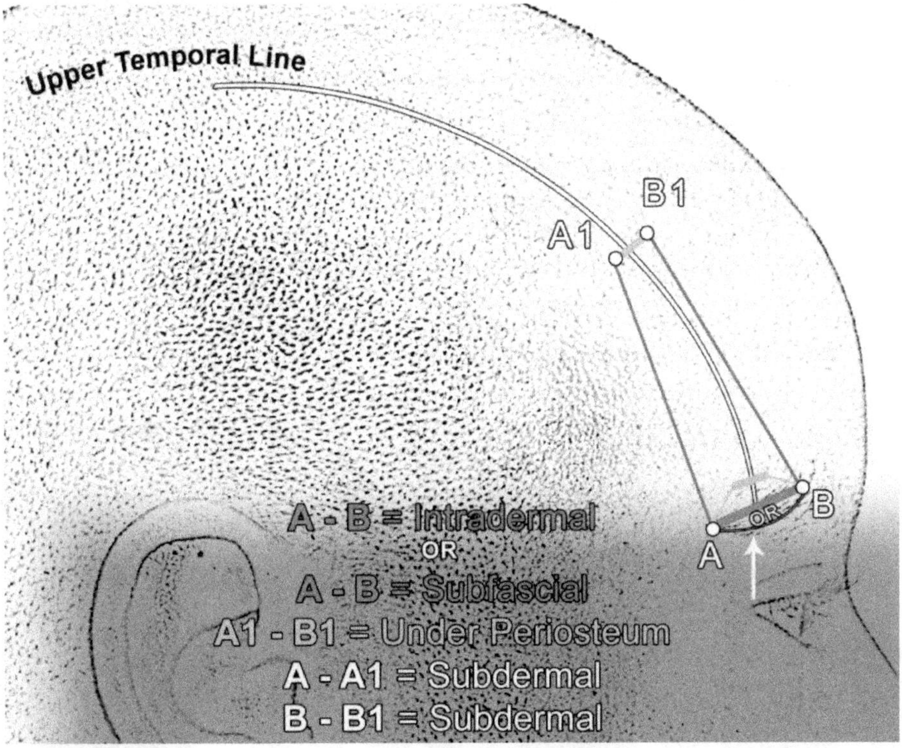

B.

Figure 5. **A.** Eyebrow lifting by suture to the upper temporal line, 1.5 cm above the superior orbital rim. **B.** Eyebrow lifting by suture to the upper temporal line at the hair line.

fixed and can be moved lateraly, it is wrongly located in a superficial tissue plane and its position should be changed deeper subperiosteal. Turning the tip up, the needle exits through the medial skin perforation - point B. **NB!** Prevent dermis fixation. The needle should not feel any resistance when passing through the skin perforation points. This could be facilitated twisting the needle gently forward and backward. Do not push or pull. After threading the needle eye, the surgical suture is introduced and positioned through the first needle pass – stable immobile subperiosteal fixation. The second needle pass is done through the lower dermis layer between the points A and B at the lower eyebrow line. After exiting through point B and re-threading the needle, the second end of the surgical suture is pulled out through the second needle pass that presents fixation of the mobile orbito-supercilliar fascia, found by the author to hold the eyebrow to the upper orbital rim. The knot of the suture is done under medium elastic tension. A symmetry check follows. Equal lift of the skin on both sides gives us symmetry in all cases. If even a slight asymmetry is noted, an additional suture is performed to solve it. Then, pressure is used to flatten the brow over the suture and stop any bleeding. Still using pressure, skin at perforation points A and B is pulled away from the suture with a mosquito clamp, in order to remove any dimpling. No bandages are necessary. A skin color tape is placed on the upper eyelid that stays on overnight to reduce (suck) swelling by the hypertensive quality of the glue.

Additionally, through a 3-mm medial brow incision, glabellar muscles can be excised or ligated.

Post-op care: Next day, tapes are removed from upper lids. Face washing is obligatory to remove residual blood. Swelling in the suture area and the upper lid is nearly invisible for observers. No bruising appears in 99% of the cases. Patients can return to social life. Wound disinfection should be performed several times in the next 2-3 days.

Video http://www.youtube.com/watch?v=cLUf6-OrMPg

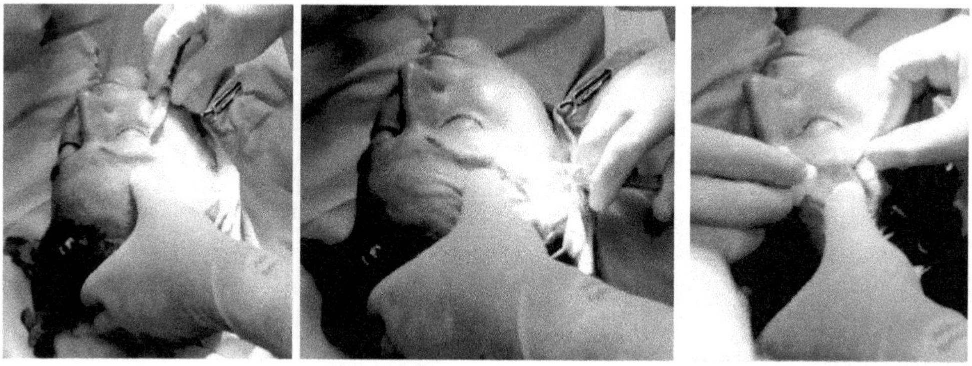

A. B. C.

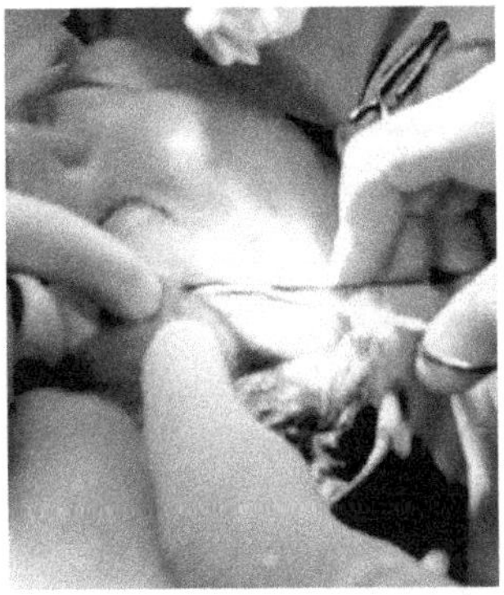

D.

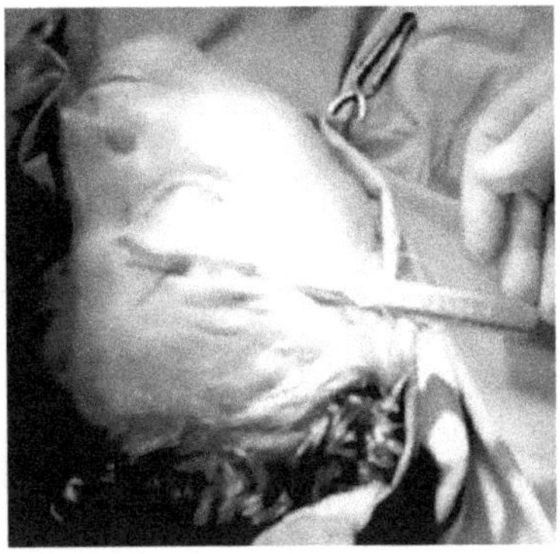

E.

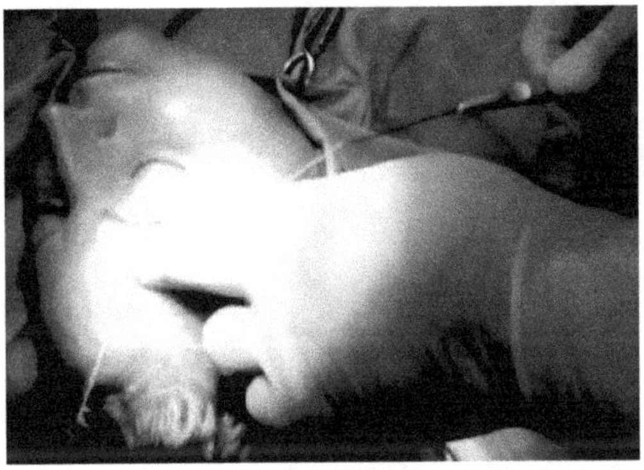

F.

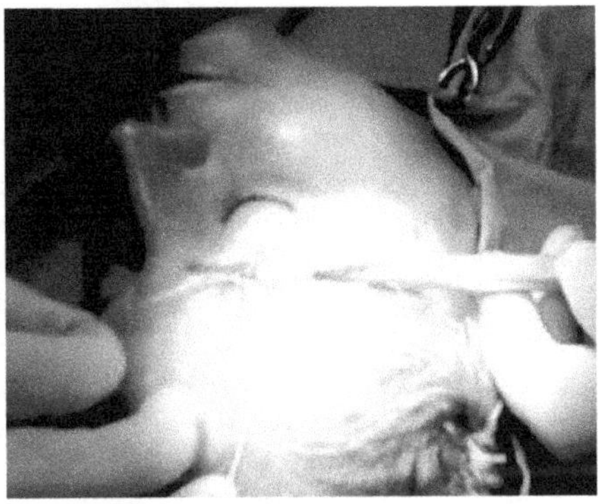

G.

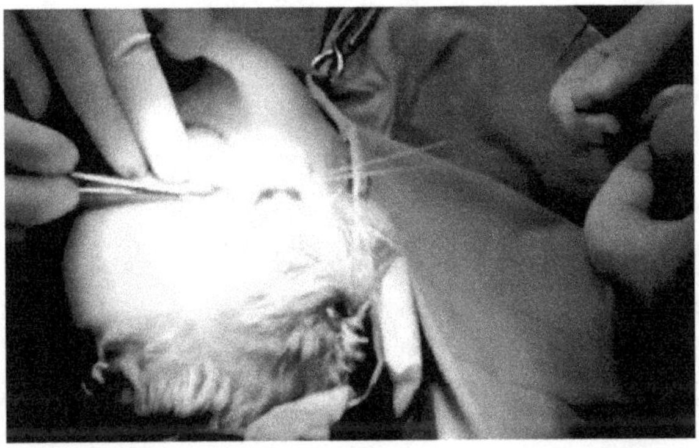

H.

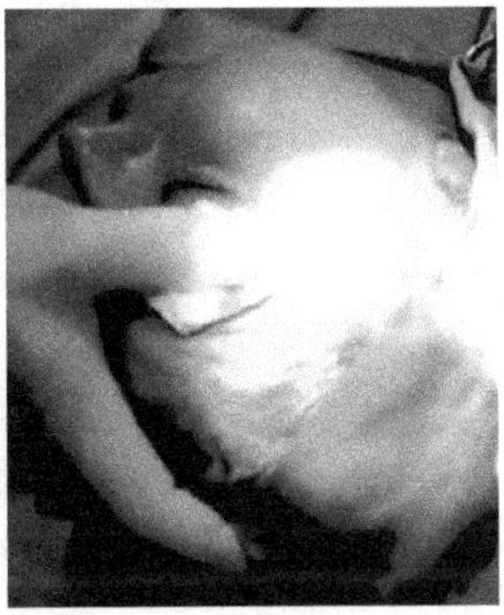

I.

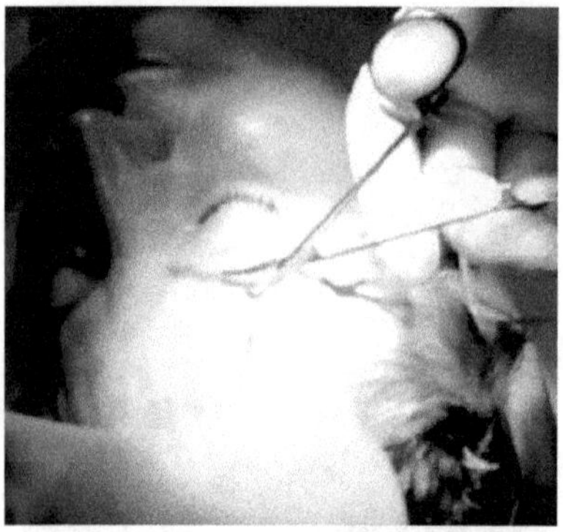

J.

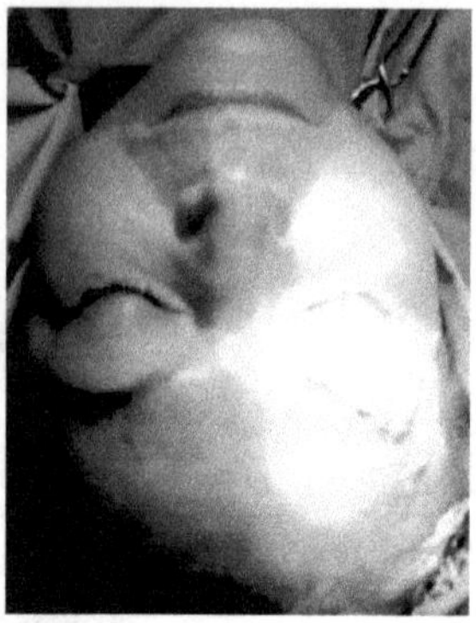

K.

Figure 6. Steps of eyebrow lift by suture. A. The needle shows where the lateral canthus line is crossing the brow. Skin perforation points A and B are located on both sides of this intersection point. Higher, on the lateral canthus line, the upper temporal line (rim) can be palpated with the thumb. Locate your thumb on the rim, 1 cm higher than the eyebrow; **B.** Lift the eyebrow with the thumb maximally and hold the brow in this position. Infiltrate point A and B, then the periosteum between, and also intradermally. Use a small amount of local anesthesia, injecting a few drops per line, to prevent swelling; **C.** Still holding the thumb in the same position, perforate points A and B with a No. 11 blade; **D.** Perforate the subdermal fascia at points A and B with the tip of a thin mosquito clamp; **E.** Still holding the brow in maximum lifted position, introduce the Serdev® needle 50mm subperiosteally between A and B. To test for proper placement, release your hand from the skin and the needle. If the needle stays in the proper subperiosteal position without moving, it is properly fixed. If needle moves, repeat this pass subperiosteally; **F.** Load the needle tip and introduce the USP 0 surgical suture subperiosteally in the line B-A; **G.** Second A-B needle pass is just subdermal, just below the brow line i.e. below the Serdev orbito-supercilliar fascia. Load the needle and introduce the second end of the surgical suture into the subcutaneous line B-A; **H.** The suture circle is finalized; **I.** Press for a minute and a half to stop any bleeding; **J.** Remove dimples at points A or B; **K.** The brow lift result is immediate. Perform the same steps the other side, holding the skin maximally lifted at the upper temporal line (rim), 1 cm higher that the brow. If the traction with the thumb is equal on both sides, the eyebrows will be lifted equally. Flex the head to check for equality.

2. Fixation of the orbito-supercilliar fascia to the periosteum of the upper temporal line at the hairline

Rarely, the author performs eyebrow fixation to the upper temporal line at the hair line (Fig .5B) – Video: http://www.youtube.com/watch?v=71n9oveGapc.

It is more traumatic and the author uses it only if higher lifting of the eyebrows is requested and only if the particular face permits aesthetic proportions with higher eyebrow position.

This technique consists on: Subdermal suture pass A-B (just below the line of the eyebrow), in order to attach the mobile Serdev orbito-superciliar fascia; two Connecting subdermal passes – A-A1 and B-B1; and Subperiosteal pass A1-B1: immobile subperiosteal attachment to the upper temporal line

2.3. Clinical cases

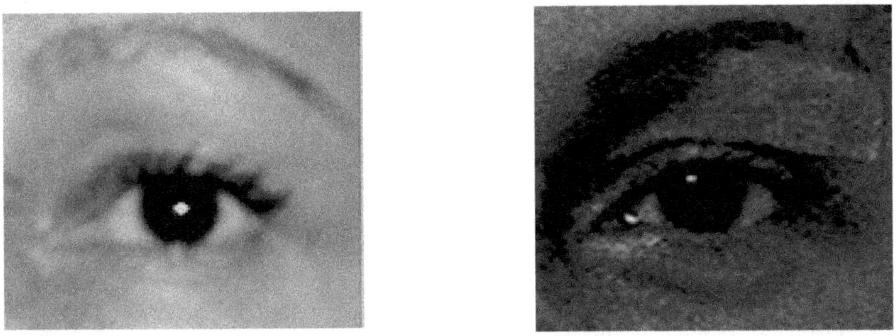

A. B.

Figure 7. A., B. Before and after brow lift by suture. A skin color tape is placed on the upper lid below the eyebrow to reduce swelling.

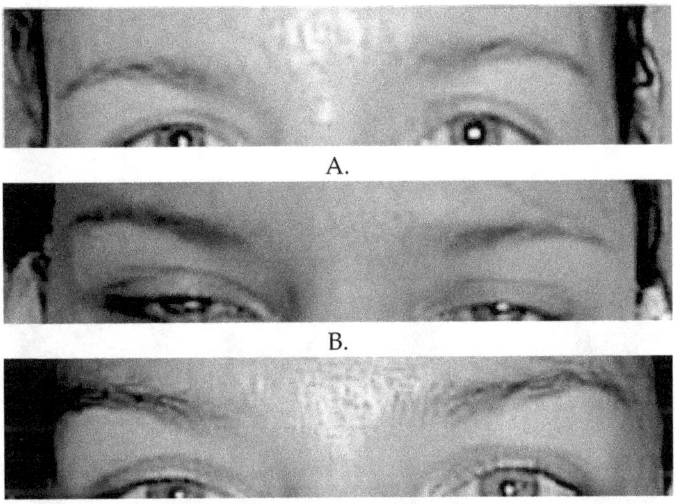

A.

B.

C.

Figure 8. A. Before, **B.** Intraop: right eyebrow is lifted without visible scars. Visible lift of the lateral canthus of the right eye, **C.** After: both eyebrows are lifted at the end of the operation. No visible scars. No operated-on appearance. No down time.

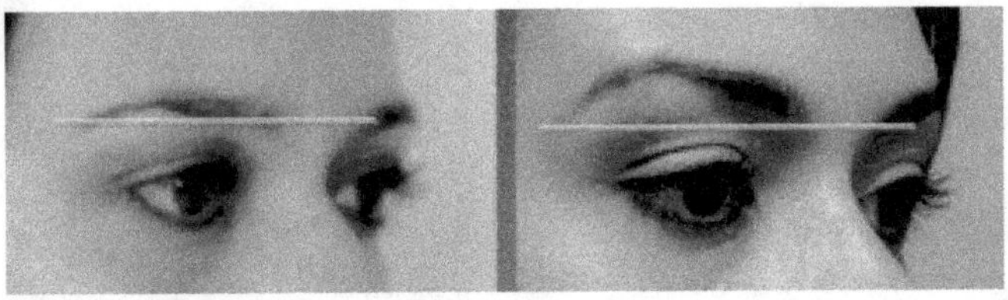

A. B.

Figure 9. A. Before and after Brow lift by Serdev Suture®. Artistic lifting and positioning of the eyebrow in a young lady.

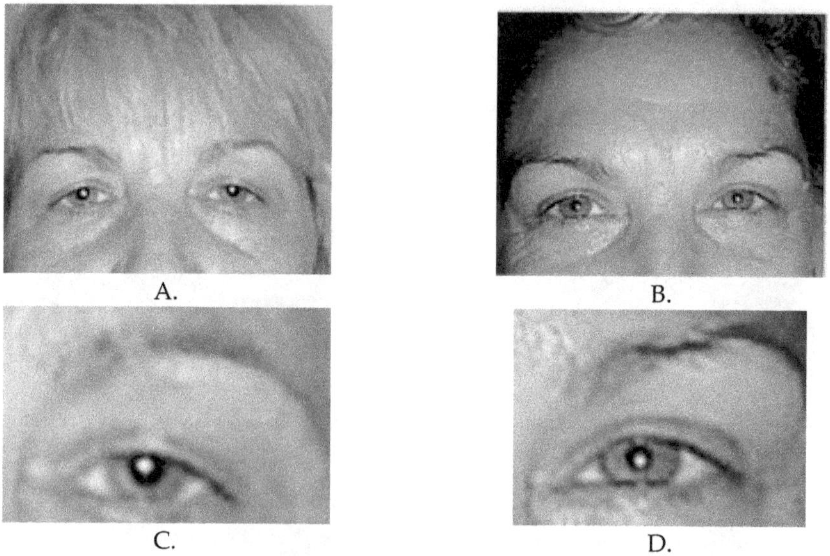

Figure 10. **A., C.** Before and **B., D.** 3 years after brow lift by suture. Visible lift of the eyebrow and lateral eye canthus.

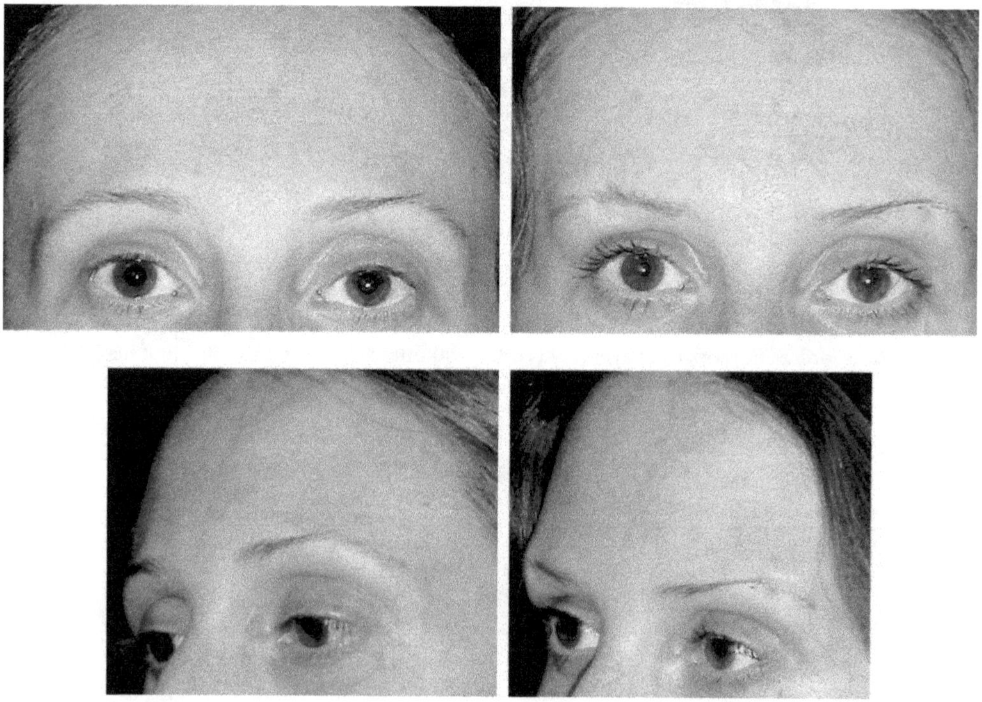

Figure 11. Eyebrow lift enhances appearance of the eyes.

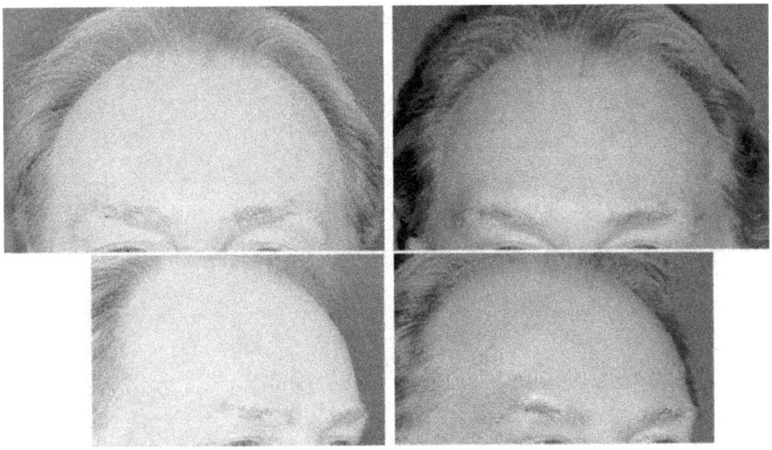

Figure 12. Lifted eyebrows solve the problem with proportions in high fronts and baldness.

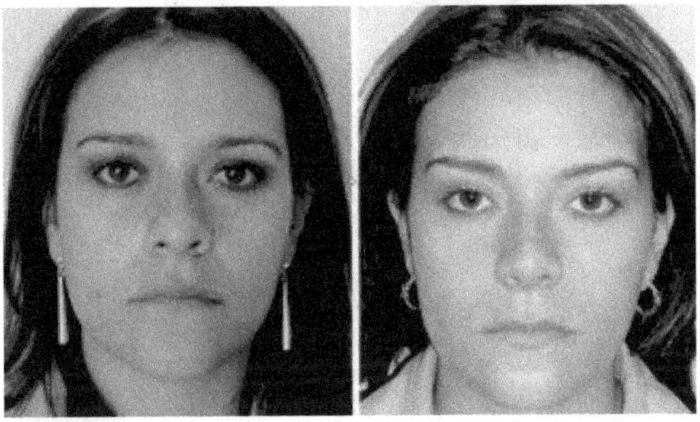

Figure 13. Total face beautification in the above 22 years young female obtained by a combination of operations: Brow lift + Nasal tip and allar base narrowing by suture + Chin enhancement + Cheekbone lift – all done by sutures + nasal hump removal. Result 4 days after surgery.

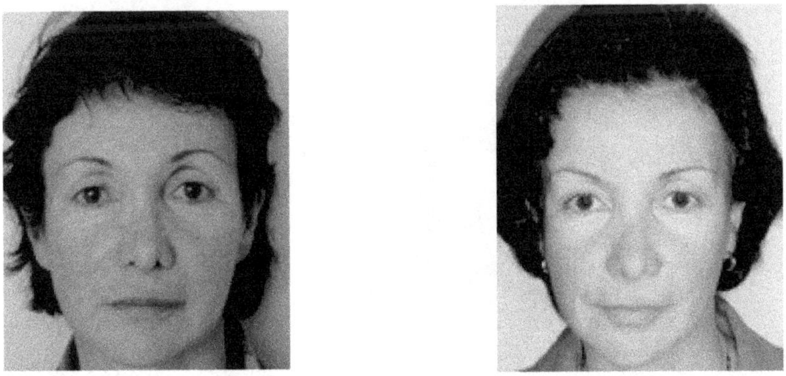

A. B.

Figure 14. A. Before and **B.** After Brow lift and Temporal SMAS lift by suture

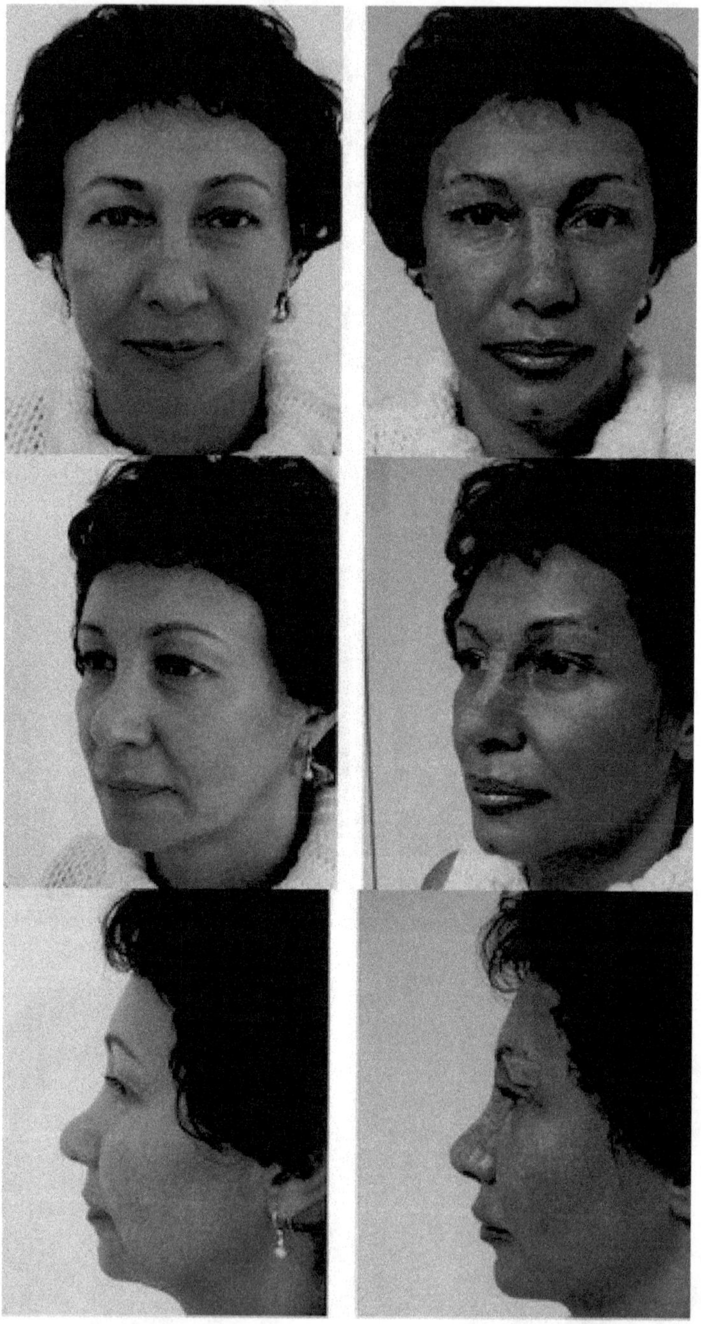

Figure 15. Beautification is mostly obtained by a combination of multiple operations – in this case: Brow lift + Chin enhancement + Chin dimple – all done by suture +secondary Rhinoplasty + Lip wy-plasty augmentation – immediate result

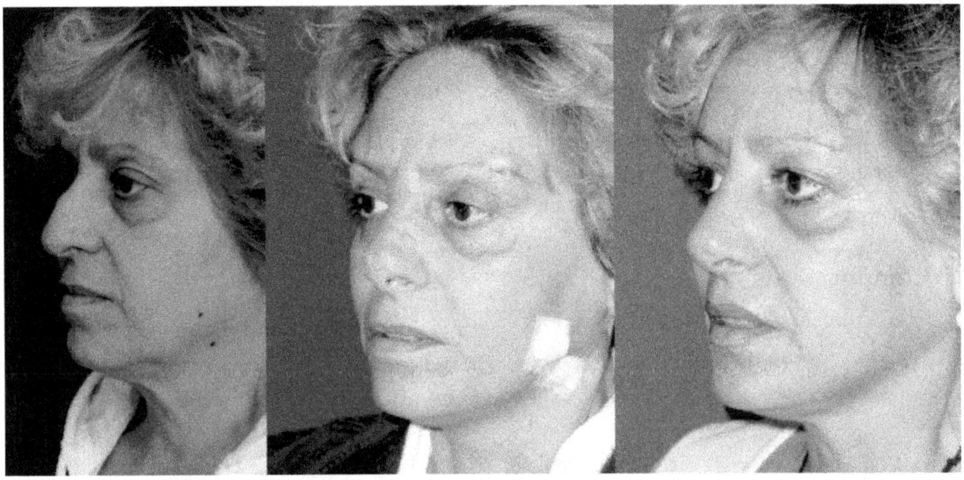

Figure 16. Beautification and rejuvenation obtained by a combination of operations: Brow + Temporal + Lower SMAS lifts by sutures + Rhinoplasty – Immediate and late result.

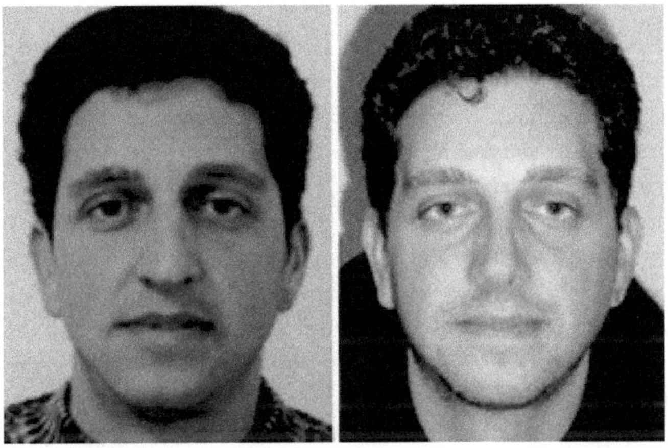

Figure 17. Total face beautification in a young male: Brow lift + Chin enhancement by sutures + Rhinoplasty. Brow lift in male patients has to be a bit lower than in female patients.

2.4. Results

During the period from 1994 to 2012, brow elevations using sutures were carried out in 982 patients. The follow up period varies from one month to 15 years. 96% of the patients reported excellent results, while 4% experienced good results. 68 % of the patients were followed during the first 5 years after surgery with very good rates of satisfaction. Only one 59 years old patient experienced aesthetic lack of satisfaction due to differences in appreciation of aesthetic proportions and angles in her age group. Complications were minimal – only 2 cases of infection in the lateral skin punctures which were treated by wound cleaning and disinfection for 2-3 days.

There were no instances of scarring, skin problems, or hair loss. The post operative period is characterized by a small percentage of swelling, no bleeding or bruising, no nerve injury, no scars, near to zero complications, immediate return to social life, preservation of facial expressive function.

In the patients with more than one year of follow up, the author has observed stable results and no ptosis was discovered with the years during follow up.

2.5. Complications

Two complications, infection in the lateral perforation point, 2 and 3 weeks after surgery, were treated by wound cleaning and disinfection and healed in 2 to 3 days. There were no cases of suture removal. No nerve damage has been noted in any patient.

2.6. Discussion

The purpose of this section is to present new trends in brow lifting philosophy and techniques.

There are a lot of procedures for brow lift that can have some negative effects for patients in modern society life: scars on the face that are only partially acceptable or non acceptable, asymmetries, increased tension across the healing wound, tension-related trophic skin changes, alopecia, paresis, ptosis etc. We can devide the proposed methods into invasive and mini-invasive surgeries. This chapter aims to describe an innovation in scarless brow lifting without any incision, without undermining but through suturing in situ the brow subdermal fibrous tissue and the orbito-supercilliar fascia higher to stable periosteum, using special needles and skin punctures only between the hairs of the brow. The method was introduced in 1994, with protocol description and was presented around the world as a part of author's "fashion art" face beautification in young patients and for correction of ptotic eyebrow and rejuvenation. In his hands it has the following advantages compared to incision and excision metods: short intervention time (about 5 minutes per side), no visible scars, minimal trauma, immediate result, a short and easy post-operative period with immediate return to social life. The suture absorbs over the longer term – in 2-3 years, so that it remains until the fibrosis is finally completed in 6 to 18 month after surgery and disappears later. The results are long lasting and pleasing.

The brow lift by suture without scars is an effective and safe technique for beautification of the eye region and rejuvenation of the upper face, producing a natural result with minimal complications and high level of longevity. It is a beautification method, ambulatory, under local anesthesia and i.v. sedation, with immediate results and near to 0 complications. It is done without visible scars, preserves the expression, the movement of the brow, and also preserves the natural look. A combination of local anesthesia and intravenous sedation provides excellent patient tolerance and comfort, both intraoperatively and postoperatively. Postoperative recovery is uneventful. Complications are very rarely encountered.

The eye-eyebrow region is the center for facial expression. The position of the eyebrows expresses emotion and even a minor change in brow position can be important for the understanding and contact between individuals. Lifting the eyebrows can change the expression into a more pleasant, young and natural one. We believe that this technique provides a more permanent and stable result. This brow lift method can be one of the most beneficial surgical procedures in cosmetic surgery. This very simple procedure allows lifting in any degree and elevation of any brow point. It supports the upper lid with lateral face improvement. It may be utilized for eyebrow ptosis alone or for fashion beauty, whether unilateral or bilateral; in conjunction with other suture techniques for equalizing asymmetrical eyebrows and for further support of markedly ptotic upper lids. It has been used by the author in instances of facial paresis or paralysis in conjunction with other procedures in the face to accomplish better symmetry. The stable duration of results with this procedure depends on the tissue quality and healing, the non-traumatic surgical technique, care given to the area during healing by the patient, amount of frowning and vigorous facial muscle use by the patient, and aging. It is a useful adjunct, especially when used with temporal SMAS lift, other suture methods on the face, beautification rhinoplasty etc. to adjust proportions, volumes and angles for beautification and rejuvenation of the individual's face.

The author's experience indicates that this specific method of scarless brow lift by suture adds a great deal to appearance and satisfaction. The procedure has taken its place as an integral part of facial beautification and rejuvenation.

3. Temporal SMAS lift

Since Mitz and Peyronie described the superficial muscle-aponeurotic system, or SMAS, in 1976, the SMAS facelift has become common and has risen into an operation to which others are compared. The author's concept to lift the whole SMAS in temporal direction is realised using the scarless Serdev Suture® method for changing the "mask of tragedy" into the "mask of comedy" in cases of beautification, soft tissue laxity, early facial ptosis and revision facelifts.

The temporal SMAS lift by suture was started in 1990 using traditional surgical instrumentarium. The author's needles and semi-elastic surgical sutures were introduced in 1993. In 1994 the author firstly reported his concept of a scarless ambulatory temporal SMAS lift by sutures, as lifting of the suprazygomatic SMAS with effect on the infrazygomatic SMAS, i.e. the whole SMAS. It became a routine ambulatory procedure for beautification and rejuvenation, presented and demonstrated around the world.

Since soft tissue and skin are attached to the SMAS in the temporal region, the lifting of the SMAS in temporal direction reflects in lifting of the face and its most important elements in the same direction (Fig. 18). It affects the lower face as well.

Anatomic landmarks for this method are: 1. The upper temporal line; and 2. The crosspoint (intersection) of the upper temporal line and the coronal line.

The aim of this method is to obtain beautification in patients of any age and rejuvenation in elderly, using minimally invasive cosmetic surgery procedures. It is performed in the ambulatory setting under local anesthesia with i.v. sedation. It is scarless with immediate results and near to 0% complications.

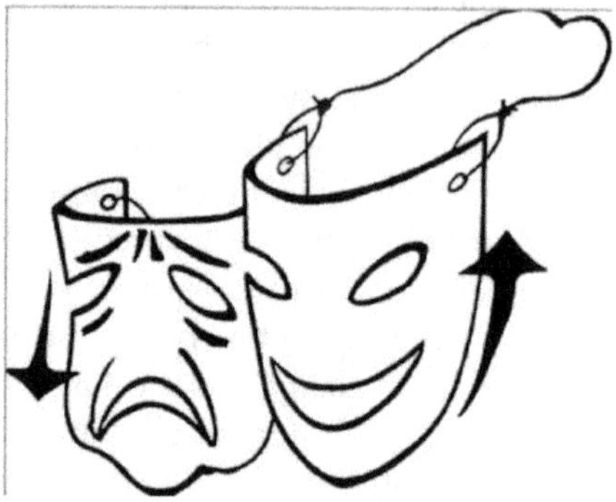

Figure 18. Mechanism of temporal SMAS lift – lifting of facial fascial mask (upper SMAS). Effect on facial structures. Transforming the old appearance into a young one. In ancient theater these masks are known as "Mask of tragedy" and "Mask of comedy".

Same idea of a temporal lift is easily created in any lady's mind, beautiful or not (Fig.19).

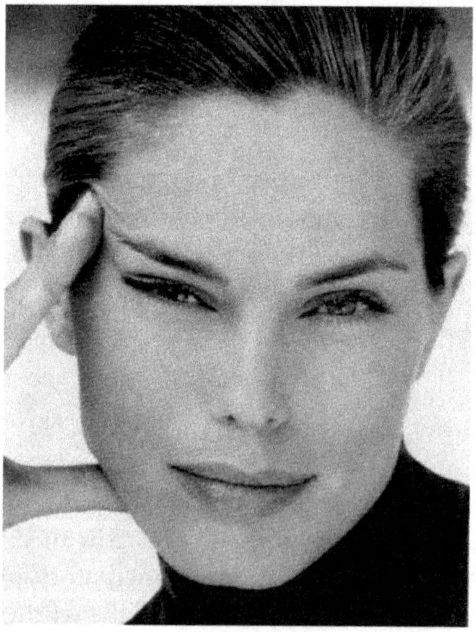

Figure 19. Ladies with no exception are thinking about temporal lift of the face.

With age, cranium volume shrinks and ptosis is reflected in the SMAS, which we can name Loose SMAS, and skin laxity changes expression into a sad and tired one. On the other hand, re-positioning of face elements could be used without restriction in face ptosis of the elderly. Aesthetically wrong face angles make young people look sad. Fixing the SMAS in a higher position allows repositioning of other soft tissue facial structures, fixed to SMAS. In young patients, the aim of the temporal SMAS lift is beautification, based on facial aesthetics.

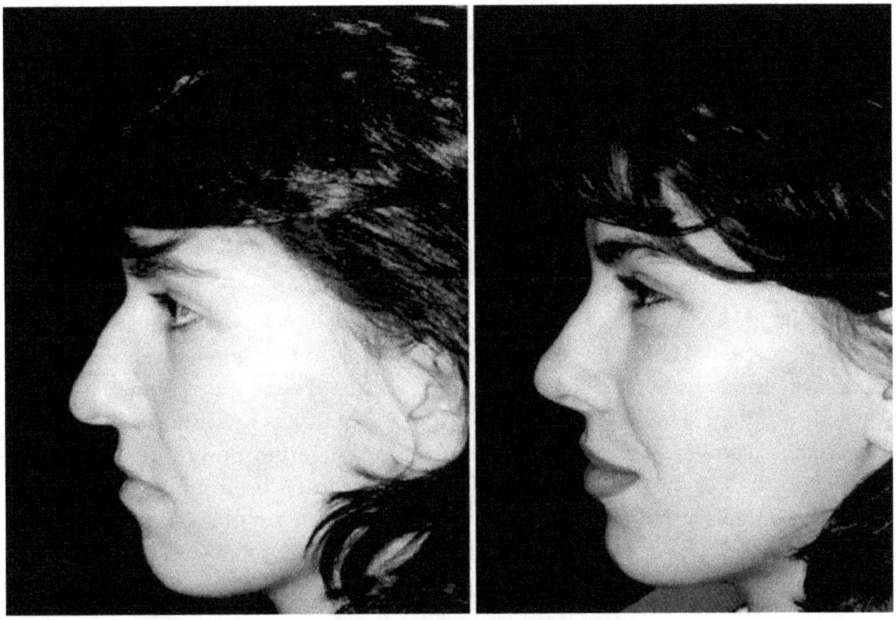

Figure 20. Before and after surgery. Temporal SMAS lift changes hanging eyebrow tail, lateral canthus angle of the eye and oral commissure. After: Better expression of cheek-bone prominence, due to the lifting of the skin and the fat pad. Additional rhinoplasty is made to correct the "golden section rule" of facial proportions in 3 equal parts; Lip augmentation to equalize lip and eye volume; Chin augmentation to obtain the "beauty triangle" and the straight line of the profile. Embellishment of the face is obtained and "smiling" expression is present ("mask of comedy" = fresh and young look).

3.1. Anatomic description of the temporal area and the SMAS

The SMAS is spread from the vertex to the platysma. It lies superficially to facial nerves. The SMAS acts as a suspension for the overlying facial skin and distributes forces of facial expression.

The Galea aponeurotica, as the upper part of the SMAS, is a muscle-aponeurotic tissue and extends from the vertex to the brow and the zygoma. It is named "superficial temporal fascia" as well, but it does not cover the temporal area solely. The temporal region, or "temporal pocket", is located over the temporal muscle, bordered by the superior temporal line above, by the lateral orbital rim in front, and by the zygomatic arch below. The layer, covering the temporalis muscle, is a bright and thick aponeurosis, the Temporalis Fascia, named also (wrongly) "deep temporal fascia". Both galea and temporal fascia are described with different names that causes confusion. At the level of the superior orbital rim, the temporal fascia (or "deep temporal fascia") splits in two layers: Superficial and Deep layer of the temporalis fascia (or /wrongly/ "deep temporal fascia"). These two fascial layers:

Superficial and Deep layer of the temporalis fascia enclose intermediate fat, including nerve and vessels. An important landmark in the temporal region is the superficial temporal artery that can be easily palpated along the hairline. The vein follows the same pattern. The frontal branch of the facial nerve, which innervates the frontalis muscle, the orbicularis oculi and corrugator supercilii lies in the intermediate fat interposed between the deep and the superficial layer of the temporalis fascia (or /wrongly/ "deep temporalis fascia"). It is considered to travel along a line connecting the base of the tragus to a point 1.5cm above the eyebrow.

3.2. The procedure

The concept of the scarless closed approach transcutaneous temporal face lift by sutures is to lift loose mobile galea and to fix it to stable immobile upper temporalis line periosteum and temporalis fascia. Skin fixed to the galea follows this repositioning in temporal direction that reflects in face lifting. To obtain such lifting, special curved semi-blunt, semi-elastic Serdev® needles with different lengths of 50 mm, 60 mm and 100 mm are used to introduce long-term absorbable, semi-elastic, braided, antimicrobial Bulgarian polycaproamide (Polycon) surgical sutures USP 2 or 4. Other surgical sutures could be used, but the short elasticity quallity of the Bulgarian suture reduces trauma to the fixated mobilised tissues. Rigid thin USP 2/0 threads work as a scalpels to mobile tissue, when under tension.

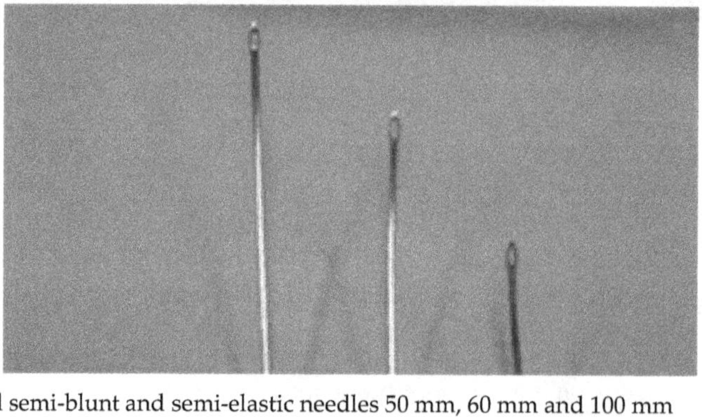

Figure 21. Curved semi-blunt and semi-elastic needles 50 mm, 60 mm and 100 mm

3.3. Surgical method

Video: http://www.youtube.com/watch?v=qFF3lr9jHqs

1. Using needle perforation only - without skin incisions

1a. First Temporal SMAS Lift Suture

Two lines A-B and A1-B1 are marked as parts of a rhombus inside the temporal area (Fig. 22 A). Line A-B represents the subperiosteal (upper temporal line) and subtemporal pass of the suture. Point A is located above the intersection point of the upper temporal line and the coronal line and point B is marked about 3-4 cm below at the coronal line. Starting from A, a line A-A1 is marked in 45 degrees angle to the line A-B in direction to the eyebrow tail. Point A1 is located at the end of that line in a distance from A, depending on the laxity, usually at 3-5 cm away from A. Line A1-B1 is the line of supragaleal fixation of SMAS. Lines A-A1 and B-B1 are subgaleal passes of the suture, connecting the two fixation lines. They mark the direction of movement of the galea to temporalis fascia. In cases of a very loose SMAS, mostly in elderly, it is advisable to perform a second suture, lower than the first one, to lift the medial and lower facial SMAS and soft tissue.

The wide spread temporal fixation (to temporal fascia) is not advisable, because temporalis fascia fibers are perpendicular and cannot hold a suture fixation with tension in distal direction. The suture will slide down and the lift will lose on longevity (Fig. 23).

1b. Second (Lower) Suture for Temporal Lift

A second line of galea fixation A2-B2 (below A1-B1) is marked (Fig. 22B) and a second suture is performed. in cases when laxity in the lower face is still presented after the first suture, mostly in elderly. The needle and surgical suture are introduced as follows: A-B – subperiosteally/subtemporally at the upper temporal line; A2-B2 – supragaleally; A-A2 and B-B2 – subgaleally.

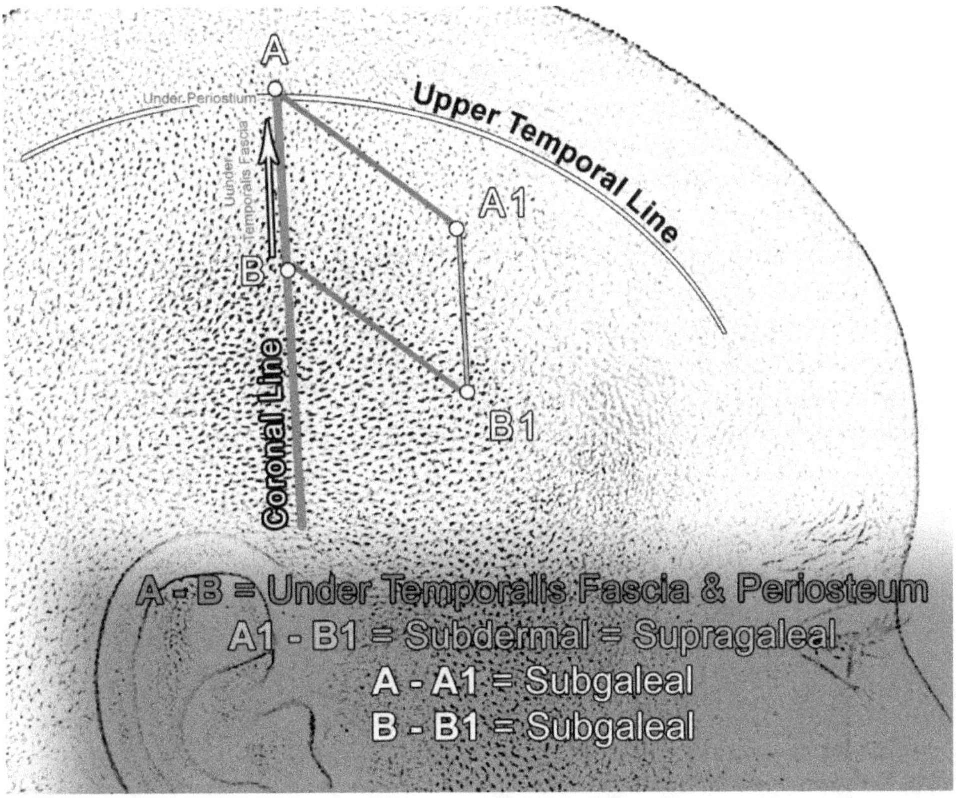

A.

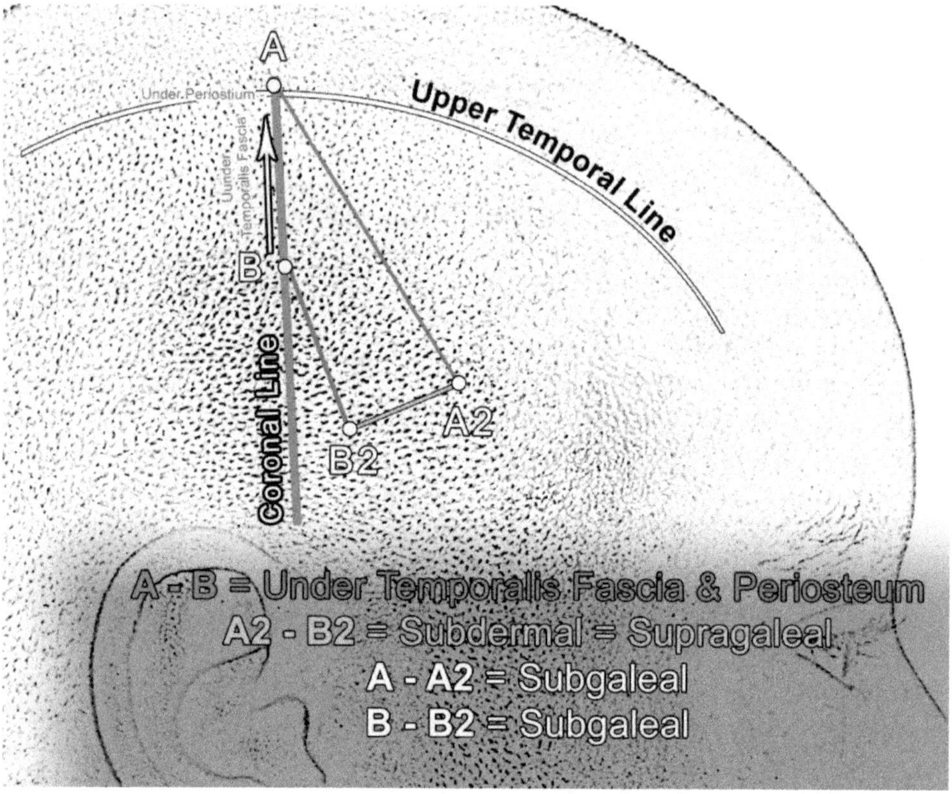

B.

Figure 22. **A.** Upper temporal line and coronal line are marked. The upper immobile fixation - subperiosteal (upper temporal line) and subtemporal pass of the suture (3-5 cm in the coronal line) is marked in red color. Line A1-B1 of supragaleal SMAS fixation will be lifted and fixed to A-B line of subperiosteal and subtemporal fixation. **B.** Same with the second lower suture in elderly: line A2-B2 of supragaleal fixation will be lifted and fixed by the suture to A-B line of subperiosteal and subtemporal fixation. Line A-A1 in direction to eyebrow and line B-B1 in direction to the cheekbone are subgaleal passes only. Lines A-A2 and B-B2 in direction to the lower face are subgaleal passes as well.

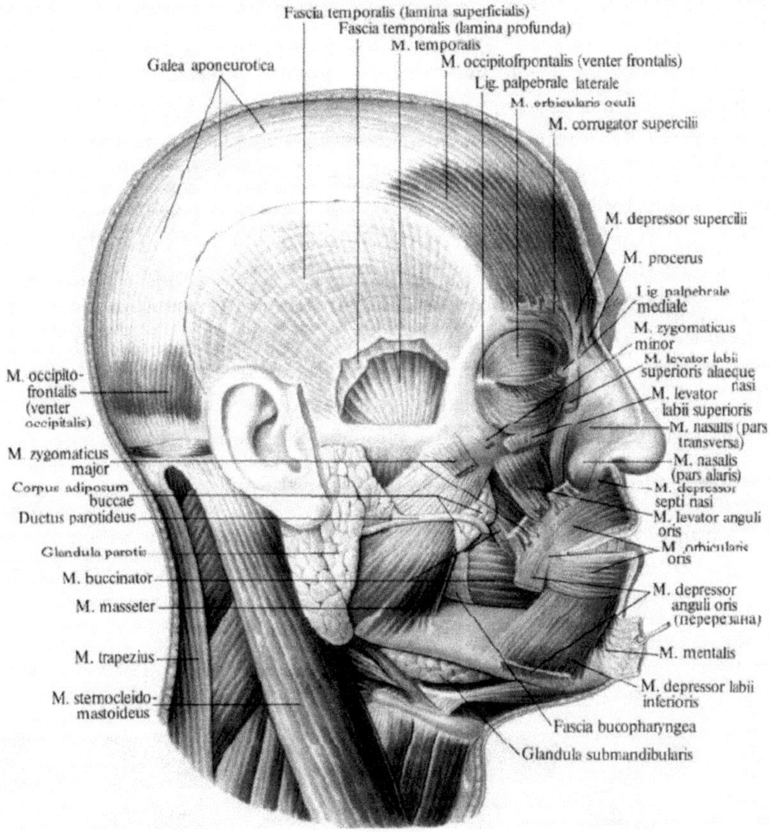

Figure 23. Temporal fascia fibers* are in distal direction and cannot hold the suture if the fixation is not attached to upper temporal line bone and periosteum. ***Anatomy figures from Sinelnikov - Atlas Of Human Anatomy, GIML, Moscow, 1963**

After local anesthesia, a No. 11 scalpel blade is used to make skin perforations at points A, B, A1 and B1. The order of needle entries should be convenient to right or left handed surgeons and could be as follows: the needle is introduced supragaleally in line A1-B1, just under the skin (between skin and galea, where a thin layer of subdermal fat allows to pass without any resistance). After threading the needle, the surgical suture is introduced in the A1-B1 supragaleal plane. The next subgaleal passes are directed from A to A1 and from B to B1 to take the suture ends. The final A-B pass is through the bone of the upper temporal line, subperiosteally and subtemporally. So, we have 3 levels of needle passes i.e. 3 levels of positioning of the surgical suture in the tissue: A1-B1 is supragaleal/subdermal (mobile fixation), A-A1 and B-B1 are subgaleal, and A-B – subperiosteal and subtemporal (immobile fixation). The location of the needle in each level has its characteristics. In the subdermal plane, the needle is not fixed by stable tissue – it is movable laterally and is covered only by a thin layer of skin. In the subgaleal plane, the needle is introduced deeper (in the tunnel of the lifted skin and galea, fixed together), and is mobile laterally again (Galea is mobile), and is covered by a thicker layer that includes skin, subdermal fat and galea. As galea is fixed to skin in that region, pulling of skin like a tunnel pulls galea as well and subgaleal entry in that tunnel is made easy. In this plane, one has to avoid taking temporalis fascia that is located below the needle. If temporalis fascia is captured with the needle, movement of the needle is impossible without movement of the entire head. Such fixation is incorrect and the needle has to be repositioned. **NB!** The needle should pass through all 4 skin perforations, in and out (or vice versa), without biting any dermal tissue, so as to prevent dimpling. The suture should not invert hair into the subdermal plane, in order to prevent foreign body reaction. When tightening, the suture dives in the subdermal tissue. Skin should not be engaged in the suture. When the circle of the suture is finished, a knot is made under medium elastic tension. The idea is to prevent trauma of the tissue. After the knot is tightened, a mosquito clamp is used to pull the skin perforations away from the suture, in order to free the skin and reduce dimpling at the perforation points. Some bulging effect (due to suture and edema) will disappear in a month, but is not visible in the temporal area, which is covered by hair.

2. Using a minimal, hidden skin incision in the coronal line:

In the very beginning, the author was using a 3 cm temporal incision in the coronal line A-B, which, working under visual control, is more comfortable for beginners to perform the subperiosteal and subtemporal fixation. In this technique we start with anesthesia and make a 2-3 cm long A-B incision along the coronal line. The skin and subdermal fat are opened and the red vascularised galea below becomes visible. After the galea is opened with a mosquito instrument, the white shiny temporal fascia is presented (Fig. 24).

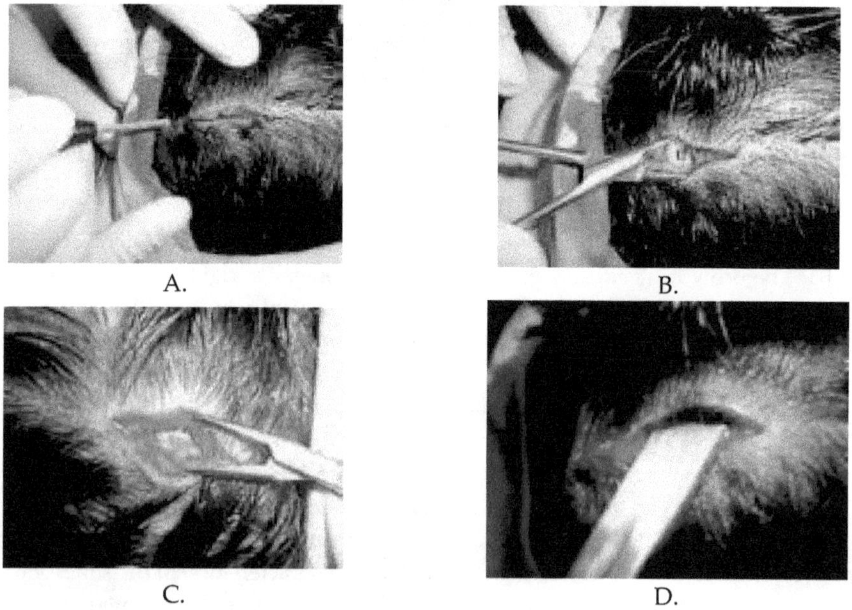

Figure 24. **A.** Skin incision, **B., C.** blunt opening of skin and red galea; then white, shiny temporal fascia is visible, **D.** Blunt dissection between galea and temporal fascia.

A blunt subgaleal dissection follows till the hairline. It should be very easy because there is no stable fixation between these two fascias – galea and temporal fascia. Further, the same surgical technique is done as described above. Lines A-A1 and B-B1 are subgaleal passes of the suture, done under visual control, A1-B1 is a supragaleal i.e. subdermal pass, and A-B is a subperiosteal and subtemporal pass under visual control as well. A very important part of the technique is prevention of hair insertion with the suture loop into the subdermal plane that will lead to granuloma formation and local infection. Deep biting of the temporal muscle instead of a subfascial pass should be avoided to prevent pain, which is described by patients as headache. The galea, presenting the SMAS, is pulled up and fixed higher to the upper temporal line with one or two sutures on each side, under elastic tension. Thus, the whole SMAS is pulled up in temporo-occipital direction. Following this, the skin is closed with single stitches and no dressing is necessary. A hair wash is recommended on the next day to remove any residual blood. Wound stitches are removed after 7 days.

3.4. Clinical cases

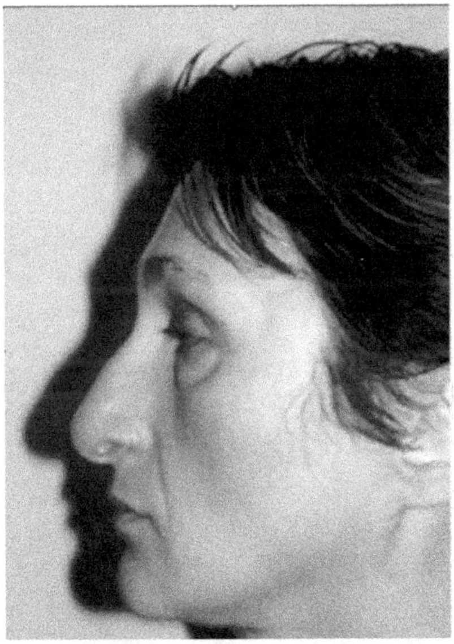

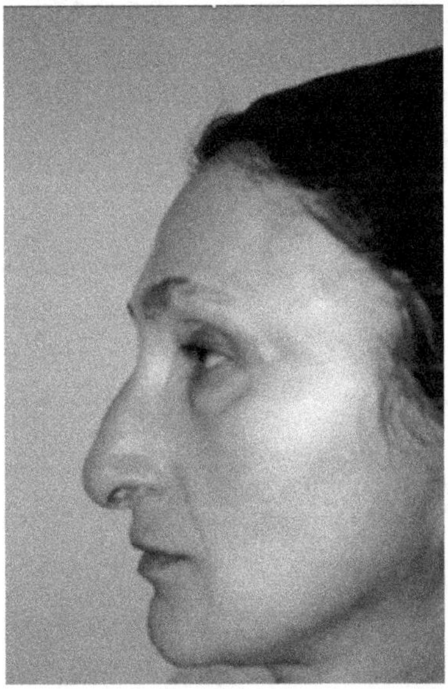

A. B.

Figure 25. **A, B**. Before and after a temporal SMAS lift. Visible elevation of the eyebrow tail and the lateral canthus of the eye, reduction of the crows-feet wrinkles, elevation of the cheeks' fat pad into a better cheekbone prominence; tightening, better texture and beautification of the skin.

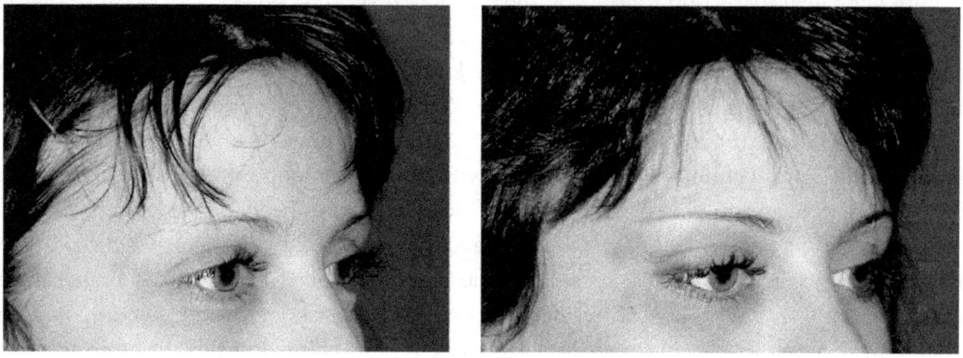

A. B.

Figure 26. **A.** before, **B.** after a temporal face lift in a young patient using Serdev Suture®. Angles of the eyes and eyebrows are changed, resulting in beautification.

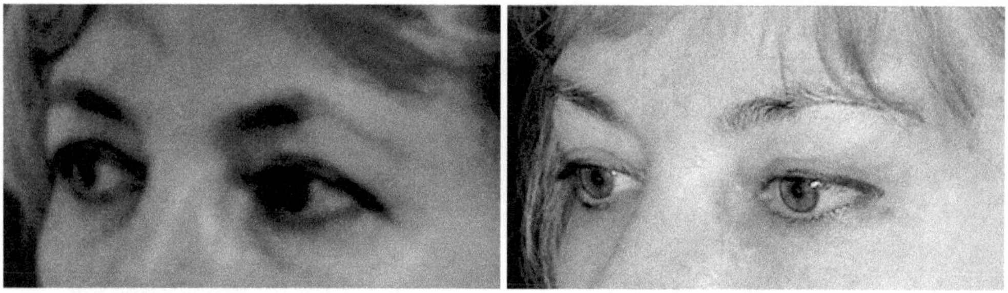

A. B.

Figure 27. **A.** before, **B.** after a temporal face lift using Serdev Suture® in an elderly patient. Angles of the eyes and eyebrows are changed resulting in rejuvenation and beautification.

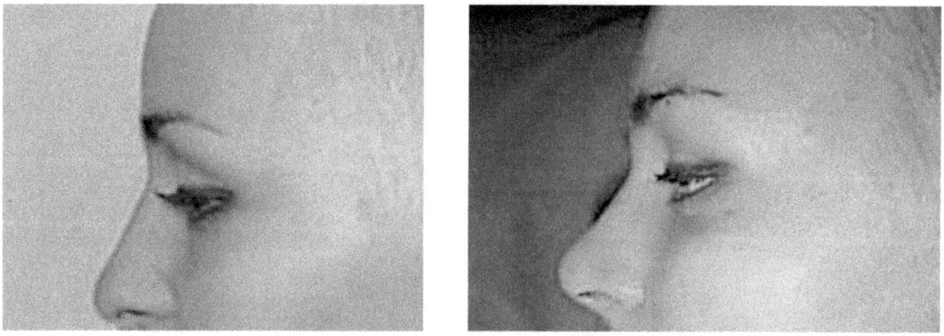

A. B.

Figure 28. **A, B.** Before and immediately after a temporal SMAS lift and tip rotation rhinoplasty. The absence of visible signs of operation permits immediate return to social life. Rhinoplasty in the author's technique does not need tampons and plaster fixation. No bruising when tip rotation only.

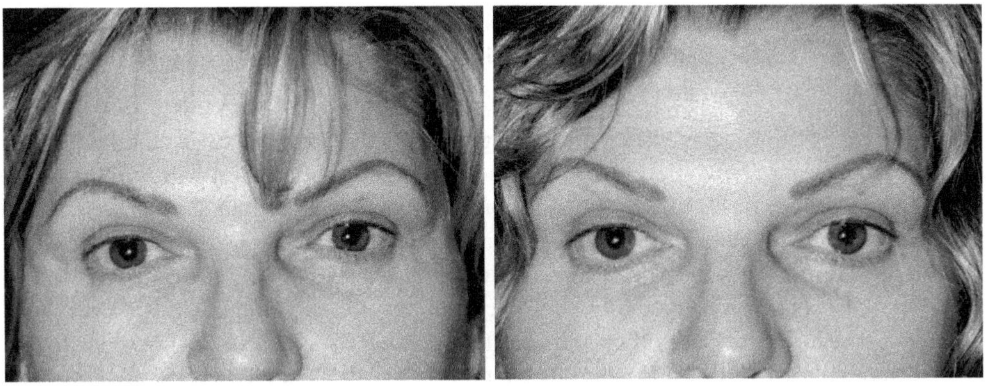

A. B.

Figure 29. A. Before. Asymmetric ptosis of the face with aging, **B.** After a temporal face lift using Serdev Suture®. The whole face is lifted resulting in beautification and rejuvenation, solving the different flabbiness on both sides. The face symmetry is equalized.

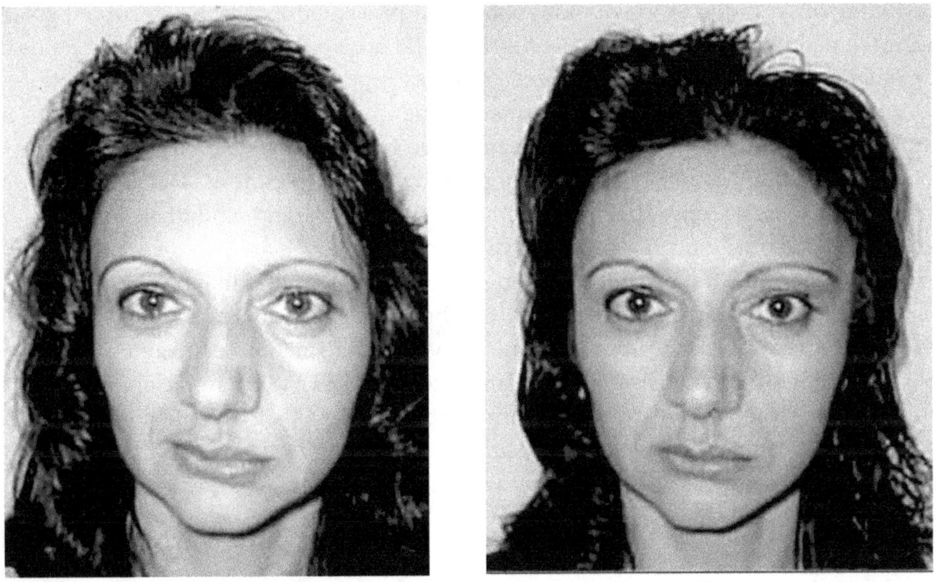

A. B.

Figure 30. A, B. Before and after unilateral temporal SMAS lift in facial paralysis. A 4-years result. The whole left side is elevated and the nose is repositioned in the middle by the temporal SMAS lift. Further equalization is possible using mid-face and cheekbone lifts, as well as chin movement to the left (see mid face and lower face chapters).

3.5. Results

1427 patients were followed up for more than 3 years, operated from 1993 to 2001, using the Temporal lift suture method, firstly with a minimal incision in the coronal line and later with needle perforations only. Patients' age ranges from 19 to 68 years. The operation was performed in ambulatory settings. After washing and styling the hair, patients could return to their social life next day, if necessary on the same day.

The temporal SMAS lift has effects on the suprazygomatic area: it reduces the lateral and forehead wrinkles; raises the eyebrow tails and the lateral canthus of the eyes; reduces the crows-foot wrinkles, raises the cheekbone prominence and tightens the skin. The effects on the lower face are collateral. The SMAS elevates the lateral canthus of the eyes, and the oral commissure. It improves the skin texture, reducing cheek flaccidity; gives a clearer outline of the jaw. Generally, the method gives excellent results in younger and middle aged patients whose lower face flacidity is minimal to medium. The facial tissues are repositioned to the desired higher youthful location. The temporal hair is preserved. There are no visible scars, no signs of operative intervention, and no "operated-on" appearance. A moderate feeling of tension in the face could be present for hours or days. The feeling is mostly pleasing. Only 7 patients described the tension as uncomfortable for one or two days. During the first week 12 patients reported headache. Lower eyelid swelling could appear on day 3 after surgery due to gravity and should be prevented by resting in supine position during the first two days. Five patients had lower lid bruising on the 3rd day on one side and four other patients – on both sides. Seven patients reported a crust formation with liquid under the crust. The reason was subdermal position of hair by the suture sling. After hair removal, the wounds healed in approximately two to four days. One patient had the same problem in another country and the surgeon removed the suture. Due to the fibrosis formation, no ptosis appeared after removal of the suture. No other infections, no hematomas or damage on the facial nerve were observed. Some palpable bulging in the temporal area could be present for some weeks. Most important in face lifting is its longevity. Numerous factors act against face stability, such as gravity and facial movements. The longevity of the result is improved due to the SMAS fixation to periosteum. This is best seen years after surgery in cases of a unilateral temporal SMAS lift in facial paralysis, post traumatic and postoperative canthal abnormalities etc. (Fig. 30). Two patients could not see the difference, despite the photograph demonstrations, contesting the aesthetic result. The effect of lifting angles was not satisfactory with 5 patients. With 3 of them the operation was repeated after 3 to 5 years.

3.6. Discussion

Currently, there are plenty of techniques used for face-lifts: conventional rhytidectomy, composite face-lifting, deep layer rhytidectomy, sub-SMAS, extended face-lifting, subcutaneous temporofacial lift combined with SMAS suspension, medial SMAS lift with aggressive temporal skin removal, temporal lift via blepharoplasty approach. Stretching the skin solely is obsolete. New techniques were proposed, such as endoscopic, subperiosteal, extended face lifts etc. There is no general agreement and no definitive answer as to which operative technique is most effective or preferable for each specific case. This is due to the subjective nature of aesthetics, aspirations and to the variability of skills and anatomy.

In the last years, an increasing number of patients ask for non-invasive or minimally invasive surgery for beautification or rejuvenation with minimal trauma and short recovery downtime, corresponding to the modern lifestyle. The suture method for temporal SMAS lift is the most preferred option by author's patients as an optimal solution for upper (and total) face beautification and rejuvenation, which preserves the natural look.

The temporal SMAS lift is a nice, weekend ambulatory procedure that gives a pleasing rejuvenation and beautification of the skin, eyes, brows, cheekbones, and most importantly - changes the expression. Complications rate is very low and the methods to solve the complications are easily performed. In young ladies, only one suture per side is usually enough to lift the lateral canthus of the eye, the eyebrow and to pull the ptotic malar fat into place, which restores and forms a nice malar eminence. It is also possible to combine the temporal lift by suture with other suture procedures: the author uses additional suture methods for brow, mid-face, cheekbone, and lower SMAS lift, simultaneous rhinoplasty, chin and lip augmentation, fat reduction and/or augmentation, skin resurfacing or blepharoplasty to obtain facial beautification and or rejuvenation. The closed approach Serdev Suture® method for temporal SMAS lift provides a safe and effective beautification, as well as rejuvenation in early laxity and face ptosis, and in some revision facelifts.

4. Supra-temporal lift

Supra-temporal lift presents fixation of the mobile galea aponeurotica at the hairline to the upper temporal line periosteum.

5. Glabella muscle ligation for permanent glabella relaxation

Video: http://www.youtube.com/watch?v=F7r-W7-kK20

5.1. Directions

1. Mark the glabella muscles: 1. Corrugator supercillii muscle; 2. Procerus muscle; 3. Depressor supercillii muscle. The glabella muscles are V-shaped. Select and mark A , B and C skin perforation points to tie and ligate that muscles in 3 lines: A-B line to ligate the Procerus muscle and Depressor supercillii muscle, A-C and B-C lines to ligate the Corrugator and Depressor supercillii muscles (Fig. 31).

2. Local anesthesia in points A, B and C intradermal and in direction A-B, A-C and B-C at periosteum and subdermally. Note: Inject local anesthesia sparingly, drop by drop as necessary, to prevent from visible swelling.

3. Perforate points A, B and C using a No. 11 scalpel blade. Using a mosquito clamp, perforate bluntly the subdermal fascia in the points A, B and C. **NB!** If not previously perforated, superficial fascias will be engaged in the suture, forming a dimpling effect on the skin surface.

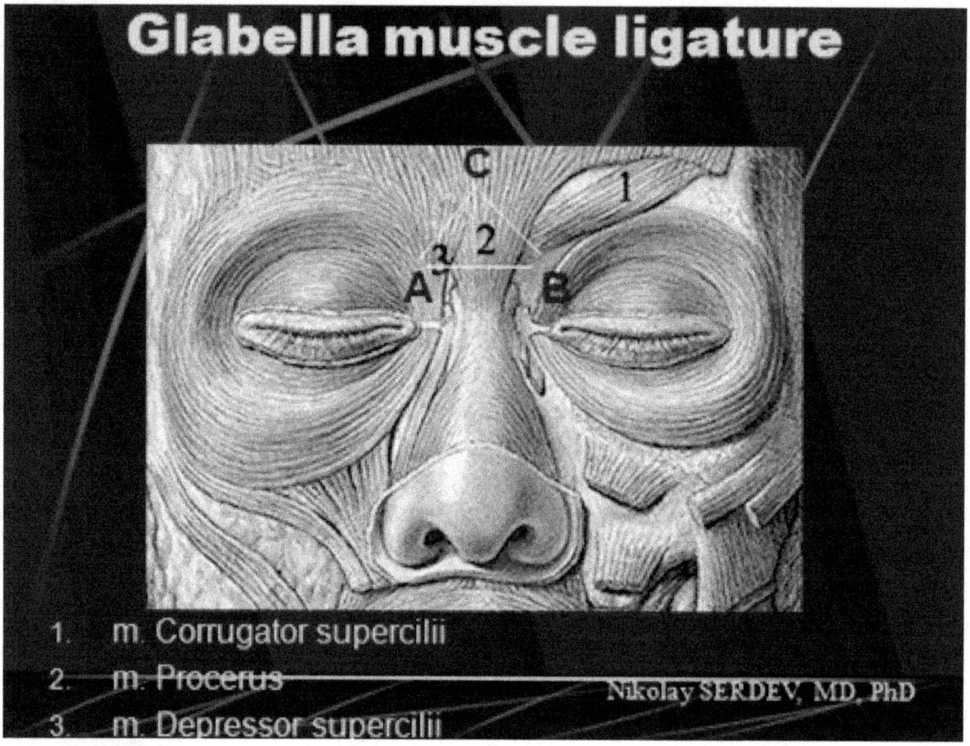

Figure 31. Suture lines A-B, B-C and A-C to ligate glabella muscles

5.2. A-B Suture - procerus & depressor supercilii muscle ligation

A. Introduce an unloaded "mini mini" Serdev® 50 mm needle from point A to point B, below the Procerus muscle, touching the periosteum. Load the needle with a surgical suture USP 3/0 and introduce it on the way of the needle pass A-B. **NB!** In skin perforation points, pass the needle perpendicularly to the skin surface, without resistance in front (to prevent engagement of dermal and fibrotic tissue), by smoothly twisting the needle. Do not push to bite dermis as this will result in a dimple. Do not push, do not pull – twist the needle smoothly forward and backward.

B. Introduce the unloaded needle from point A to point B subdermally, above the muscles. Feed the second suture end into the Serdev® needle at point B and introduce it toward A to finalize the circle of the suture. **NB!** The needle tip is always in direction to the suture end - to reach and load it.

C. Tie strongly at point A to ligate the muscles and obtain muscle necrosis at that place. After securing the knot, release any dimpling with a hemostat at point A and B.
NB! Serdev Sutures® should not engage skin.

5.3. A-C suture - corrugator supercilii & depressor supercilii muscle ligation

A. Introduce an unloaded "mini mini" Serdev® needle from point C to A, below the muscles Corrugator supercillii and Depressor supercillii, touching periosteum. Load the needle with suture USP 3/0 and introduce it on the way of the needle pass A-C.
B. Introduce the unloaded Serdev® needle from point C to A subdermally, above the muscles. Feed the second suture end into the Serdev® needle at point A and introduce it from A to C to finalize the circle of the suture.
C. Tie strongly at point C to ligate the muscles and to obtain muscle necrosis at that place. After securing the knot, release any dimpling with a hemostat at point A and C.

5.4. B-C suture - corrugator supercilii & depressor supercilii muscle ligation

A. Introduce an unloaded "mini mini" Serdev® needle from point B to C, below the muscles Corrugator supercillii and Depressor supercillii, touching periosteum. Load the needle with surgical suture USP 3/0 and introduce it on the way of the needle pass C-B.
B. Introduce the unloaded Serdev® needle from point B to C subdermally, above the muscles. Feed the second suture end into the Serdev® needle at point C and introduce it at B to finalize the circle of the suture.
C. Tie strongly at point B to ligate the muscles and to obtain muscle necrosis at that place. After securing the knot, release any dimpling with a hemostat at point B and C.

5.5. Results

20 patients were followed up to 3 years after operation with the suture ligation method to block glabella muscles. 3 years results show 80-95% relaxation of the glabella muscle function that is permanent.

Serdev Sutures® glabella muscle ligation provides a minimally invasive, scarless glabella muscle ligation, necrosis and relaxation with no downtime and near to zero complications. Longevity is very satisfactory. Aesthetic results often exceed patient expectations.

6. Lateral canthus lifting

There are 2 methods for lateral canthus lifting:

1. Fixation to the lateral orbital rim. Using 2 skin perforation points, the needle passes once below the lateral canthus and perforates orbital rim periosteum, and second time it passes above the orbital rim, subcutaneously. The suture fixes the lateral canthus to the lateral orbital rim periosteum.

2. Fixation to the upper temporal rim and temporal fascia.

First pass: Two skin perforation points are necessary on both sides of the lateral canthus to pass below or through the lateral canthus (using the 50 mm "mini mini" Serdev® needle), and introduce the surgical suture through that sub- or trans-canthal line.

Second pass: Then, a small (100 mm) or medium (140 mm) Serdev® needle is introduced through a third skin perforation point in the temporal line area to perforate the periosteum of the upper temporal line and the temporal fascia, take one of the suture ends and introduce it subtemporally and subperiosteally.

Third pass: This pass is subdermal, in order to take the second end of the suture, pull it through subdermally and fulfill the suture.

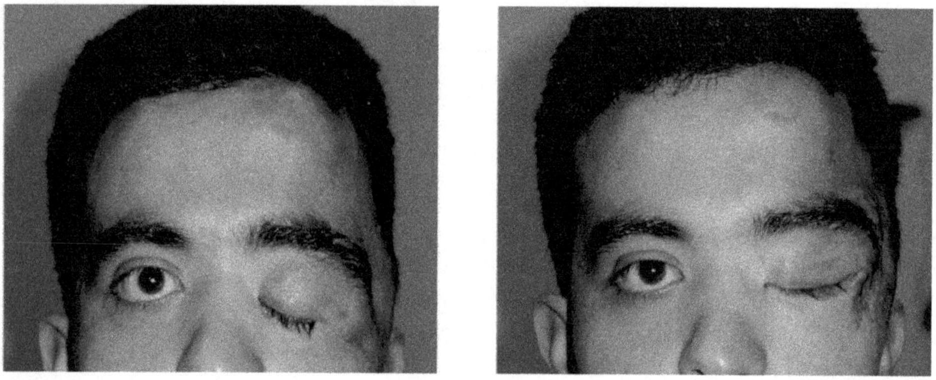

A. B.

Figure 32. **A.** After eye tumor enucleation, **B**. After lateral canthus fixation to upper temporal line and temporal fascia.

Lateral canthus repositioning is performed mostly in reconstructive surgery. Serdev Suture® lift permits beautification as well. Another possibility for lateral canthus lifting is the Serdev Suture® brow lift, which also reflects in a lateral canthus lifting.

Author details

Nikolay Serdev
New Bulgarian University, Sofia, Bulgaria

7. References

[1] Serdev, N.P. Year 1994, Suture Suspensions For Lifting Or Volume Augmentation In Face And Body (English version), presented at the 2nd Annual Meeing of the National Bulgarian Society for Aesthetic Surgery and Aesthetic Medicine, Sofia, 18 March 1994, Int J Aesth Cosm, 2001,1:1, 2561-2568

[2] Serdev, N.P. Eyebrow lifting by suture (from "Serdev Sutures. Scarless face and body liftings"), Int J Aesth Cosm, 2011,11:3, 1-2

[3] Serdev, N.P. Brow lifting to the upper temporal line 1.5 cm, Int J Aesth Cosm, 2012,12:1, 1-62

[4] Serdev, N.P. Brow lifting with fixation to the upper temporal line at the hairline, Int J Aesth Cosm, 2012,12:1, 3-6

[5] Paul MD. The evolution in aesthetic cosmetic surgery. Plast Reconstr Surg 2001 Oct;108(5):1409-24

[6] Wang TD. Rhytidectomy for treatment of the aging face. Mayo Clin Proc 1989 Jul;64(7):780-90

[7] Cook TA, Musgrave-Zwetsch J. Adjuncts to face lifting procedures. Otolaryngol Clin North Am 1980 May;13(2):321-35

[8] Forrest CR, Phillips JH, Bell TA, Gruss JS. The biomechanical effects of deep tissue support as related to brow and facelift procedures. Plast Reconstr Surg 1991 Sep;88(3):427-32

[9] Rafaty FM. Elimination of glabellar frown lines. Arch Otolaryngol 1981 Jul;107(7):428-30

[10] Liebman EP, Webster RC, Berger AS, DellaVecchia M. The frontalis nerve in the temporal brow lift. Arch Otolaryngol 1982 Apr;108(4):232-5

[11] Webster RC, Gaunt JM, Hamdan US, Fuleihan NS, Giandello PR, Smith RC. Supraorbital and supratrochlear notches and foramina: anatomical variations and surgical relevance. Laryngoscope 1986 Mar;96(3):311-5

[12] Whitaker LA, Bartlett SP.Skeletal alterations as a basis for facial rejuvenation. Clin Plast Surg 1991 Jan;18(1):197-203

[13] Fogli A. Orbicularis oculi muscle and crow's feet. Pathogenesis and surgical approach Ann Chir Plast Esthet 1992 Oct;37(5):510-8

[14] Yeatts RP. Current concepts in brow lift surgery. Curr Opin Ophthalmol 1997 Oct;8(5):46-50

[15] Bruck JC, Baker TJ, Gordon H. Facial mimics and the coronal brow lift. Aesthetic Plast Surg 1987;11(4):199-201

[16] Bruck JC, Baker TJ, Gordon H. Facial mimics and the coronal brow lift. Aesthetic Plast Surg 1987;11(4):199-201

[17] Freund RM, Nolan WB 3rd. Correlation between brow lift outcomes and aesthetic ideals for eyebrow height and shape in females. Plast Reconstr Surg 1996 Jun;97(7):1343-8

[18] Arteaga DM, Taylor CO. Esthetic evaluation and treatment of the upper one third of the face. J Oral Maxillofac Surg 1991 Jan;49(1):27-32/

[19] Quantitative analysis of facial motion components: anatomic and nonanatomic motion in normal persons and in patients with complete facial paralysis. Plast Reconstr Surg 1997 Jun;99(7):1894-902; discussion 1903-4/

[20] Elkwood A, Matarasso A, Rankin M, Elkowitz M, Godek CP.National plastic surgery survey: brow lifting techniques and complications. Plast Reconstr Surg 2001 Dec;108(7):2143-50; discussion 2151-2

[21] Matarasso A, Elkwood A, Rankin M, Elkowitz M. National plastic surgery survey: face lift techniques and complications. Plast Reconstr Surg 2000 Oct;106(5):1185-95; discussion 1196

[22] Forrest CR, Phillips JH, Bell TA, Gruss JS. The biomechanical effects of deep tissue support as related to brow and facelift procedures. Plast Reconstr Surg 1991 Sep;88(3):427-32

[23] Webster RC, Fanous N, Smith RC. Blepharoplasty: when to combine it with brow, temple, or coronal lift. J Otolaryngol 1979 Aug;8(4):339-43
[24] Adamson PA, Cormier R, McGraw BL. The coronal forehead lift -modifications and results. J Otolaryngol 1992 Feb;21(1):25-9
[25] McKinney P, Mossie RD, Zukowski ML. Criteria for the forehead lift. Aesthetic Plast Surg 1991 Spring;15(2):141-7
[26] Rafaty FM, Goode RL, Fee WE Jr. The brow-lift operation. Arch Otolaryngol. 1975 Aug;101(8):467-8.
[27] Ortiz-Monasterio F, Barrera G, Olmedo A. The coronal incision in rhytidectomy--the brow lift. Clin Plast Surg. 1978 Jan;5(1):167-79.
[28] Ellenbogen R. Transcoronal eyebrow lift with concomitant upper blepharoplasty. Plast Reconstr Surg. 1983 Apr;71(4):490-9.
[29] Fett DR, Sutcliffe RT, Baylis HI. The coronal brow lift. Am J Ophthalmol 1983 Dec;96(6):751-4
[30] Riefkohl R. The forehead-brow lift. Ann Plast Surg 1982 Jan;8(1):55-63
[31] Nassif PS, Kokoska MS, Homan S, Cooper MH, Thomas JR.Comparison of subperiosteal vs subgaleal elevation techniques used in forehead lifts. Arch Otolaryngol Head Neck Surg 1998 Nov;124(11):1209-15
[32] Troilius C. A comparison between subgaleal and subperiosteal brow lifts. Plast Reconstr Surg 1999 Sep;104(4):1079-90; discussion 1091-2
[33] Dempsey PD, Oneal RM, Izenberg PH. Subperiosteal brow and midface lifts. Aesthetic Plast Surg 1995 Jan-Feb;19(1):59-68
[34] Riefkohl R, Kosanin R, Georgiade GS. Complications of the forehead-brow lift. Aesthetic Plast Surg 1983;7(3):135-8
[35] Gasperoni C, Salgarello M, Bajaj-Luthra A, Mueller T, Johnson PC. Karabulut AB, Tumerdem B. Forehead lift: a combined approach using subperiosteal and subgaleal dissection planes. Aesthetic Plast Surg 2001 Sep-Oct;25(5):378-81
[36] Camirand A, Doucet J. A comparison between parallel hairline incisions and perpendicular incisions when performing a face lift. Plast Reconstr Surg 1997 Jan;99(1):10-5
[37] Holcomb JD, McCollough EG. Trichophytic incisional approaches to upper facial rejuvenation. Arch Facial Plast Surg 2001 Jan-Mar;3(1):48-53
[38] Johnson CM Jr, Waldman SR. Midforehead lift. Arch Otolaryngol 1983 Mar;109(3):155-9
[39] Johnson CM Jr, Anderson JR, Katz RB. The brow-lift 1978. Arch Otolaryngol 1979 Mar;105(3):124-6 The We discuss the surgical technique in detail.
[40] Lewis JR Jr. A method of direct eyebrow lift. Ann Plast Surg 1983 Feb;10(2):115-9
[41] Byrd HS, Andochick SE. The deep temporal lift: a multiplanar, lateral brow, temporal, and upper face lift. Plast Reconstr Surg 1996 Apr;97(5):928-37
[42] Miller TA, Rudkin G, Honig M, Elahi M, Adams J.Lateral subcutaneous brow lift and interbrow muscle resection: clinical experience and anatomic studies. Plast Reconstr Surg 2000 Mar;105(3):1120-7; discussion 1128
[43] Gasperoni C, Salgarello M, Gargani G. Subperiosteal lateral browlift and its relationship to upper blepharoplasty. Aesthetic Plast Surg 1993 Summer;17(3):243-6

[44] Gargani G. Subperiosteal lateral browlift and its relationship to upper blepharoplasty. Aesthetic Plast Surg 1993 Summer;17(3):243-6

[45] Ramirez OM. Transblepharoplasty forehead lift and upper face rejuvenation. Ann Plast Surg 1996 Dec;37(6):577-84

[46] Ramirez OM. Endoscopically assisted biplanar forehead lift. Plast Reconstr Surg 1995 Aug;96(2):323-33

[47] Dayan SH, Perkins SW, Vartanian AJ, Wiesman IM. The forehead lift: endoscopic versus coronal approaches. Aesthetic Plast Surg 2001 Jan-Feb;25(1):35-9

[48] Pakkanen M, Salisbury AV, Ersek RA. Biodegradable positive fixation for the endoscopic brow lift. Plast Reconstr Surg 1996 Nov;98(6):1087-91

[49] McKinney P, Celetti S, Sweis I. An accurate technique for fixation in endoscopic brow lift. Plast Reconstr Surg 1996 Apr;97(4):824-7

[50] Namazie AR, Keller GS. Current practices in endoscopic brow and temporal lifting. Facial Plast Surg Clin North Am 2001 Aug;9(3):439-51

[51] Byrd HS. The extended browlift. Clin Plast Surg 1997 Apr;24(2):233-46

[52] Putterman AM. Intraoperatively controlled small-incision forehead and brow lift. Plast Reconstr Surg 1997 Jul;100(1):262-6

[53] Kikkawa DO, Miller SR, Batra MK, Lee AC. Small incision nonendoscopic browlift. Ophthal Plast Reconstr Surg 2000 Jan;16(1):28-33

[54] Graziosi AC, Beer SMC. pp Browlifting with thread: the technique without undermining using minimum incisions. Aesthetic Plast Surg 1998 Mar-Apr;22(2):120-5

[55] Ahn MS, Catten M, Maas CS. Temporal brow lift using botulinum toxin A. Plast Reconstr Surg 2000 Mar;105(3):1129-35; discussion 1136-9

[56] Serdev, N. Accessories to Face Lifting. II International Symposium of Updating on Skin Aesthetic, Sao Paolo, Brazil, 6-8 May, 1994

[57] Serdev N. Live Surgery Workshop, SMAS Lifting of the face by minimal incision – Brow, Temporal, Medial, Lower - the Serdev Technique. The International Academy of Aesthetic Surgery and Aesthetic Medicine, The Krulig Clinic, Caracas, Venezuela, Nov. 1999

[58] Serdev, N. Scarless Brow Lift Using A Special Suture. Presentations – 3rd World Congress of Cosmetic Surgery with Live Surgical Demonstrations. Int. J. Cosm. Surg. 2002, Volume 2, Number 4

[59] Serdev, N. P. Forehead Subperiosteal Masklift in Combination with McIndoe Facelift Technique and Profile Correction. The 7th IPRAS Congress European Section, Berlin, Germany, June 2-5, 1993.

[60] Serdev N. P. Temporal SMAS lift without skin excision In: Lip Augmentation During Mask and SMAS Lift Procedure, AAARS Annual Meeting, New Orleans, USA, October 5-9, 1994

[61] Serdev, N.P. Temporal SMAS Lifting of the Face. Life Surgery Workshop. Unidad Medica Clinica Del Country, Bogota D.C., Colombia, November 8-10, 1999

[62] Serdev, N. P. SMAS Lifting of the Face by Minimal Incisions – the Serdev Technique. Life Surgery Workshop sponsored by International Academy of Cosmetic surgery and

the Balkan Academy of Cosmetic Surgery, held at the Krilig Clinic in Caracas, Venezuela, November 12-18, 1999.

[63] Serdev, N. P. Principles of Face Beautification, Ier Congresso Internacional de Cirurgia Cosmetica, Buenos Ares Argentina, 31 Octubre – 1 de Noviembre 1999

[64] Serdev, N.P. Temporal SMAS lift, Lecture and Life Demonstration, 1st World Congress of Cosmetic Surgery with Life Demonstrations, Edsa Shangri-La Manila and Quezon City Medical Center, February 25-27, 2000.

[65] (http://www.mpint.co.jp/apacs/Congress2000/con007.htm).

[66] Serdev, N.P. Temporal SMAS Lifting of the Face, Combined with Liposuction and Chin Augmentation Using Suture. Life Surgery Workshop, Tel Aviv, Israel, April 20-24, 2000.

[67] Serdev, N. P. Principles of face beautification, The 3-rd World Congress of ISAS, Tokyo, April 8-10, 2000 , 9W58

[68] Serdev, N.P. Lifting del SMAS con Una Pequenna Incision Temporal, VIIIas Journadas Mediterraneas de Confrontaciones Terapeuticasen Medicina y Cirurgia Cosmetica, Sitges, Barcelona, March 16-19, 2000

[69] Serdev, N.P. Facial Rejuvenation by Minimal Skin Incisions, International Congress "Refinements in Aesthetic Surgery" Oradea, Romania, June 22-24

[70] Mitz, V, Peyronie M. The superficial musculoaponeurotic system (SMAS) in the parotid and cheek area. Plast. Reconstr. Surg. 1976; 58: 80.

[71] Miura Y, Moura PD, Ramasastry S, Hochberg J. Can we simplify the nomenclature of the fascial lyers of the temporo parietal region? OnLine J Plast Reconstr Surg, Nov 1997;1: 1.

[72] Stuzin, J. M., Baker, T. J., Gordon, H. L., and Baker, T. M. Extended SMAS dissection as an approach to midface rejuvenation. Clin. Plast. Surg. 1995; 22: 295.

[73] Connell, B. F., and Marten, T. J. The male foreheadplasty: Recognizing and treating aging in the upper face. Clin. Plast. Surg. 1991; 18: 653.

[74] Aston, S. J. Platysma-SMAS cervicofacial rhytidoplasty. Clin. Plast. Surg. 1983;10: 507.

[75] Barton, F. E., Jr. The SMAS and the nasolabial fold. Plast. Reconstr. Surg. 1992; 89: 1054.

[76] Bosse, J. P., and Papillon, J. Surgical Anatomy of the SMAS at the Malar Region. In Transactions of the 9th International Congress of Plastic and Reconstructive Surgery. New York: McGraw-Hill, 1987: 348.

[77] Cardoso de Castro, C. The role of the superficial musculoaponeurotic system in face lift. Ann. Plast. Surg. 1986; 16: 276.

[78] Stuzin JM, Wagstrom L, Kawamoto HK, Wolfe SA. Anatomy of the frontal branch of the facial nerve: The Significance of the Temporal Fat Pad. Plast Reconstr Surg 1989; 83: 265-71.

[79] Ramirez OM, Maillard GF, Musolas A. The extended Subperiosteal Face lift: A definitive Soft-tissue Remodeling for Facial Rejuvenation. Plast Reconstr Surg 1991; 88:227-36.

[80] Tolhurst DE, Carstens MH, Greco RJ, Hurwitz DJ. The Surgical Anatomy of The Scalp. Plast Reconstr Surg 1991; 87: 603-12.

[81] Larrabee Jr., W.F., Makielski, K.H. Surgical Anatomy of the face. New York: Raven Press,1993: 41-48.

[82] Hochberg J, Kaufman H, Ardenghy M. Saving The Frontal Branch during a Low Fronto-orbital Approach. Aesth Plast Surg 1995; 19: 161-163.

[83] Core GB, Vasconez LO, Graham III, HD Endoscopic Browlift. Clin. Plast. Surg.1995; 22: 619-31.

[84] Bostwick III, J., Eaves, F.F., Nahai, F. Endoscopic Plastic Surgery. Quality Medical Publishing, Inc. St. Louis, MO, 1995: 86-129. S.E. The Deep Temporal Lift: A multiplanar, lateral Brow, Temporal, and Upper face Lift. Plast. Reconstr Surg 1996; 5: 928-37.

[85] Bostwick III, J., Eaves, F.F., Nahai, F. Endoscopic Plastic Surgery. Quality Medical Publishing, Inc. St. Louis, MO, 1995: 86-129.

[86] De la Fuente A, Santamaria AB Endoscopic subcutaneous and SMAS facelift without preauricular scars.Aesthetic Plast Surg1999 Mar-Apr; 23: 119-24.

[87] Kamer FM, Frankel SMAS rhytidectomy versus deep plane rhytidectomy: an objective comparison.ASPlast Reconstr Surg 1998 Sep; 102 (3): 878-81

[88] Hagerty RC, Scioscia PJThe medial SMAS lift with aggressive temporal skin takeout.Plast Reconstr Surg 1998 May; 101 (6):1650-6.

[89] Gray H, Goss CM. Anatomy of The Human Body. Philadelphia: Lea and Febiger, 1966: 375-99.

[90] Hamra ST. The tri-plane face lift dissection. Ann Plast Surg 1984 Mar; 12 (3): 268-74.

[91] Casanova R, Cavalcante D, Grotting JC, Vasconez LO, Psillakis JM. Anatomic basis for Vascularized Outer-Table Calvarial Bone flaps. Plast. Reconstr Surg 1986; 78: 300-8.

[92] Abul-Hassan, HS, Ascher, GD, Acland, RD. Surgical Anatomy and Blood Supply of the Fascial Layers of the Temporal Region. Plast Reconstr Surg 1986; 77: 17-24.

[93] Hamra ST. The deep-plane rhytidectomy. Plast Reconstr Surg 1990 Jul; 86 (1):53-61.

[94] Mitz V, Use of deep planes in surgery of rejuvenation of the face Chirurgie 1991; 117 (4): 278-86.

[95] De La Plaza R, Valiente E, Arroyo JM, Supraperiosteal lifting of the upper two-thirds of the face.Br J Plast Surg 1991 Jul; 325 :32- 44.

[96] Caix P, Goin JL, Modschiedler T. "Total SMAS lift" or deep facial lift by temporal approach. Initial eport. Ann Chir Plast Esthet 1992 Jan; 37 (1): 67-74.

[97] Bonnefon ADeep "en bloc" facial lift" Ann Chir Plast Esthet 1992 Jan; 37 (1), 85-94

[98] Hamra ST, Composite rhytidectomy.Plast Reconstr Surg, 1992 Jul; 90 (1): 1-13.

[99] Teimourian B, Delia S, Wahrman A, The multiplane face lift.Plast Reconstr Surg 1994 Jan 93; 1: 78-85.

[100] Campiglio GL, Candiani P. Anatomical study on the temporal fascial layers and their relationships with the facial nerve.Aesthetic Plast Surg 1997 Mar-Apr; 21 (2): 69-74.

[101] Byrd HS The extended browlift. Clin Plast Surg, 1997 Apr; 24 (2): 233-46.

[102] Honig JF Concepts in face lifts. State of the art Mund Kiefer Gesichtschir 1997 May; 1(Suppl): 1S21-6.

[103] Bonnefon A. Deep vertical lift and its development regarding the central facial area and lower two-thirds of the neck. Our technique, Ann Chir Plast Esthet, 1999 Dec: 609-16.

[104] Quatela VC, Sabini P. Techniques in deep plane face lifting. Facial Plast Surg 2000 May; 2: 193-209.

[105] Mittelman H, Newman J. Smasectomy and imbrication in face lift surgery.Facial Plast Surg 2000 May; 2: 173-82.

[106] Maloney BP, Schiebelhoffer J. Minimal-incision endoscopic face-lift. Arch Facial Plast Surg 2000 Oct-Dec; 4: 274-8.

[107] Achauer BM, Adair SR, VanderKam VM, Combined rhytidectomy and full-face laser resurfacing. Plast Reconstr Surg, Dec 2000; 106: 1608-11.

[108] Serdev, N. Glabella muscles ligature using Serdev Suture technique, http://www.youtube.com/watch?v=F7r-W7-kK20

[109] Edgerton, M., Wolfort, F. Technique of Value in the Surgical Treatment of Facial Palsy, Plastic & Reconstructive Surgery: January 1969 - Volume 43 - Issue 1 - ppg 42-52

[110] Montadon, D. A Modification of the Dermal-Flap Canthal Lift for Correction of the Paralyzed Lower Eyelid, Plastic & Reconstructive Surgery: April 1978 - Volume 61 - Issue 4 - ppg 555-557

[111] Yip C-Chew, McCann J. D., Goldberg R. A. The Role of Midface Lift and Lateral Canthal Repositioning in the Managementof Euryblepharon, Arch Ophthalmol. 2004;122(7):1075-1077.

Chapter 2

Serdev Sutures® in Middle Face

Nikolay Serdev

Additional information is available at the end of the chapter

http://dx.doi.org/10.5772/55674

1. Introduction

Scarless, closed approach Serdev Suture® liftings, suspensions and tissue volumising in middle face present skeletal fixation with skin punctures, without incisions. They are a first and in many cases -superior alternative to classic excision lifts, implants etc. Author's contribution is that his closed approach suture techniques can be used in areas, where access is difficult or impossible for other surgeries; they lift SMAS and fascias without traditional incisions; cheekbone augmentation and lifting is possible without implants and transplants. Operations are ambulatory, with excellent results, as reported by the patients. Trauma is minimal and the follow-up period is not longer than a few hours to 3 days with fast, sometimes immediate return to work and social life. There are no visible scars, only needle perforations on the skin, which disappear within 2-3 days. The techniques consist of passing closed sutures, by needle perforations only, to lift movable fascias and fix them to non-movable skeletal structures in several mid-facial areas.

2. Cheekbone lift

2.1. Introduction

Scarless, closed approach Serdev Suture® techniques for augmentation and lifting of cheekbones were introduced by the author in 1994. They use the **mobile cheek SMAS flap** or **fascial tube of the buccal fat pad** (also called Bichat's fat pad) to elevate and attach it to the **immobile, stable zygoma periosteum**, and in selected rare cases - to the **orbital rim periosteum**, or **temporoparietal tendon insertion and underlying periosteum,** or the **upper temporal line periosteum and temporal fascia**. The idea is to lift the SMAS and fat pad via its fascial tube at the level of the zygomatic bone; restore cheekbone fullness; volumize and elevate the cheekbone; eliminate the tear trough fold; improve facial expression; and achieve a youthful elongation of the so-called "beauty triangle". To achieve the cheekbone lift, the author uses special semi-blunt and semi-elastic curved needles with lengths of 50 mm, 60 mm, 100 mm, and 140 mm with an eye at the tip, and prefers semi-elastic Bulgarian polycaproamide (Polycon) USP 2 sutures with prolonged resorption (2-3 years). The Serdev Suture® lifting techniques are ambulatory, performed under local anesthesia, very well tolerated by patients, produce immediate results, with an extremely short post operative period, fast recovery and nearly immediate return to social life. Complications are under 0,1% and patient satisfaction is high, especially in the aesthetic aspects of rejuvenation and beautification.

There were no known specific surgical methods for simultaneous direct cheekbone lifting, enhancement and volumising without the use of implants or transplants before 1994. The superficial muscle-aponeurotic system, or SMAS, was described by Mitz and Peyronie in 1976 and the SMAS facelift became the gold standard. Earlier procedures developed into a large rotation-advancement skin flap for indirect lifting of this area. Classic rhytidectomy progressed into sub-fascial, tri-plane, deep-plane, composite, subperiosteal, multiplane, "en-bloc" and other extended surgical methods, with a progressively increasing rate of complications and downtime. Nowadays, minor operations with reduced risks and faster recovery time have become more common, but the SMAS lifts without undermining remain the best long-term suspension, affecting the overlying skin. Later techniques, such as barbed "thread lifts", are placed subdermally and naturally cannot include the SMAS in the lift. They are free floating, not sutured, nor stabilized by attachment to immobile anatomical structures. Therefore, in the author's opinion, they are different from suture lifts and cannot guarantee a safe prolonged outcome.

2.2. Procedure

Anesthesia

Only local anaesthesia, or in combination with i.v. sedation, is used. It is preferable to general anaesthesia, due to the benefits of decreased intervention time and for preferences expressed by the surgeon and patient.

Anatomical guidelines

A **"Fascial tube"** was found by the author to envelop the Bichat's fat pad at the nasolabial fold. He captures this mobile fascial tube and uses it to lift the included fat pad to the zygoma periosteum, for a cheekbone lift.

A **"Danger area"** is described by the author, where the frontal branch of the facial nerve is believed to cross the zygomatic bone, traveling along a line that connects the tragus base to a point 1.5 cm above the eyebrow. The topographical anatomy forms a square – 3 cm anterior to the tragus and 3 cm above the zygomatic bone (danger area). **NB!** Needle perforation and attachment to the zygoma in a cheekbone lift should not be performed in this area! Do not perforate the zygoma periosteum in the first 3 cm anterior to the tragus! When performing a cheekbone lift in this zone, the needle must be in a superficial, subgaleal mobile plane. If the needle gets blocked in the "danger area", it means that it has perforated the deeper non-mobile lamina superficialis of the temporal fascia, which is a potentially dangerous situation (see the anatomical description in "Temporal face lift"), because of possible vessel perforation. In such case, prolonged direct pressure is described to stop bleeding in this area.

The temporoparietal tendon is attached to and above the spina suprameatica of the meatus acusticus externus. Its insertions, together with the underlying periosteum are stable, immobile and in rare cases are used by the author for mid-face lift. **NB!** Temporalis fascia and tendon fibers are directed downwards and aren't suitable for attachment in middle face lift, nor for a temporal lift (Fig. 1).

The SMAS has a fascial extension, attached to the zygoma (called zygomatic SMAS exptension), which can move up and down, permitting facial movement and flaccidity. The author captures and stretches this mobile extension in a temporoparietal direction, thus lifting the mid and lower face SMAS.

The cheekbone lift, using a transcutaneous closed suture approach, without excision of skin, was created initially (1990-1993) due to an increasing demand by young (as well as elderly) patients, who declined classic scarring lifts, associated with a month-lasting recovery, and also by people who could not afford to skip their work for a long time. Exploring topographic anatomy, designing new instruments and semi-elastic sutures allowed the author to lift loose SMAS and fat pads, using patients' own fascial structures, and attach them to stable, immobile anatomical structures, zygomatic periosteum and in rare cases – to temporoparietal tendon insertion and underlying periosteum, or upper temporal line periosteum with temporal fascia. To achieve the objective of scarless lifting, the author uses needle perforations only. In order to attach the different subdermal fascial layers, he has created special curved, semi-blunt and semi-elastic needles with different lengths. For the cheekbone lift, 50 mm, 60 mm, 100 mm or 140 mm Serdev® needles are used. They can

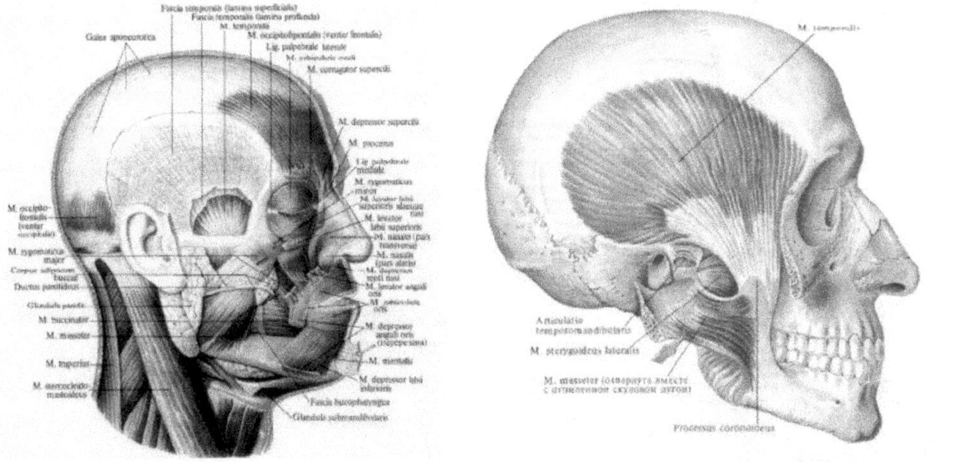

A B

Figure 1. A, B. Temporal tendon and fascia are not suitable for mid-face fixation and lifting, because of their direction. Sutures slide down due to distal fibers direction. ***Anatomy figures from Sinelnikov - Atlas Of Human Anatomy, GIML, Moscow, 1963**

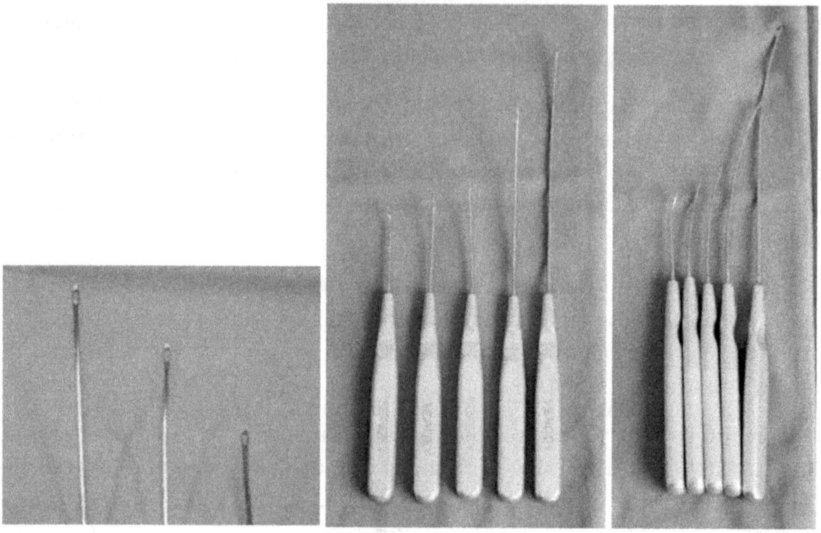

Figure 2. Curved, semi-blunt and semi-elastic needles, with lengths of 50 mm, 60 mm, 100 mm and 140 mm and hollow tip.

introduce long-term absorbable (in 2-3 years), semi-elastic Polycon USP 2 surgical sutures, for suturing the fat pad fascial tube and attaching it to the stable zygomatic periosteum. Suture selection is the surgeon's responsibility; nevertheless, a proper diameter semi-elastic surgical suture is recommended to obtain long-term results. Sutures with a diameter of 3/0 and 2/0 are too thin for the middle and lower face heaviness and act like a scalpel (cutting through the tissues) and fail to securely immobilize facial tissue. They are not acceptable or appropriate for satisfactory and stable results.

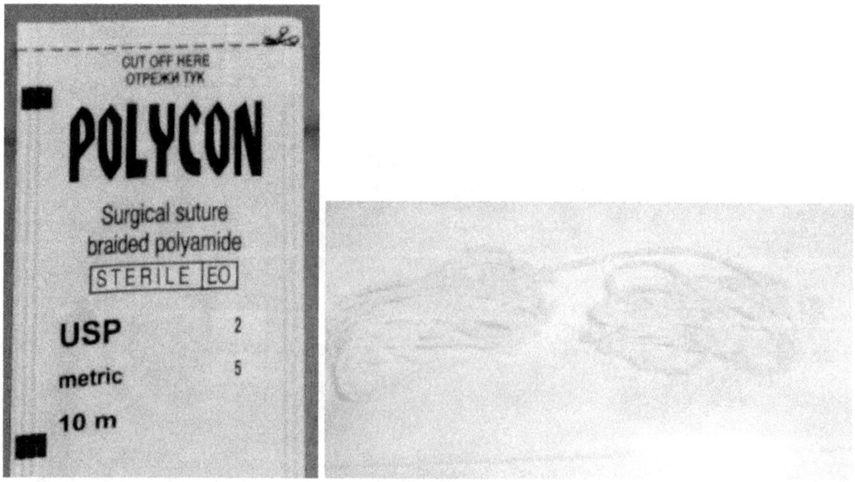

Figure 3. Long-term absorbable (in 2-3 years), semi-elastic, braided, antimicrobial Bulgarian polycaproamide (Polycon) USP 2 surgical sutures for suture cheekbone lift.

Surgical methods

For any of the cheekbone lifts described below, the author uses 2 or 3 skin perforations to introduce the needle and place the suture at the desired anatomical level.

Most important attachments:

- **immobile attachment**: to the zygomatic periosteum; or the temporoparietal tendon insertion and the periosteum underneath; orbital rim periosteum; upper temporal line periosteum and temporal fascia.
- **attachment of mobile** Bichat's fat pad fascial tube, cheek SMAS and zygomatic SMAS extension to be lifted to an immobile attachment. The author has found a fascial tube to envelop the Bichat's fat pad.

Skin perforation point A:

The skin perforation point A can be positioned differently in young and in elderly patients, in order to obtain a secure attachment of the suture to the zygoma periosteum or the temporoparietal tendon insertion and periosteum below, or the upper temporal line and temporal fascia, or the border of the orbit.

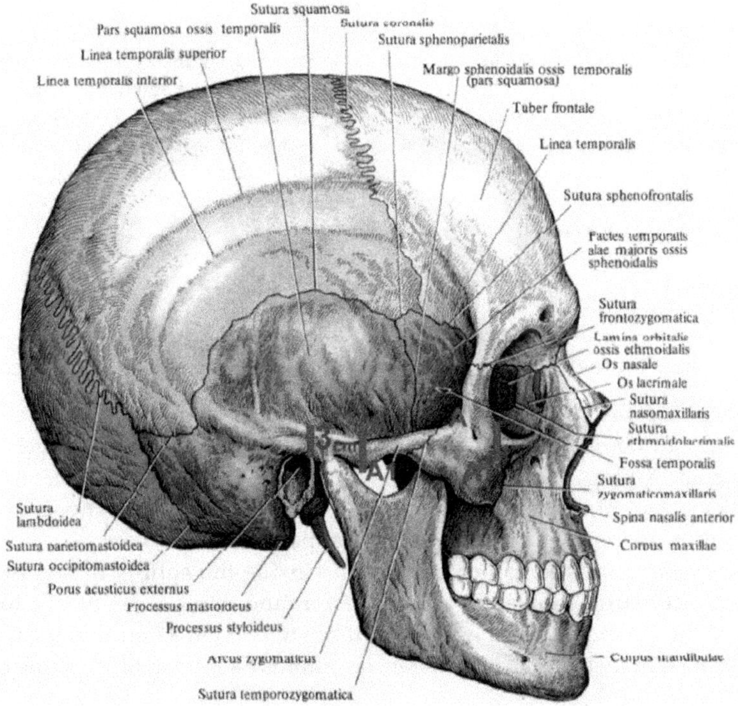

Figure 4. The main suture fixation is to zygoma periosteum. There is a limitation for perforation of the zygoma periosteum in the "danger area" – the first 3 cm in front of the tragus. **Anatomy figures from Sinelnikov - Atlas Of Human Anatomy, GIML, Moscow, 1963.**

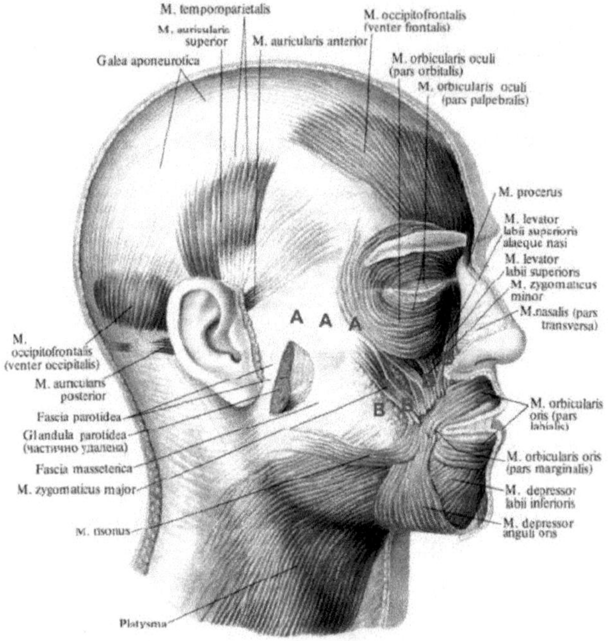

Figure 5. Skin Perforation Point A can be located along the length of the zygoma, except in the danger area - the first 3 cm in front of the tragus. Perforation point B is located about 3 mm laterally to the nasolabial fold. This allows the nasolabial fold to be stretched and flattened. Point B could be planned at any point along the length of the nasolabial fold, from the nasolabial angle up to the oral commissure and smiling point. The smiling dimple location is at the intersection of the following lines: 1. The line, connecting the oral commissure and the tragus; 2. The lateral canthus line. ***Anatomy figures from Sinelnikov - Atlas Of Human Anatomy, GIML, Moscow, 1963**

1. At the zygoma

Point A can be located along the length of the zygoma, except in the danger area, which is the first 3 cm anterior to the tragus and should not be used to attach the sutures.

- **In young and middle aged patients: At the intersection of the lateral canthus line with the upper zygoma line.** This is the preferred point to catch the zygoma periosteum. Young people do not have a large quantity of tissue to enhance the cheekbones, but many of them have a marked tear trough fold. Higher cheekbones are always nice, giving a young and attractive appearance.
- **In elderly the aim is to gather more tissue inside the suture, flatten the tear trough fold and lift marionette and jaw lines. Perforation point A can be at a lower, anterior angle of the sideburn hairline.** This point has to be 1 cm anterior to the presumed path of the frontal branch of the facial nerve, i.e. minimum 3 cm anterior to the tragus.

2. Other rare anatomical immobile fixations (point A)

- **at the temporo-auricular angle - in bald patients,** to catch the temporoparietal tendon insertion and the periosteum underneath.

- **at the upper temporal line - in selected cases, mostly in open surgery.**
- **at the orbital rim - in selected cases, mostly in open surgery.**

Skin perforation point B. Attachment of Bichat's fat pad fascial tube and/or the cheek SMAS:

Point B is located about 3 mm lateral to the nasolabial fold. This allows the nasolabial fold to be stretched and flattened. It can be placed at any point along the length of the nasolabial fold – from the nasolabial angle to the oral commissure and smiling point. The smiling point is located at the intersection of lines: 1. connecting the oral commissure and the tragus and 2. the lateral canthus line.

- **at the nasolabial angle** - in young patients: 2 variations:
  - **Skin perforation** at 3 mm laterally from the nasolabial fold, or
  - **Transmucosal in the nostril** (Fig. 7). **NB!** To protect the suture and needle from the nostril mucosa, the author uses plastic cannulas with openings at both ends. They are easily made from needle caps, by cutting the closed end.
- **at the mid point of the nasolabial fold** - in middle aged or elderly patients: 3mm laterally from the nasolabial fold
- **at the lower point of the nasolabial fold** - in elderly patients with a pronounced nasolabial fold, 3mm laterally from the nasolabial fold in 2 variations:
  - **Skin perforation** at 3 mm laterally from the nasolabial fold, or
  - **Transmucosal in the oral cavity. NB!** To protect the suture and needle from the oral mucosa, use plastic cannulas with 2 open ends.
- **at the smiling point – in elderly patients,** for cephalic traction of "hanging" jowls and fat pads in elderly patients to gather more soft tissue and correct marionette and jaw lines. **NB!** In all variations, the Bichat's fat pad fascial tube has to be captured along its entire length using one or two skin perforation points. If two skin perforation points at B are used, their location should be: 1. at the nasolabial angle and 2. at the level of the oral commissure, 3 mm lateral to the nasolabial folds or at the smiling point.

The traction **vector** is in a cephalic or temporoparietal direction.

2.3. Medial cheekbone projection. Mostly using 2 perforation points

1. **Fixation at anterior zygoma.** Perforation Point A at the lateral canthus line, 1 cm lower than lateral canthus, Point B at nasolabial angle in 2 variants: Perforation point B through skin or through nasal mucosa

Option 1. Lifting of buccal fat pad fascial tube

Video: http://www.youtube.com/watch?v=jbi3hHxUdcw

First pass: After local infiltration, the skin perforation points are punctured using a No. 11 scalpel blade and widened with the tip of mosquito clamp. **NB!** The superficial fascia should be perforated as well, otherwise the suture will involve it in traction, forming dimples.

Using skin perforations:

A semi-blunt, curved 50 mm or 60 mm Serdev® needle is introduced at point A at the lateral canthus line, 1 cm below the lateral canthus on the cheekbone prominence; the pass is first made subperiosteally, engaging the anterior zygoma periosteum. **NB!** At that stage, check whether the needle is locked under the periosteum. If positioned subperiosteally, the needle can lift the entire head, due to the strength of the zygoma periosteum. If the needle moves freely, it means the needle is not inserted at the sub-periosteal level. This is a common beginner's error and the needle should be repositioned deeper, under the periosteum. Then, the needle passes deep in the soft tissue flap, following the lower cheek line. When it arrives at the distal end of the nasolabial fold, distal to perforation point B, it should perforate the fascial tube of buccal Bichat's fat pad. After changing direction (while still inside the fat pad fascial tube), the needle tip arrives under point B. Turn the tip upward towards the opening B, then fold the skin against the needle tip at a 90^0 angle and move the needle upwards with a gentle twisting movement until it exits from point B. The specially designed needle surface prevents cutting the periosteum in line A-A1 and allows all subsequent movements. **NB!** Avoid catching the dermis as you enter or exit through the skin perforation points, in order to prevent skin dimpling. If you feel that the needle is encountering resistance, it means that the needle has caught the dermis. Twist the needle, while withdrawing it, and repeat the maneuver. Do not push or pull – twist the needle gently forwards or backwards.

The suture is then introduced in the needle eye and the first suture end is pulled out through line A-B (Fig.6).

Transmucosal perforation point B: Perforation point B could be done inside the lateral nostril. The surgical suture and needle should be protected from nostril mucosa (using a cannula), in order to prevent contamination. The author uses needle caps with a cut dead end (Fig. 7).

Second pass: It is performed above the zygoma, mid-deep in the soft tissue (do not touch zygoma periosteum): The needle is introduced through point A. It passes medium deep in the soft tissue flap, just above the upper zygoma line. **NB!** This pass is made in mobile tissue. Avoid making this pass too deep – the needle can become blocked in the supraperiosteal fibrotic tissue. After perforation of the fat pad fascial tube at its upper part, the needle direction is changed (while still inside the fat pad fascial tube) and exits at point B (in skin perforation or trans-mucosal). The second suture end is introduced in the needle eye and pulled out through the second needle pass A-B. The suture circle is now completed, attaching the buccal fat pad fascia to the zygoma periosteum, and a knot is tied under medium tension. **NB!** Making the knot too tight can damage the involved tissue. Dimpling is released by pulling the suture ends upwards and the skin in perforation point B downwards, using the tip of a mosquito clamp.

Medial cheekbone lift in cephalic direction solves emptiness below the eyes in Asians, hollow eyes, tear through fold, gives volume, projects and lifts cheekbone medially (important in Asians). Soft tissue amount inside the suture provides cheekbone volume and prominence.

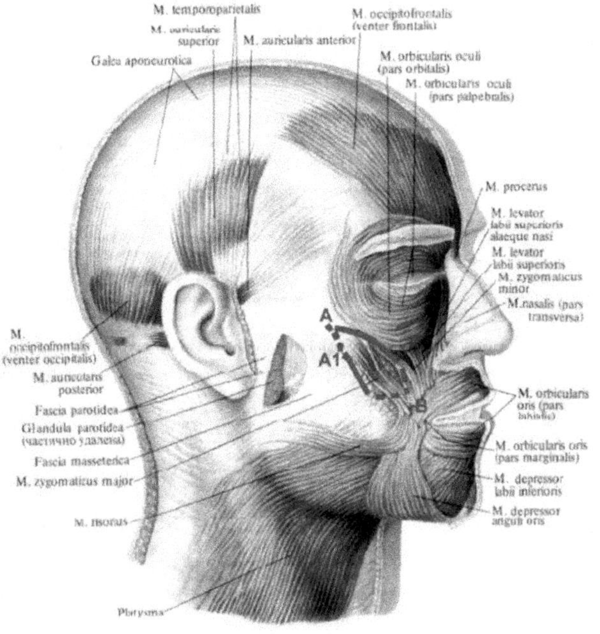

Figure 6. Traction on Bichat's fat pad fascial tube. In young, middle aged patients and Asians, to obtain medial cheekbone projection. The dotted A-A1 pass is subperiosteal. Point A1 is only a mark, not a perforation. Dotted line B marks the pass inside the fascial tube of Bichat's fat pad. ***Anatomy figures from Sinelnikov - Atlas Of Human Anatomy, GIML, Moscow, 1963**

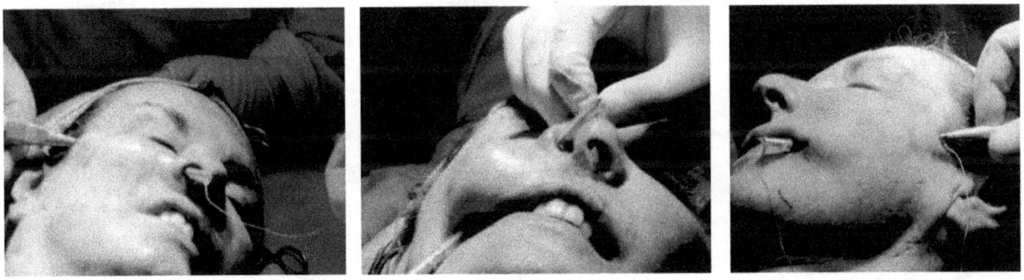

A B C

Figure 7. Transmucosal cheekbone lift. Protection of needle and suture contamination using plastic cannula from a needle cap.

Option 2: Lifting of muscle-cheek SMAS flap (Fig 8):

First (deep) pass A-B

After local anesthesia, skin perforations are made, using a No. 11 scalpel blade. A 60 mm Serdev® needle is introduced through point A, biting into the anterior zygoma periosteum, then continuing directly to point B, deep into the cheek SMAS. The needle passes through

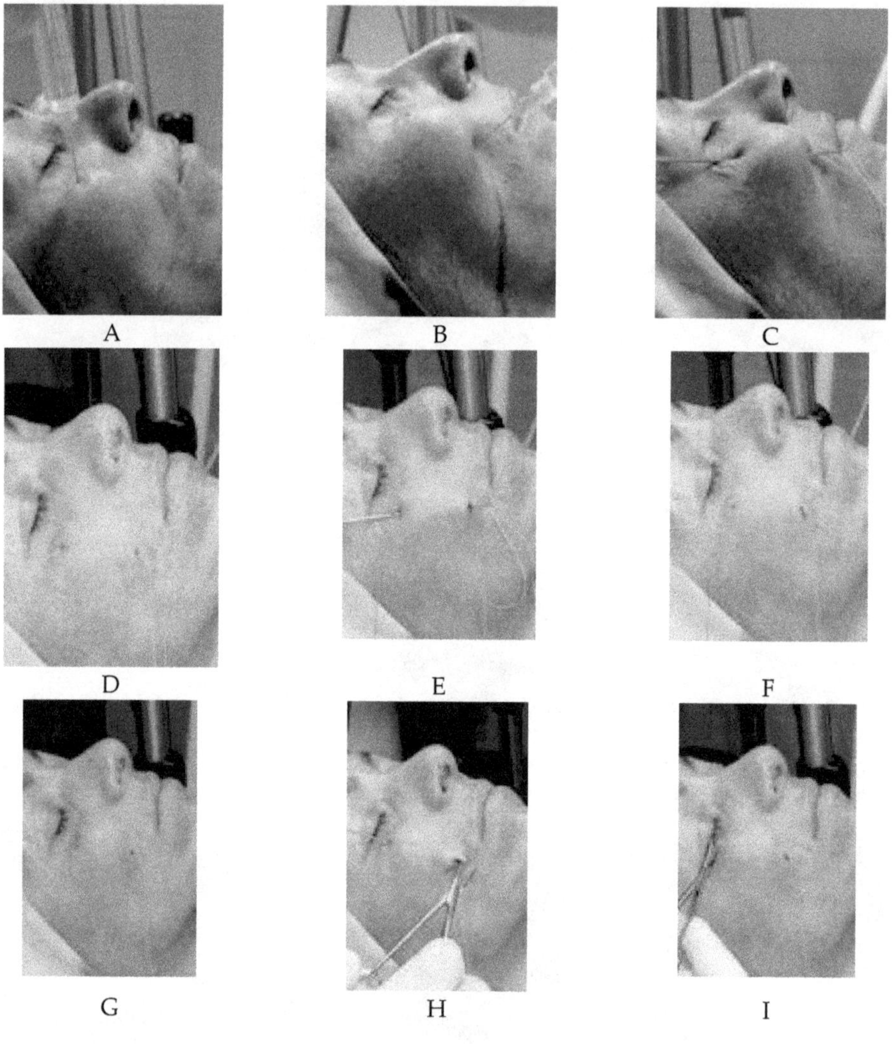

Figure 8. Lifting of muscle-cheek SMAS flap using 2 perforation points. Steps: A., B. intradermal infiltration at skin perforation points A and B; subdermal infiltration in deep and middle deep lines A-B; skin perforations made with a No. 11 blade; widening of the perforations using the tip of a mosquito clamp; **C.** Serdev® needle is introduced through 1. perforation point A, 2. anterior zygoma periosteum, 3. deeper cheek SMAS flap, 4. the buccal fat pad fascial tube; exits through point B. The needle is threaded; **D.** Semi-elastic Polycon suture is introduced through the first needle pass A-B; **E.** Second needle pass A-B is more superficial, but deep enough not to form dimpling on the skin surface, the needle is treaded at point B; **F.** The second end of the suture is introduced in the second, more superficial needle pass A-B; **G.** The suture circle is completed and knotted. The lifting and volumising of the cheekbone is immediately visible; **H.** Any skin dimpling is removed using the tip of a mosquito clamp instrument. Suture and skin perforation are pulled in opposed directions; **I.** Any dimpling in perforation point A should also be removed using a mosquito clamp.

the buccal fat pad fascial tube, point B, and is treaded. Then, it is introduced through the first (deep) needle pass A-B.

Second (more superficial) pass A-B

The second needle pass A-B is more superficial (again directed from A to B). **NB!** Avoid a too superficial pass. If dimples appear on the skin surface above the needle position, it means that it is located too superficially and should be introduced deeper.

In point B, the needle is threaded and the second suture end is introduced in the more superficial needle pass A-B. The suture circle is completed. Both suture ends at point A and the skin perforation B are pulled in opposite directions to remove any skin dimpling. Remove any dimpling at perforation point A as well.

In both options the zygomatic SMAS extension is also included in the lift.

Medial cheekbone lifting in cephalic direction resolves the flat emptiness below the eyes in Asians, hollow eyes, tear trough folds; adds volume, projects and lifts the cheekbone medially. The amount of soft tissue inside the suture provides cheekbone volume and prominence, without implants and transplants. In Asians the procedures for medial cheekbone lift can remarkably reduce lateral bulging of the zygoma, soften the facial oval and give a Caucasian type appearance.

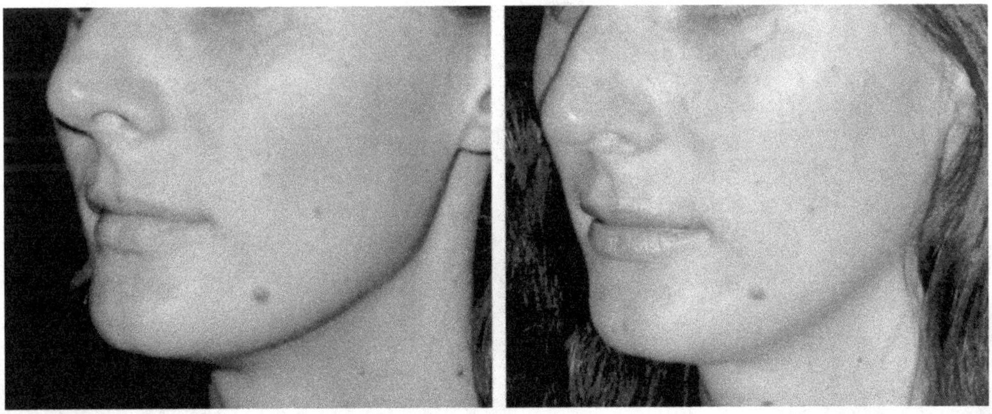

Figure 9. Medial cheekbone lift to fulfill the emptiness below the eyes. Better definition of the beauty triangle.

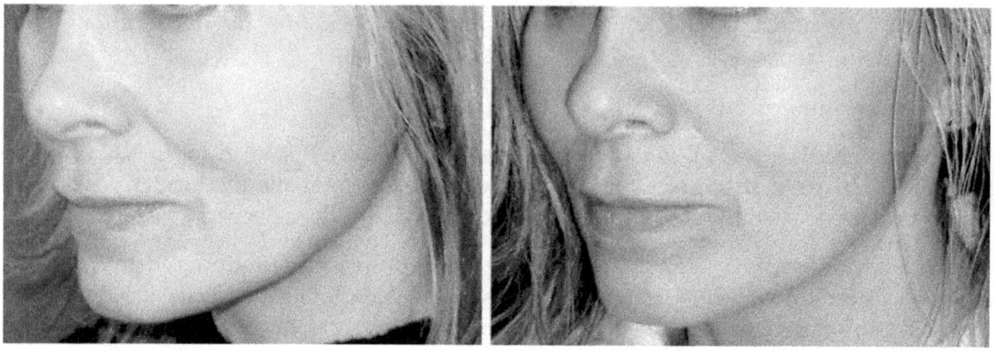

Figure 10. Medial cheekbone lift. Higher cheekbones and better definition of the beauty triangle

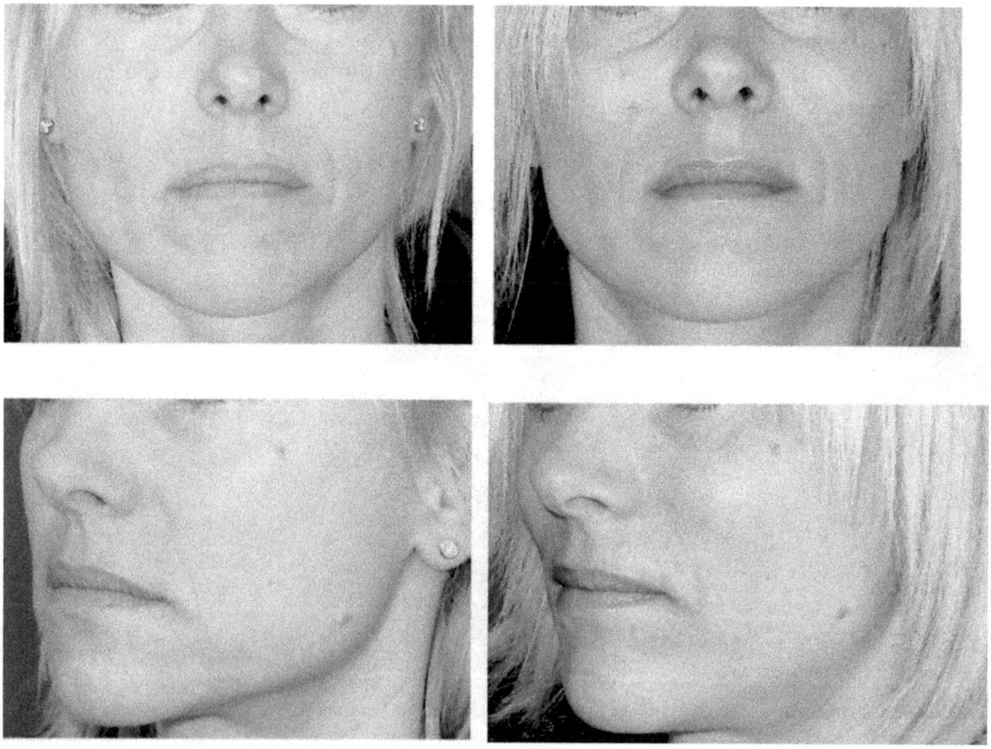

Figure 11. Before and after simultaneous cheekbone SMAS lift and chin enhancement by suture to obtain the "beauty triangle". Lifting of muscle-cheek SMAS flap, using 2 perforation points in a 49 y.o. patient.

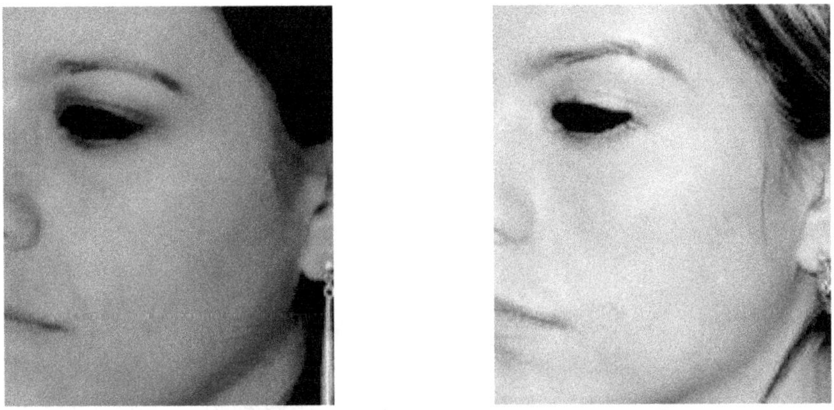

A B

Figure 12. Cheekbone augmentation and lifting. **A.** Before; **B.** After cheekbone lift and simultaneous brow lift by suture.

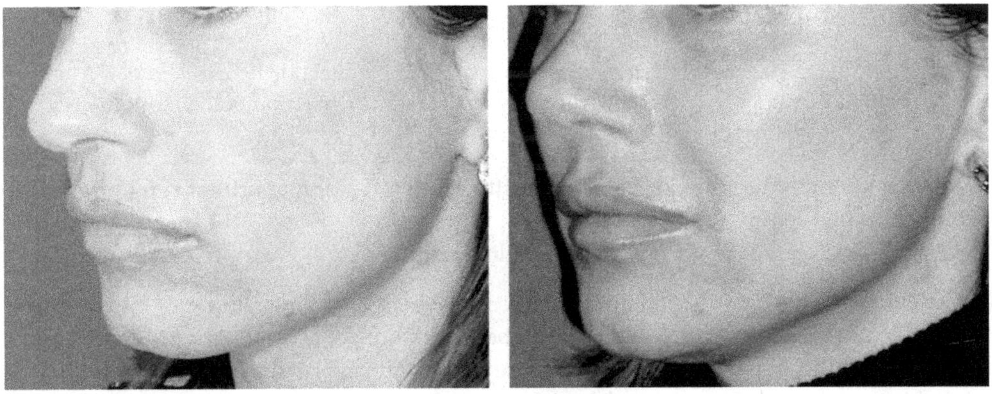

Figure 13. Medial cheekbone lift in a 45 y.o. patient to fulfill the tear trough fold, lift and volumize the cheekbones. Better definition of the beauty triangle. Simultaneous nasal tip rotation by suture aligns the tip at the line of the cheekbones (part of beauty triangle).

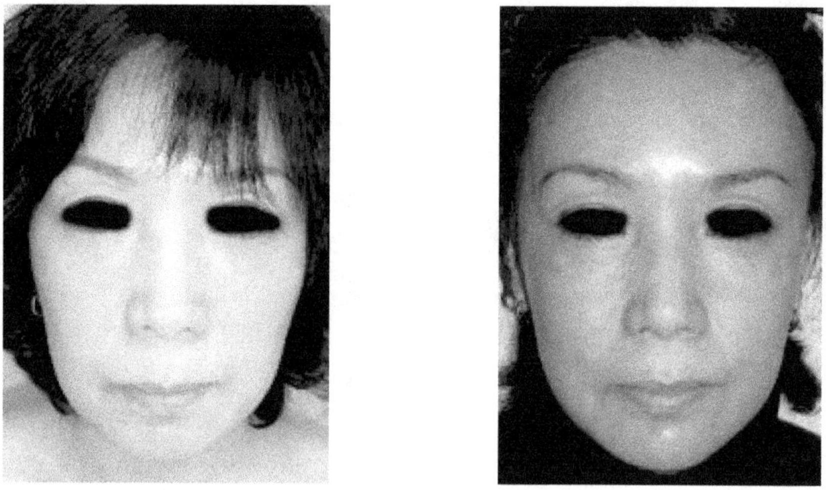

A B

Figure 14. Medial cheekbone lift in an Asian patient, **A.** Before, **B.** After. Medial cheekbone enhancement and simultaneous chin down lift (moving the chin down) for proportion correction by suture change Asian face into a Caucasian oval appearance.

2. Another possibility for medial cheekbone lifting is the **fixation at orbital rim periosteum.** Skin perforation point A at desired orbital rim position, Point B at any point of the nasolabial fold, 3 mm lateral from it, or at smiling point:

The technique is the same as the one described above, in 2 variants: lifting of muscle-cheek SMAS flap or facial tube of buccal fat pad. In both variations, the zygomatic SMAS extension is also included in the lift. The older and more flabby the patient, the lower the point B. It is advisable to include Bichat's fat pad fascial tube in the suture in both variants. This is a very rarely used modification, only in cases where higher fixation is needed, usually in cases with smaller lower face proportion and mostly in open surgery, combined with blepharoplasy. For cases of facial disproportions in the lower face and especially in microgenia and retrogenia, the author has in his hands the suture method to elongate and enhance the chin (see Fig. 14 and Serdev Sutures® in Lower Face) that is a better technique to adapt proportions.

2.4. Lateral cheekbone projection

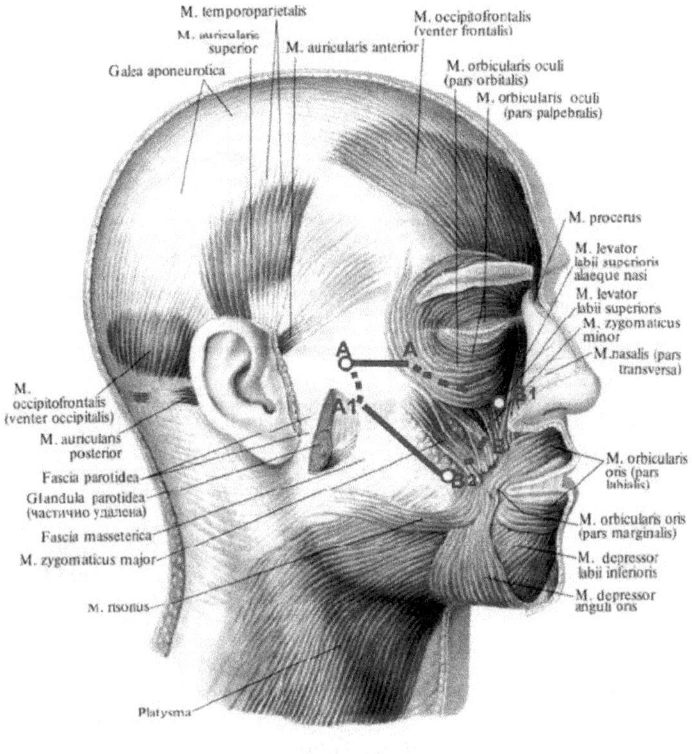

Figure 15. Skin perforation point A is located at lower, anterior sideburn hairline angle. Using 1 or 2 perforation points B. A) In elderly patients two B points are used to collect more soft tissue and to obtain the lateral cheekbone projection. Pass A-A1 is subperiosteal. A1 is only a mark, not a skin perforation point. All the B perforation points are 3mm lateral to the nasolabial fold. The dotted A-B1 line is located in deep soft tissue, below the lower lid. The dotted B1-B2 line is located inside the fascial tube of Bichat's fat pad. B) If only one perforation point B is used, points B1 and B2 are only marks (not perforated). ***Anatomy figures from Sinelnikov - Atlas Of Human Anatomy, GIML, Moscow, 1963**

1. Fixation to posterior zygoma periosteum. Using 2 perforation points. Skin perforation point A at lower anterior sideburn hair line angle, point B at any point at nasolabial fold, 3 mm lateral from it **or at smiling point** (Fig.15).

The older and more flacid the patient, the lower point B should be located. Bichat's fat pad fascial tube should be included in the suture. At the lower part of the nasolabial fold, perforation point B can be made through the skin or the oral mucosa. This suture presents: Combined traction on SMAS zygomatic extension and fat pad fascias; Collection of all the cheekbone soft tissue.

First Pass A-(A1)-(B2)-B – deep in the tissue flap (see Fig.15)

Variation 1 - Perforation point B through the skin: a 140 mm Serdev® needle is introduced in point A, at the lower anterior sideburn hairline angle; at the start the pass is subperiosteal, biting anterior zygoma periosteum (line A-A1). Point A1 is only a mark, not a perforation point. **NB!** At that point check whether the needle is locked under the periosteum. If it moves freely, it is not inserted at the subperiosteal level and should be repositioned deeper, under the periosteum. After that, the needle passes deep in the soft tissue, following the lower cheek line. When the fascial tube of Bichat's fat pad is reached, it should be perforated at the distal part (marked, but no skin perforation at point B2). Subsequently, the direction of the needle is changed toward point B (while still inside the fat pad fascial tube). Fold the skin against the needle tip at a 90^0 angle and with a gentle twisting motion move the needle upward until it exits from point B. **NB!** Try to avoid engaging the dermis as you enter or exit through the perforation points, in order to prevent creation of skin dimpling. If you feel the needle facing any resistance it means that the needle has caught the dermis. In such case, pull the needle backwards by twisting it, and repeat the maneuver. Do not push or pull – twist the needle gently forwards or backwards. The needle is threaded and the first suture end is pulled out through the A-B needle pass.

Variation 2 - Transmucosal perforation point B: At the lower nasolabial fold, point B is made through the oral mucosa. The needle and suture should be protected from the mucosa with a cannula (cut needle cap), to prevent contamination.

Second pass A-(A)-(B1)-B

The needle is introduced through point A, without catching periosteum, and continues in a medium deep level above the zygoma to the lateral canthus line (line A-A). If a dimple appears on the skin surface above the needle position, it means that the needle is located too superficially and should be repositioned deeper. At the lateral canthus line, the needle changes direction below the lower lid and perforates the fascial tube of Bichat's fat pad at its upper point B1 (B1 is only a mark). Then, the needle direction is changed (while still inside the fat pad fascial tube) and exits at perforation point B (through the skin or trans-mucosal). The second suture end is threaded and pulled out through the needle pass A-B (A-(A)-(B1)-B). This completes the suture circle, attaching the buccal fat pad fascia to the zygomatic periosteum. A knot is tied under medium tension (suturing too tightly damages the tissue). The vector is in a temporoparietal direction. The zygomatic SMAS extension is engaged in the suture. This corrects the tear trough fold, gives optimum volume while projecting and lifting the lateral cheekbone. The soft tissue inside the suture gives cheekbone volume and prominence, without using implants or transplants. Dimpling at perforation point B is released by pulling the skin at this point with a mosquito clamp and the suture ends at A in opposite directions. Eventual dimpling at point A should be removed as well.

2. Fixation at posterior zygoma. **Using 3 perforation points.** **Perforation Point A is at sideburn lower anterior hairline angle. Point B1 at nasolabial angle, Point B2 at lower nasolabial fold or at smiling point.** Perforation point B2 could be through skin or oral mucosa. **TYPE: Combined traction on SMAS zygomatic extension and fat pad fascias.** Collection of whole cheekbone soft tissue in elderly or in cases of overly regressed cheekbone soft tissue (Fig 15).

The surgical technique is the same as the one described above.

The author uses skin or mucosal perforation point B1, and skin or mucosal perforation point B2.

The pass between the B1 and B2 must be located in the fat pat fascial tube (Fig. 16). Otherwise, traction will occur on unstable fat and soft tissue.

Using trans-mucosal perforation points: When perforation points B1 and B2 are trans-mucosal (intra-nasal at nasolabial angle or in oral mucosa at lower nasolabial fold area and smiling point), needle and suture should be protected using a cannula (Fig. 7). All collected soft tissue included in the suture is tractioned in temporoparietal direction. Skin and tissue impressions at perforation points should be managed using a mosquito clamp.

Cheeks will be augmented laterally, which is recommendable mostly in Caucasians. Vice versa, Asians have laterally projected cheekbones but their faces are more flat medially and hollow below their eyes. In Asians, the author recommends medial cheekbone enhancement.

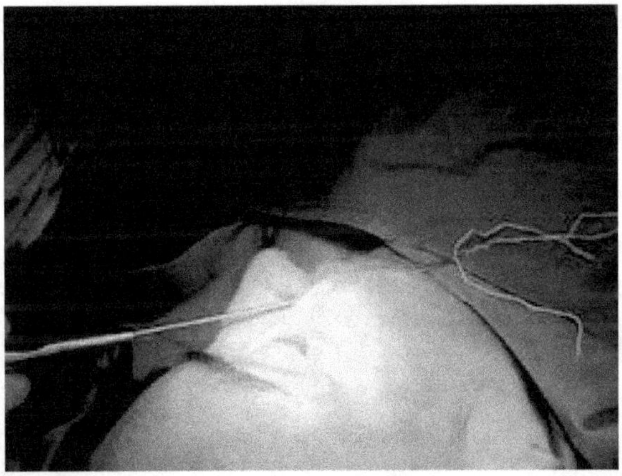

Figure 16. Pass between perforation point B1 and B2 is located inside of fat pad fascial tube.

3. Fixation at temporoparietal tendon and underlying periosteum. Perforation Point A at temporoauricular angle to fix the suture to immobile temporoparietal tendon insertion and periosteum below it. Point B1 at nasolabial angle, Point B2 at lower nasolabial fold or at smiling point. Perforation points B1 and B2 could be through skin or mucosa. TYPE: Combined traction on SMAS zygomatic extension and fat pad fascias. Collection of whole cheek-bone soft tissue in elderly or in cases of overly regressed cheek-bone soft tissue. Used mostly in bald male patients to prevent from scaring in the lateral cheekbone area. It is a very rarely used modification.

4. Fixation to upper temporal line and temporal fascia. 2 or 3 perforation points in selected cases. Perforation Point A at upper temporal line just above intersection point between: 1. Upper temporal line and 2. Coronal line. **Perforation point A1 may exist about 1-2cm lateral and lower than lateral canthus to facilitate the long pass**. Skilled surgeons may surpass this perforation point. TYPE: Combined traction on cheekbone lateral canthus and temporal region. It is a very rarely used modification in closed technique. The author has used it in open techniques of face and mid-face lift. We train plastic surgeons using open techniques to use it to prevent wide dissections.

Clinical cases

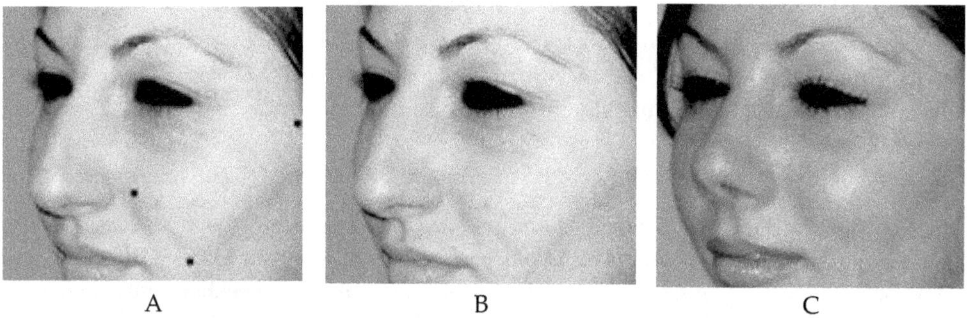

Figure 17. Lateral cheekbone lift. Fixation at posterior zygoma. Combined traction on SMAS zygomatic extension and fat pad fascias using 3 perforation points with trans-nasal, trans-mucosal perforation point B1, and trans-dermal B2; **A.** Perforation points, **B.** Before, **C.** After simultaneous cheekbone lift and beautification rhinoplasty to place the tip at the cheekbone line and produce 3 equal facial proportions.

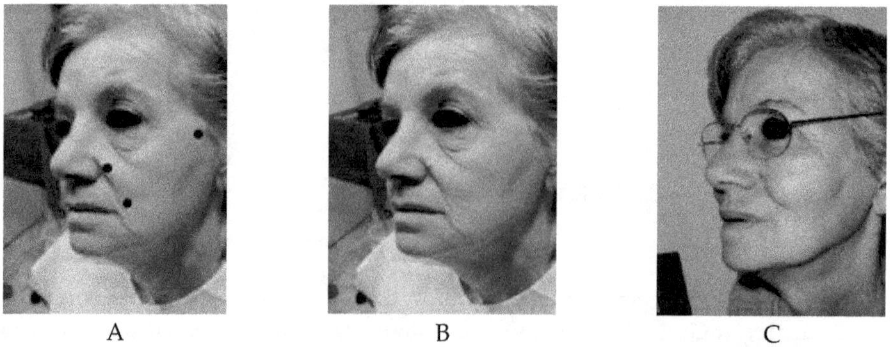

Figure 18. Lateral cheekbone lift. Fixation at posterior zygoma. Using 3 perforation points. Combined traction on SMAS zygomatic extension and fat pad fascias. **A.** Perforation points, **B.** Before, **C.** After cheekbone lift. Collected tissue gives a new cheekbone volume; nasolabial, tear through and marionette folds are managed; lower lid is changed – orbital fat is located under the lifted cheekbone flap.

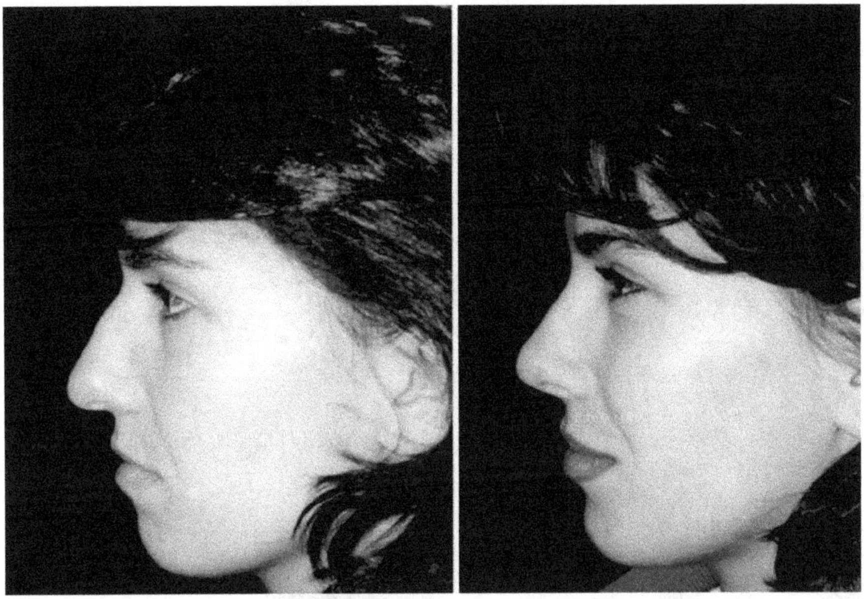

A B

Figure 19. Medial cheekbone lift. Fixation to anterior zygoma, using 2 perforation points. **A.** Before, **B.** After simultaneous temporal cheekbone SMAS lift, rhinoplasty, chin enhancement by suture, and WY lip augmentation.

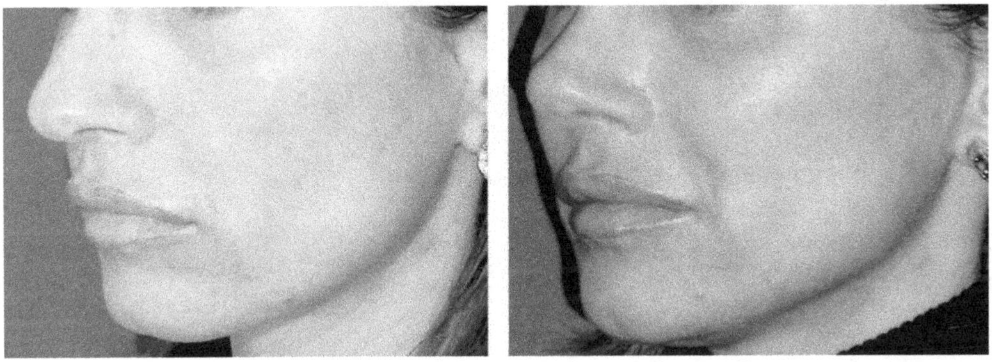

A B

Figure 20. Medial cheekbone lift to eliminate the tear through fold. Fixation to anterior zygoma, using 2 perforation points. **A.** Before, **B.** After simultaneous temporal cheekbone SMAS lift, rhinoplasty, chin enhancement by suture.

2.5. Cheek dimple formation

1. In combination with cheekbone lift. Using 2 or 3 perforation points. Point A - fixation at the zygomatic arch, at desired point, Point B at smiling point with biting and engaging dermis.

Formation of cheek dimple at smiling point is easy, engaging dermis in the suture at skin perforation point B, located at the smiling point (Fig 21).

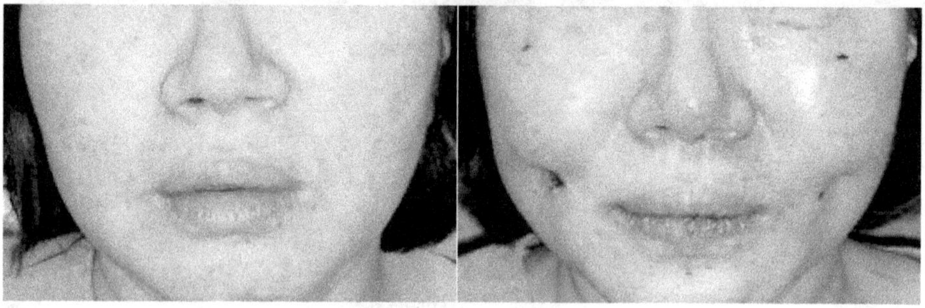

A B

Figure 21. Cheekbone lift with cheek dimple. Using 2 points in an elderly patient. **A.** Before, **B.** immediately after operation

2. Cheek dimple only. Using 2 perforation points: Skin perforation point A at anterior zygoma. Perforation point B at smiling point (Fig. 22).

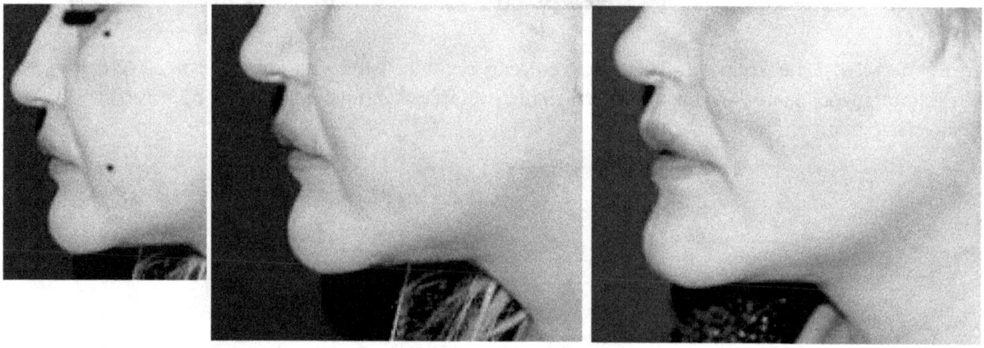

A B C

Figure 22. Traction on dermis at smiling point, which forms cheek dimple. Using 2 points in an elderly patient. **A.** Perforation points, **B.** Before, **C.** After.

2.6. Results

1280 patients with suture cheekbone lifts were followed from 3 to 18 years. The procedures took place during the period between 1993 and December 2012 to enhance, lift and improve the checkbones, as well as to solve problems of an ageing face, such as nasolabial folds, tear trough folds, marionette folds, hollow area, skin wrinkling etc. 92% of these patients had simultaneous suture lifts and other treatments of face or body. In the face, the author combines the cheekbone lift mostly with temporal lift, brow lift, lower SMAS-platysma lift, chin enhancement and beautification rhinoplasties. Early and late results are mostly satisfactory to excellent. Patient satisfaction, apart from consideration of rejuvenation and beautification outcomes, is mostly connected to local anesthesia, absence of pain, short operation time, immediate or very rapid recovery and fast return to social activities and work. Patients' aesthetic satisfaction goes beyond pre-operative expectations. In the first 7-10 days an expected sensation of tension in the operated area is present, which is normal. In fact, most patients love this "lifting sensation" and describe it as pleasant and expected.

2.7. Complications

In 1 patient, after cheekbone lifting with dimple formation, the dimple on the left cheek had disappeared 3 days after the operation, due to pillow pressure. Immediate re-suturing was performed, which successfully reconstructed the symmetry and the smiling dimple.

Four patients had post-operative bruising at the lower lid.

The author has had no nerve injuries, no hematomas, no seromas, and no infections in the follow-up clinical cases.

In 2 patients, on the first post-operative day, an additional pull on the skin was performed to obtain lifting-level symmetry on both sides. The correction was performed under local anesthesia.

In the first 3-4 days, five patients complained about having a perception of an overcorrection or an exceedingly high lift and projection of the cheek-bones. This is normal during the maximum swelling period. These complaints disappeared in 5 to 10 days. One Asian patient did not feel comfortable with the new cheekbones and the sutures were removed 30 min after operation. **NB!** The sutures are easy to remove – the knot is at the point of the stable immobile attachment at the periosteum in skin perforation point A. A mosquito clamp is introduced in the opening at point A, the knot is pulled outside of the skin, the suture is cut and removed.

Serdev Sutures® can be placed, removed and replaced at any time with nearly no down time.

There were 12 cases of late secondary repetition after 5 to 12 years, as part of a total face maintainance, combined with suture lifts in neighboring facial areas.

2.8. Discussion

Except lifting and augmentation, the cheekbone lift forms nice, young looking "hungry" cheeks. In elderly patients, the cheekbone lift gathers tissue, resolves the tear trough fold, projects and lifts the cheekbone (as part of beauty triangle), lifts, flattens nasolabial and marionette folds, and stretches the jaw line. In young patients it projects, enhances and elevates cheekbones. Cheekbone volumizing is part of the beauty triangle formation (projected cheekbones and chin). Additional chin enhancement using sutures is always advisable if the chin is not projected enough. Patient satisfaction is closely related to the individual possibility of obtaining correct proportions, volumes and angles of the face, including cheekbones.

To date, there are not many methods for cheekbone lifting and volumizing without implants and transplants. Classic rhytidectomies do not correct volume and do not change proportions even with modern endoscopic methods. Simultaneous suture SMAS lifts, even in open surgery during rhytidectomy, can improve the cheekbones, lower face and jowls. This method, especially the suture tissue volumizing without the use of implants or transplants is unique. Classic rhytidectomies cannot lift cheekbones in a medial direction and most of the time use implants. This also demonstrates the pre-eminence of the author's method. Complications in scarless closed approach suture techniques are rare (less than 0,1%). In other invasive surgeries, the rate increases with the extension of the surgery.

Cheekbone lift using the scarless, transcutaneous, closed approach Serdev Suture® method is ambulatory, very well tolerated by patients, with immediate effect. The recovery period is very short and patients can return to their social life and work almost immediately. Complications are less than 0,1% and patient satisfaction is extremely high, especially with regards to aesthetics. A particularly positive advantage in suture lifts is the possibility to select the position, volume and level of cheekbone enhancement and lifting. Patients prefer the possibility of total facial improvement, in combination with neighboring facial areas, as part of the mini-invasive procedure.

3. Mid-face lift

In the face, Serdev Suture® techniques lift the mobile SMAS and fix it to stable immobile anatomical structures. Scarless Serdev Suture® mid-face lift sutures loose zygomatic SMAS extension to firm temporoparietal tendon insertion and underlying temporal periosteum. Such a lift results in lifting the mid and lower SMAS, restoring cheekbone into a higher position, resolving the tear trough, nasolabial and marionette folds, stretching mid-face SMAS and attached skin in a temporoparietal direction. Lower face and neck are also improved. Serdev Suture® lifting techniques are ambulatory, performed under local anesthesia, very well tolerated by patients, with an immediate effect, with an extremely short post operative period, fast recovery and nearly immediate return to social life. Complications are about 0% and patient satisfaction is very high, especially in the aspect of aesthetics.

The concept of a mid-face lift by sutures, without skin incisions and excisions, is to lift loose zygomatic SMAS extension and fix it to stable temporoparietal tendon, it's insertion and underlying temporal periosteum. For the purpose of scarless lifting the author has created an innovative design that uses needle perforations only.

The author has created special, curved, semi-blunt and semi-elastic needles of different lengths, with an eye at the tip (Fig. 23). For mid-face lift, needles with lengths of 50 mm, 60 mm, and 100 mm are used to introduce long-term absorbable (in 2-3 years), semi-elastic Polycon surgical sutures USP 2 and 4.

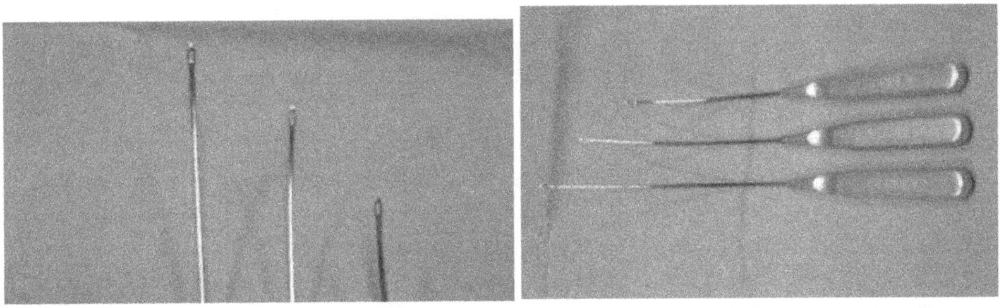

Figure 23. Curved, semi-blunt and semi-elastic needles with different lengths of 50 mm, 60 mm, and 100 mm and an eye at the tip.

Anesthesia

Local anaesthesia with i.v. sedation is used instead of general anaesthesia, in order to shorten intervention time, along with both surgeon and patient preference.

Important fixation lines:

A-B – stable fixation to immobile temporoparietal tendon insertion and underlying periosteum.

A1-B1 – fixation of mobile zygomatic SMAS extension.

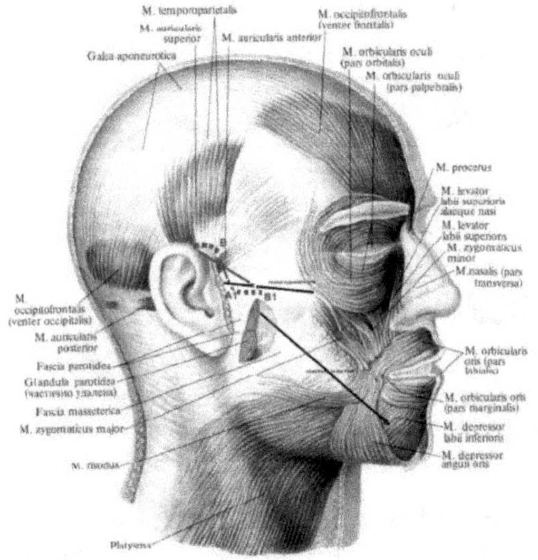

Figure 24. Scheme of mid-face lifting – fixation of zygomatic extension of SMAS (line A1-B1 below zygoma) to temporoparietal tendon and temporal periosteum (line A-B), just above the ear at temporoauricular angle. The vector is from chin to temporoparietal tendon - in temporoparietal direction. Thus, the mid-face SMAS and marionette lines will be stretched. Connection lines A-B1 and B-A1 are crossed to reduce bulging. ***Anatomy figures from Sinelnikov - Atlas Of Human Anatomy, GIML, Moscow, 1963**

Anatomy guidelines

The fibro-muscular layer, described as Superficial Muscle Aponeurotic System (SMAS), connects the vertex and platysma and acts as suspension for the overlying facial skin. SMAS is fixed to the zygoma by the zygomatic SMAS extension that permits movement of the lower SMAS. In direction towards the zygoma, at the superior orbital rim level, the immobile temporalis fascia (or deep temporalis fascia in some textbooks) splits in two immobile layers: superficial and deep layer. These two immobile fascial layers enclose an intermediate fat pad and within - frontal branches of facial nerve, artery and vein. The frontal branch of the facial nerve is considered to cross the zygomatic bone, traveling along a line, connecting the tragus base to a point 1.5 cm above the eyebrow.

So, the anatomic topography forms a square - 3 cm front of the tragus and 3 cm above the zygomatic bone that is described by the author as a **"danger area"**. There, the frontal branch of the facial nerve is considered to cross the zygomatic bone at about 1.5 cm anterior to the tragus. **NB!** Fixation to zygoma in cheekbone suture lift should not be done in the danger area – do not perforate zygoma periosteum in the first 2-3 cm in front of the tragus.

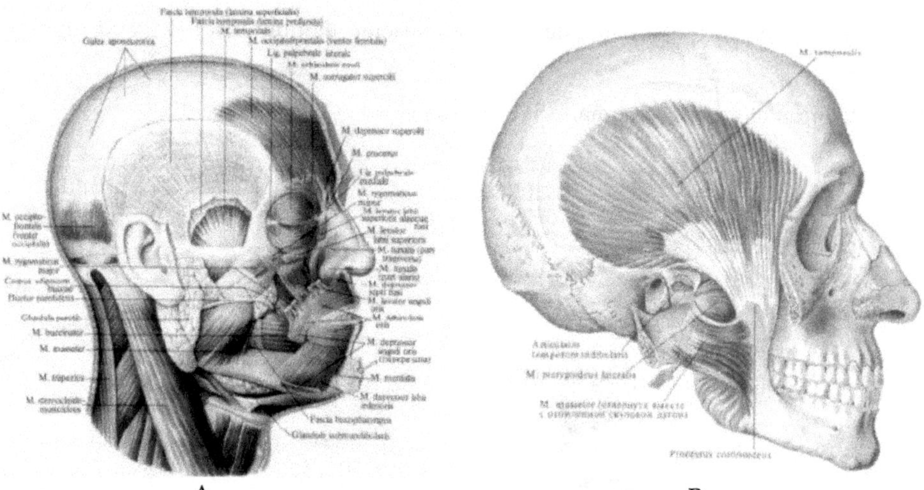

A B

Figure 25. A, B. Temporal tendon and fascia are not suitable for mid-face fixation and lift, because of their direction. Sutures slide down due to fibers' distal direction. ***Anatomy figures from Sinelnikov - Atlas Of Human Anatomy, GIML, Moscow, 1963**

Temporoparietalis muscle tendon is fixed to spina suprameatica of meatus acusticus externus. It is stable, immobile and is used by the author for firm cephalic fixation of the suture in mid-face lift. **NB!** Temporalis fascia and tendon directions are not suitable for this particular fixation (Fig. 25A, B). If fixed to the temporalis fascia, the suture will slide down and loosen.

SMAS zygomatic extension is a mobile fascia which is used by the author to lift mid and lower SMAS.

The mobile A1-B1 SMAS fixation to zygoma will be lifted to the immobile A-B line at the temporoparietal tendon insertion and underlying temporal periosteum. **NB!** In the **"danger area"** (connecting lines B-A1 and A-B1) the needle should pass carefully (superficially), just below the mobile tissue (skin and galea aponeurotica, fixed together). If the needle becomes fixed, it has perforated deeper immobile superficial layer (lamina superficialis) of temporal fascia that is dangerous, because of possible vessel perforation. Prolonged pressure in such cases can stop bleeding in the "danger area".

Directions

Pass B-(A1)-B1. Point A1 is only a mark. It should be drawn for orientation and should not be perforated. **NB!** Needle pass B-A1 is in the "danger area" – it should be superficial, just below galea and skin, i.e. supratemporal. Passing below the lower line of zygoma, the needle catches the mobile zygomatic SMAS extension.

Pass A-B1 is a connecting pass, located in "danger area". The needle should pass superficially/subgaleally i.e. supratemporally, to take the suture from point B1 to A.

Pass A-B is the stable fixation under temporoparietal tendon insertion and underlying temporal periosteum.

Vectors: 2 vectors are effective with this lift:

- Temporoparietal direction from chin to temporoauricular angle - point A, with strong effect of traction on cheek SMAS, on the marionette folds and additional effect on the nasolabial folds,
- Dorsal direction from cheekbone to point A, with strong effect on the nasolabial and tear trough folds and additional effect on marionette folds.

Video: http://www.youtube.com/watch?v=S51JZOCfLfg

FIRST SUTURE PASS: consists of connecting line B-A1 and movable zygomatic SMAS fixation at line A1-B1

Mark perforation points A, B and B1 for skin perforations. Entry point A is placed just above the ear, in the temporoparietal angle, and point B - approximately anteriorly to A, at the hairline. Point A1 is only a mark and should be not perforated. Point A1, line A1-B1 and point B1 should be below the lower line of zygomatic arch, i.e. lower than the mobile SMAS zygomatic extension. Perforation point B1 is placed at intersection point of chin to temporoauricular angle line and lower zygomatic line.

Line A-B is the subperiosteal immobile fixation to temporoparietal tendon insertion and underlying temporal periosteum. A1-B1 is the line of fixation below mobile SMAS zygomatic extension.

Local anesthetic is introduced intradermally at points A and B, then subperiosteally at the line A-B, just subdermally in connection lines B-A1 and A-B1, and deeper subdermally in line A1-B1. Use only a small amount of anesthetic – a few drops per line. Larger amounts will result in visible post-op swelling. **NB!** In the "danger area" (connection lines

B-A1 and A-B1), the needle should be supratemporal, just below skin and galea aponeurotica.

The skin is perforated with a No. 11 scalpel blade in points A, B, and B1 (respect Langer lines) and then, using the thin tip of a mosquito clamp, the skin perforations at point B1 will be widened and deepened. **NB!** If superficial fascia is not perforated at point B, it could produce dimpling when engaged and lifted with the suture.

Introduce a "mini" 60 mm Serdev® needle in a perpendicular fashion through point B (do not engage dermal tissue), then slide it strictly subgaleally/supratemporally in direction to point A1, then rotate it toward B1. When the needle tip reaches a position below point B1, direct the tip upward toward opening B1, then fold the skin against the needle tip at a 90^0 angle and with a gentle twisting movement direct needle upward, until it exits from point B1. Try to avoid engaging dermis as you are exiting, in order to prevent creation of skin dimples. **NB!** If at point B1 the needle is facing any resistance, this means that it has caught dermis, in which case twist the needle backwards and repeat the maneuver. Do not push or pull – twist needle forwards and backwards.

After the needle is threaded at point B1, it is pulled back until it exits through point B, bringing the suture with it. This represents the pass, which fixes the movable SMAS zygomatic extension.

SECOND SUTURE PASS: supratemporal A-B1 connecting line. Connection lines A-B1 and B-A1 are crossed to reduce bulging.

The second needle pass is subdermal, between points **A** and **B1.** Avoid deeper perforation of superficial layer of temporal fascia. To facilitate needle advancing, locate the needle laterally and use a gentle twisting movement, until you reach point B1 (exit point).

After exiting perpendicularly through point **B1,** the free end of suture is threaded through the needle eye and pulled backward to exit through point A.

Important! At this stage, take both ends of the suture, pull them in temporoparietal direction and at the same time pull the dermis in perforation point B1 in opposite direction to the chin, using a mosquito clamp, until any dimpling is released. You could feel a "click" when releasing the suture from the trabecular attachments and dimpling will disappear. If dermis at point B1 is attached to the suture through carelessness, it will not be possible to release the dimpling. Then the suture has to be removed and previous steps - repeated.

THIRD SUTURE PASS: Line A-B - Subperiosteal fixation at temporoparietal tendon insertion

Introduce a specially bended "mini mini" 50 mm Serdev® needle in a perpendicular fashion through point A (do not touch or engage dermal tissue!). Once the needle touches the bone, slide it subperiosteally to point B. **NB!** Check whether the needle is locked under periosteum. If it moves freely laterally, it means that it is not inserted at sub-periosteal level. This is a common beginner's mistake. If locked under periosteum, the tissue is so stable that it is possible to lift the patient's entire head with the needle. If movable, it should be repositioned deeper under periosteum.

When the needle tip reaches a position below point B, direct the tip upward towards opening B, then fold the skin against the needle tip at a 90^0 angle and with gentle twisting movements direct needle upward until it exits from point B. Avoid engaging dermis as you are exiting, in order to prevent creation of skin dimpling. If you feel that the needle is facing any resistance, it means that the needle has caught the dermis, in which case move the needle backwards and repeat the maneuver.

NB! Do not push or pull – gently twist needle forwards or backwards.

After threading the needle at point B, it is pulled back towards point A until it exits, bringing the suture with it. This will complete the suture circle formation and a surgical knot is performed, using optimum tension. Use one branch of a mosquito clamp to release dimpling at the perforation points.

The author does not use stitches to close perforation points A, B or B1. They are taped for overnight. On the next day, patients should take a shower with shampoo to remove blood residuum at the perforation points. Multiple disinfections are applied by the patient on a daily basis, for 3-4 days. Some swelling (like soft bulging) in the area can be visible for 3-4 weeks and then disappears. Patients usually cover it with their hair.

3.1. Results

520 patients were followed up from 3 to 18 years, starting in 1993. In 95% of the cases, patients had simultaneous treatment in other face and/or body areas. In the face, combinations were mostly with temporal, brow lift, lower SMAS-platysma lift, chin enhancement and beautification rhinoplasties.

Results were excellent in 96% of all cases, as reported by our patients. Patients' satisfaction is mostly connected to the immediate aesthetic result and visible rejuvenation of the medial and lower face, local anesthesia, short operation time, lack of pain, immediate or rapid recovery and speedy return to social activities or work. There is an almost complete correlation between aesthetic outcomes with pre-operative patient expectations.

In the first 7-10 days patients experience a traction sensation. Most patients find this sensation desirable and are attracted to it. Some pain was reported when pressure is applied to the area, which is considered normal.

After three years, results are reported to remain satisfactory in 85% and good in 12% of the cases.

In five years, 52% of the patients report satisfaction and 37% consider results as good.

Only in 3 cases the mid-face lift has been repeated after 4, 6 and 8 years. Such additional suture lifts and enhancements have mostly been performed to complete or maintain a good status.

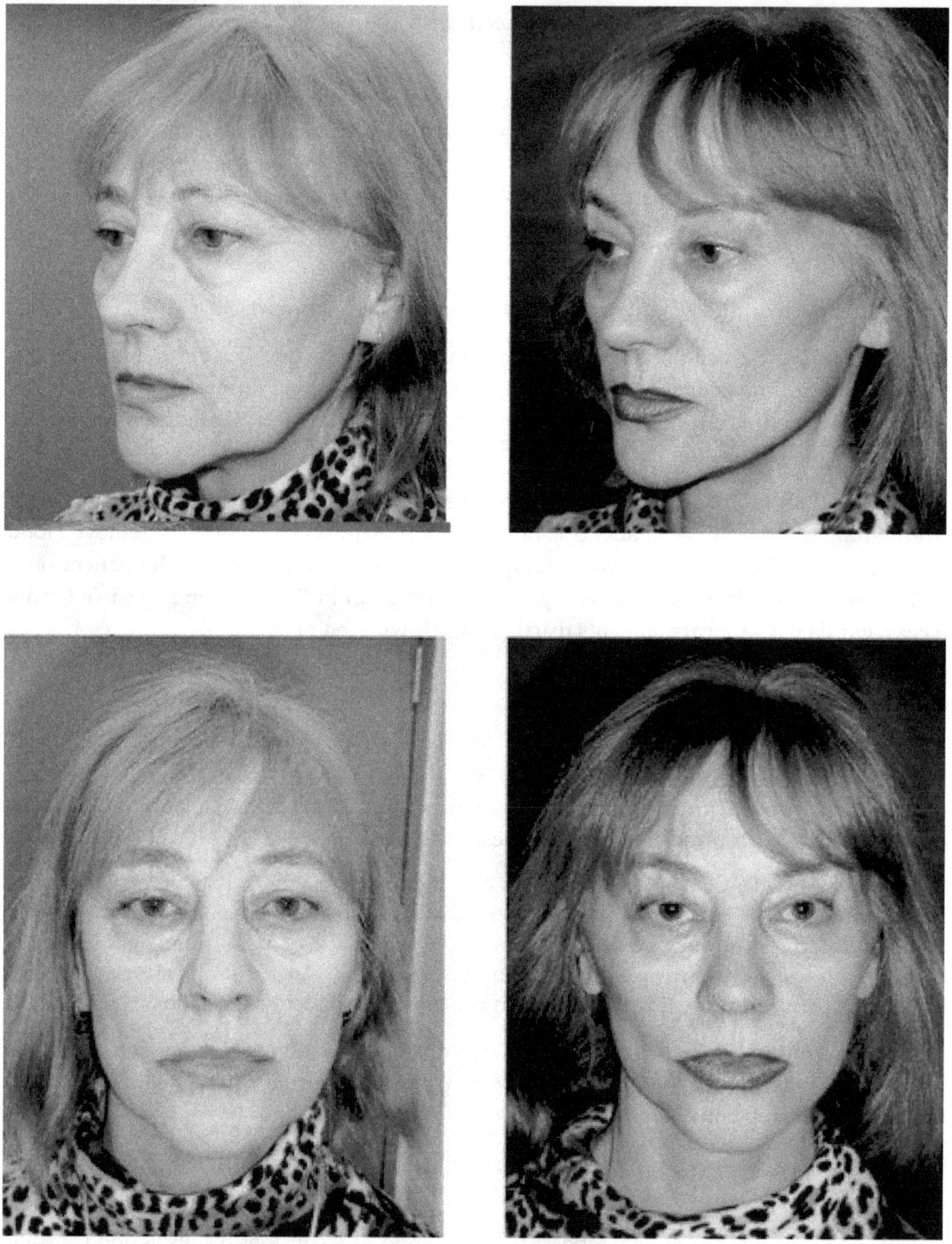

Figure 26. Before and after mid-face lift and simultaneous brow lift using Serdev Sutures®. Better cheekbone position, and jaw line, formation of so-called "hungry cheeks". Face is tightened and changed from "square" to oval.

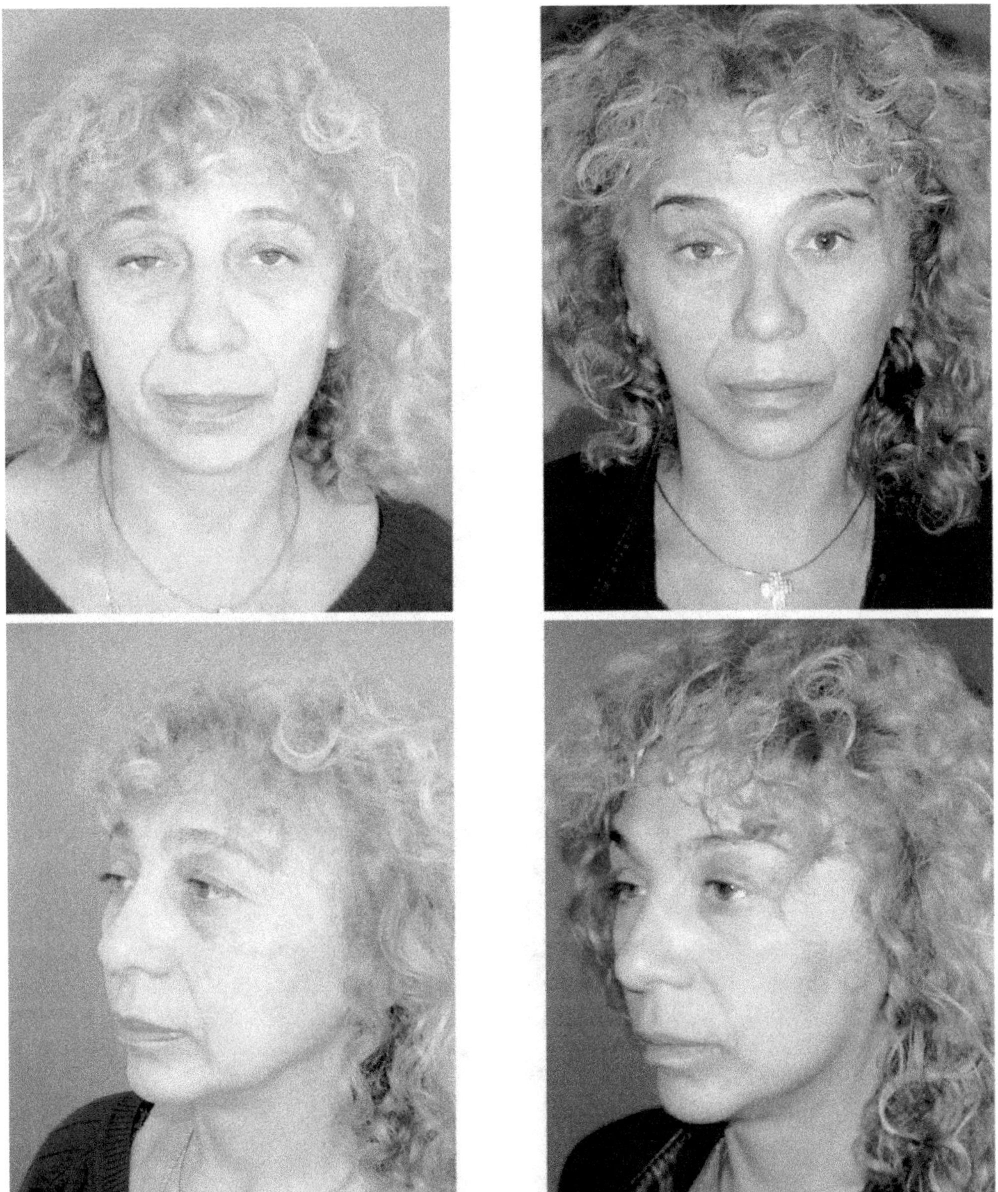

Figure 27. Before and after mid-face lift and simultaneous brow lift using Serdev Sutures®. Better cheekbone position, and jaw line. Face is changed from "square" to oval.

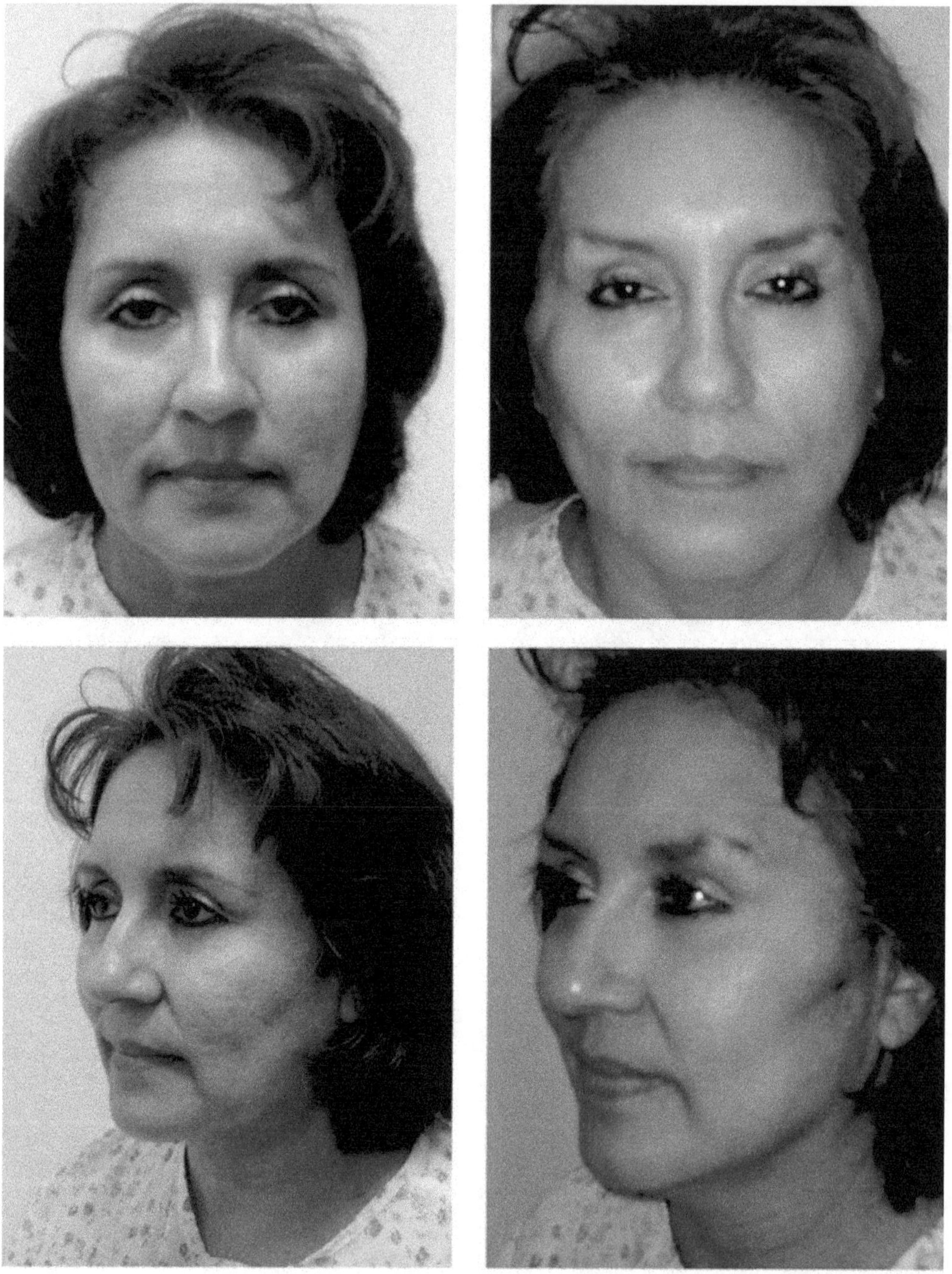

Figure 28. Before and immediately after mid-face lift and simultaneous brow lift using Serdev Sutures®. Better cheekbone position and jaw line. Face is tightened, refreshed and changed from "square" to oval.

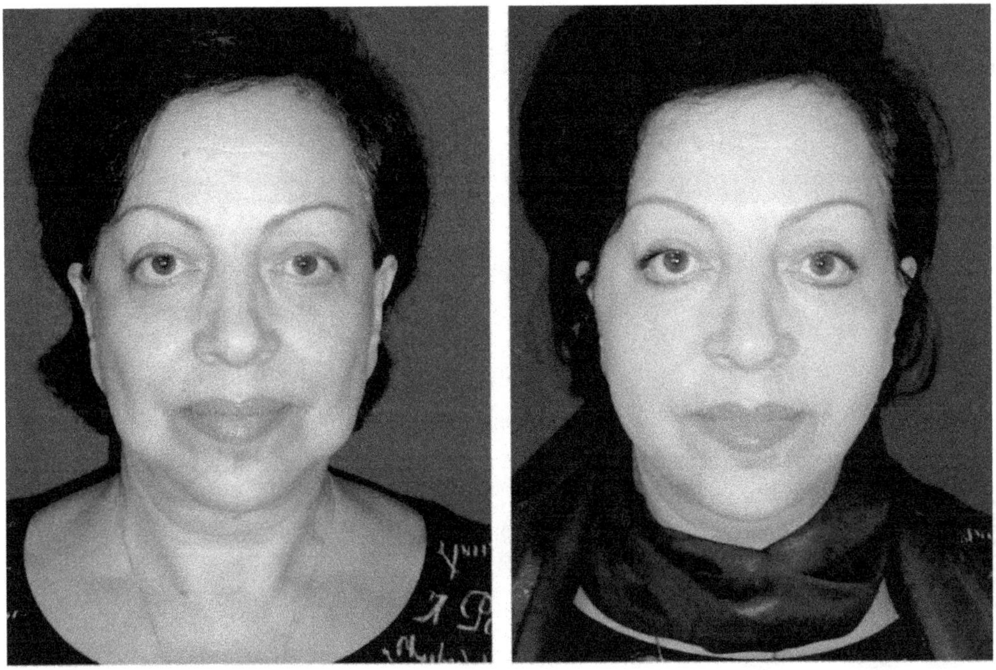

Figure 29. Before and after mid-face lift using Serdev Sutures® and simultaneous ultrasonic assisted liposculpture of buccal fat. Better cheekbone position and jawline. Face is tightened, totally refreshed and changed from "square" to oval.

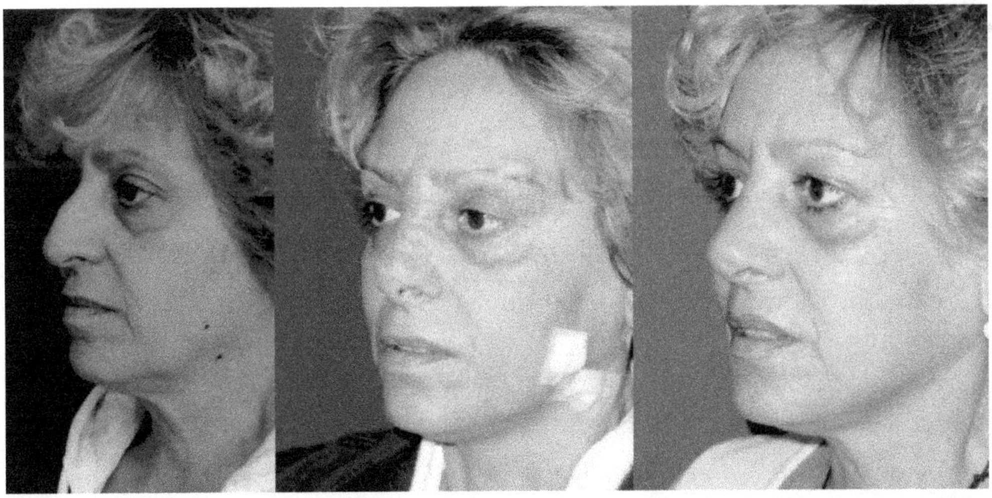

Figure 30. Before, immediately after and 4 years after mid-face lift and simultaneous temporal, brow, lower face and neck lift using Serdev Sutures®, and rhinoplasty.

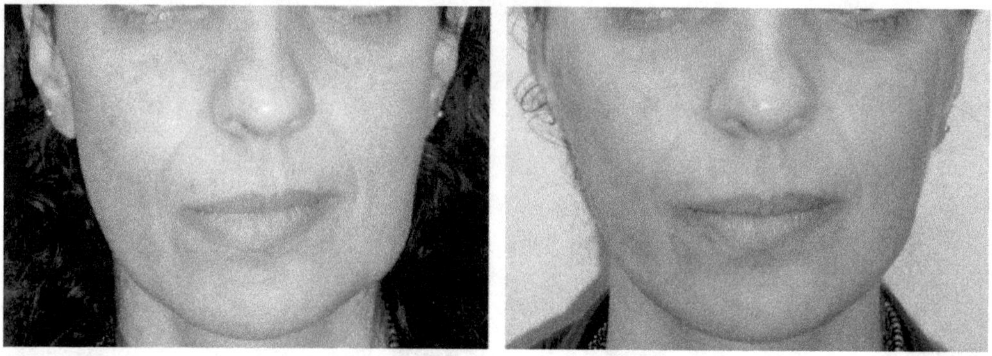

Figure 31. Before and immediately after mid-face lift to equalize both sides in a case of facial paralysis.

There was no case of secondary correction after mid-face lift except the three reported in a late stage. In one case, during hands-on training, a growing swelling was marked in a unilateral "danger area". Having in mind a possible trauma, pressure was applied for 10 minutes. This swelling successfully flattened and the operation was finalized. No bleeding, hematoma or bruising in the area was observed in the early post-operative period.

The author has had no infection, hematoma, seroma, or nerve injury after suture mid-face lifts.

3.2. Discussion

Skin lifting in classic subdermal and deep rhytidectomies does not significantly improve nasolabial and marionette folds. Flattening of marionette and nasolabial folds with the suture technique demonstrates its superiority over invasive lifting methods, where complication rates rise with extensive surgery.

Mid-face lift using Serdev Suture® methods is ambulatory, very well tolerated by patients, with immediate effect, with an extremely short post operative period, fast recovery and nearly immediate return to social life. Complications are near 0% and patient satisfaction is very high, confirming the longevity of results.

The advantages of the suture lifts include the possibility to correct and improve anatomy at any time, with nearly no down time, no trauma, and high patient satisfaction.

4. Beautification rhinoplasty – tip rotation and refinement, alar base narrowing

The author describes his experience and methods in different aesthetic disproportions of the external nose and in secondary cases.

Rhinoplasty is a part of the beautification process and has to follow anatomical proportions and beauty principles. Nose length has to occupy the middle 1/3 of the face, according to the proportions of the "golden section" rule of 3 equal thirds.

Proper nose **proportions, angles and volumes** should guide the cosmetic surgeon.

Proportional nose is one that occupies 1/3 of the face (golden dividing rule). Proper volumes are: thin dorsum, thin tip, narrow allar base. The tip of the nose prominence gives volume to the central face and its position should be in harmony with the beauty triangle (projected cheekbones and chin). The tip should be in the line of the cheekbone prominences. The nasal dorsum should be straight or slightly concave. Best angles are: 90^0 angle at the tip, 110^0 nasolabial angle, 30^0 angle of nostrils to columella, 30^0 dorsum to profile line.

The aim of Serdev Suture® techniques in beautification rhinoplasty is to improve the above mentioned aesthetic proportions, volumes and angles not only of the nose but adapted to the face as a whole. Serdev Sutures® include tip refinement, tip rotation, and allar base narrowing.

4.1. TIP REFINEMENT SUTURE TECHNIQUES on greater alar cartilages: 1. Transcutaneous domal suture of all four crura to refine bulbosity, 2. Transmucosal suture of the domal segment of the medial crura.

Earlier nasal tip techniques were based on cartilage removal that can destabilize the nasal framework and nasal tip support. Later, radical cartilage resections have been replaced by reshaping and reorienting of the nasal tip components. Suture techniques of the nasal tip in open surgery became popular with McCollough and English double-dome unit procedure to increase tip projection and refinement, using a horizontal mattress suture through all 4 crura just beneath the domes; with Goldman tip procedure for the wide or bulbous lobule, with Daniel domal creation suture, a horizontally placed mattress suture, which shaped separately each dome. Numerous suturing techniques appear in the open technique rhinoplasty literature. All suture techniques are used in open surgery.

Serdev Sutures® tip refinement techniques represent scarless **closed approach** techniques. They are: 1. transdermal methods to suture all 4 crura beneath the domes, or 2. transmucosal medial crura mattress suture.

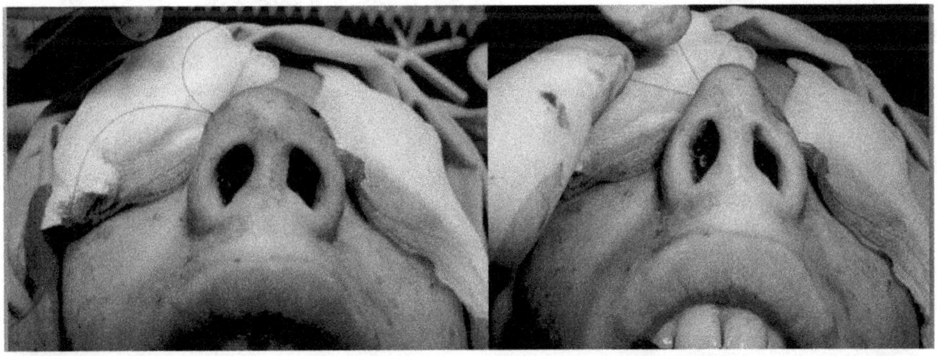

Figure 32. The suture is made through the domal part of the lower alar cartilages. The traction during knotting the suture is visibly tractioning the tip by the side. Be careful not to enter through the nostril as this will cause suture contamination.

4.1.1. Transdermal suture - all 4 crura domal fixation

The suture consists of 2 needle passes, using 2 skin perforations, without engaging skin. Each needle pass uses a different but parallel path through the cartilages. The transdermal suture is diving, buried below the skin, attaching only cartilages, without including skin in the suture. Skin perforations can be moved per side with each pass, in order to obtain parallel passes with a 2-3mm distance between. Both needle passes have to be placed in the domal area, without perforating the nostril, in order to prevent contamination and compromising the result.

4.1.2. Transmucosal suture – domal medial crura fixation

This method is usually combined with other author's closed rhinoplasty techniques, such as T-excision and columella sliding. The suture should be placed as high as possible to fix the domal medial crura. There is no need for this suture to be buried below the nasal mucosa, as the latter is involved on each side. Using absorbable sutures, the fibrosis stabilizes the effect after the first 3 - 4 weeks. If suture is not absorbable, it has to be removed after 3 weeks.

Both transdermal and transmucosal sutures give good refining definition and at the same time a projection effect. In cases of bulbous tip, transdermal suture of all 4 crura is preferable. Both sutures can be used separately, combined, or as a part of a rhinoplasty.

4.2. Tip Rotation – lifting of the greater alar cartilage medial crura with fixation to the periosteum of the nasal bones –

Video: http://www.youtube.com/watch?v=nRh8NDSgDck

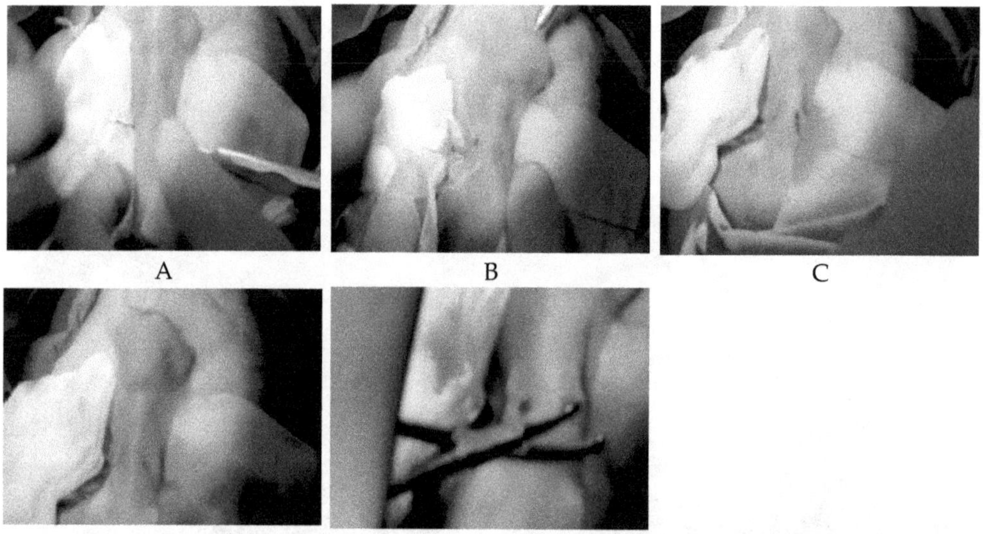

A B C

D E

Figure 33. **B**. fixation to medial crus of the right greater alar cartilage and taking the suture from the right side, **C**. fixation to medial crus of the left greater alar cartilage and taking the suture from the left side, **D**. Suture is tied. **E**. removal of dimpling -http://www.youtube.com/watch?v=nRh8NDSgDck

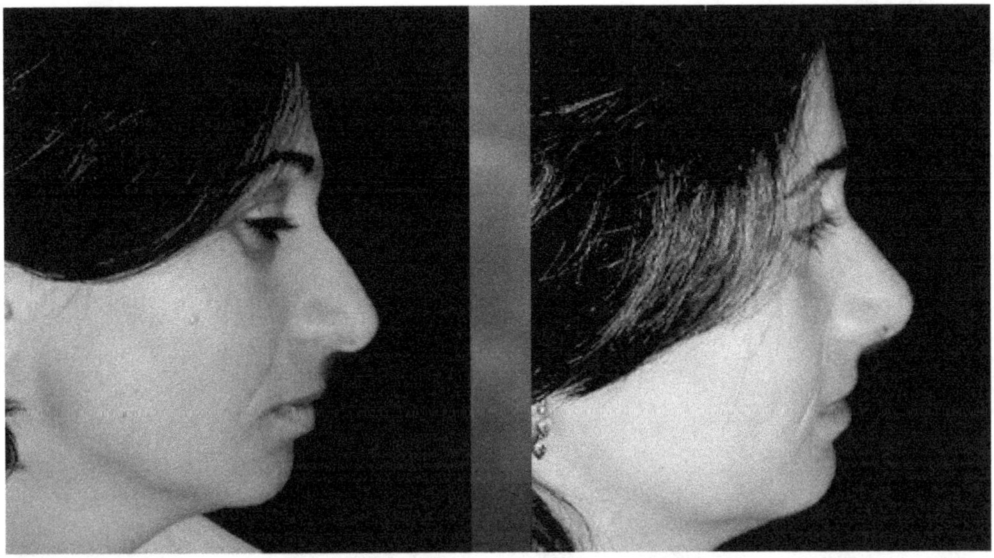

Figure 34. Nasal tip rotation in a Caucasian patient with properly sized septum and excess of skin at the tip.

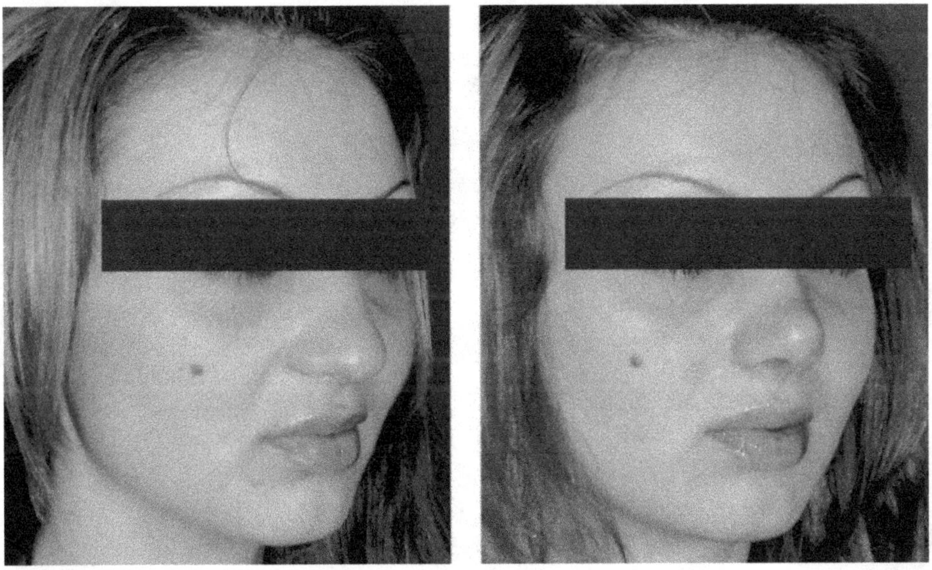

Figure 35. Nasal tip rotation for proportional beautification in a young patient. Nasal tip at the line of the cheekbones results in beautification

Two lines of the suture are important: the nasal bone subperiosteal pass that represents the immobile fixation and the subdermal pass in columella, fixing the mobile medial crura of the greater alar cartilages. Using 2 subdermal connecting passes, the circle of the suture is fulfilled and knotted. In each skin perforation point, the suture dives without engaging skin.

Nasal tip rotation by suture is mostly useful in Asians and Afro-Americans, having softer septum and unstable columella. In Caucasians, such suture lift is possible if the soft tissue is hanging over a normal length septum. In cases with a hard and elongated septum the tip cannot be lifted by suture and another author's technique is performed – the T-excision and columella sliding, which could be supported by that suture. This suture is very helpful to align the dorsum, especially in irregular dorsum and secondary rhinoplasties.

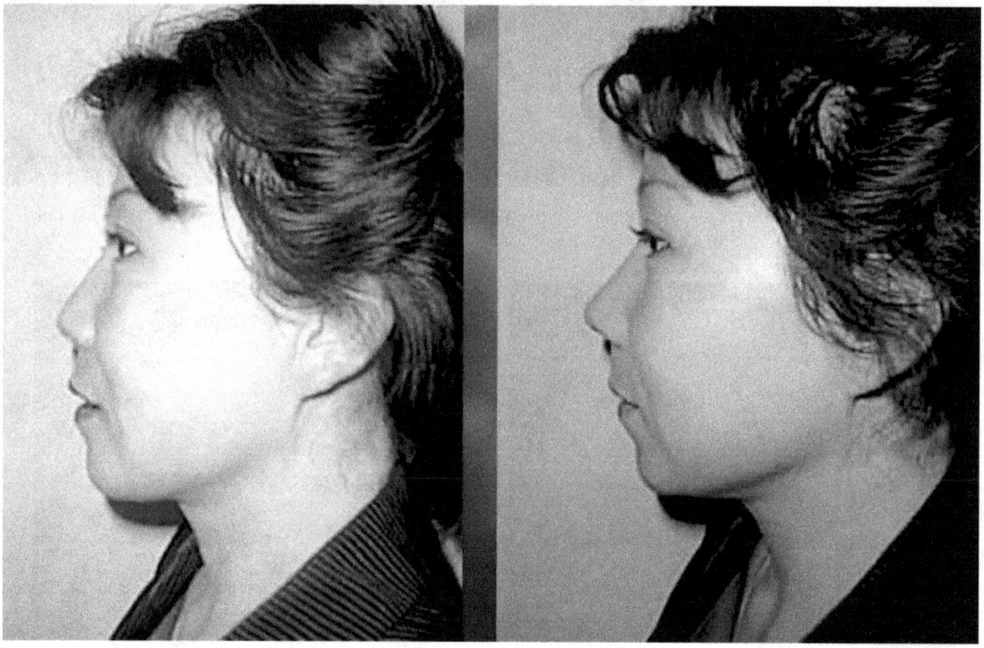

Figure 36. Nasal tip rotation for projection in an Asian patient with unstable septum columella.

4.3. Alar base narrowing

The suture represents 2 parallel passes (1-2 mm distance between them), using 2 skin punctures at both nasolabial angles. The cartilages are engaged to stabilize the suture on both sides. The suture lines should pass subdermally, exactly below the nostrils and nasal spine. **NB!** Do not perforate into the nostrils to avoid contamination.

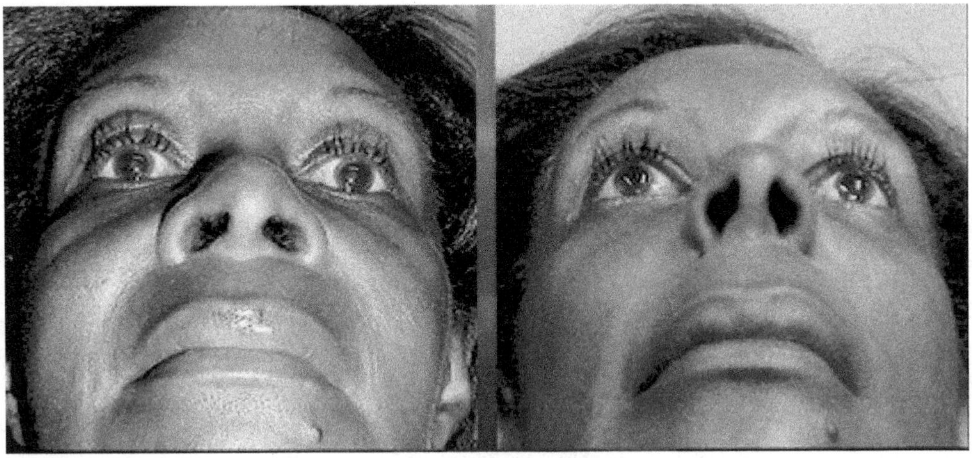

Figure 37. Before and after alar base narrowing in an Afro-American patient.

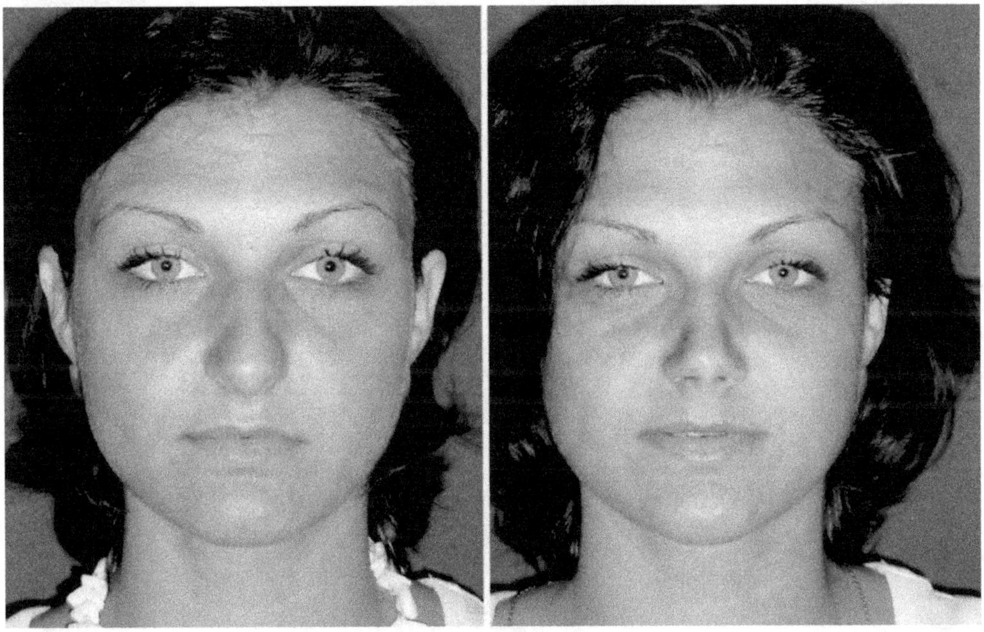

Figure 38. Tip rotation using T-excision and Columella sliding in a young Caucasian female to form the golden section rule (3 equal parts of the face) and obtain beautification. Tip refinement by suture is performed to reduce the volume of the tip.

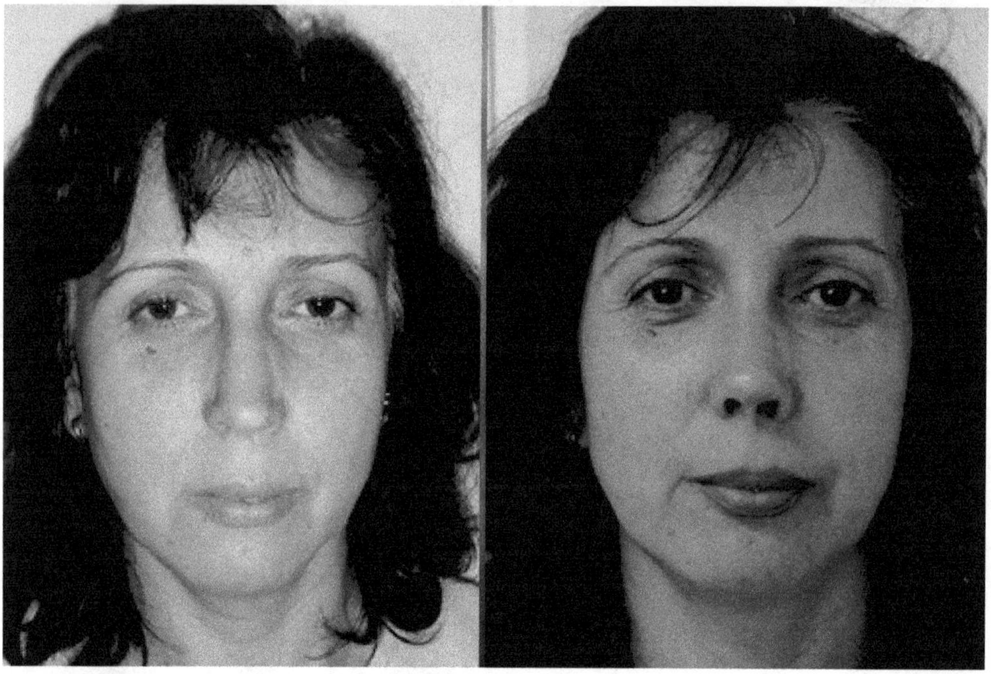

Figure 39. Tip Rotation and refinement by suture.

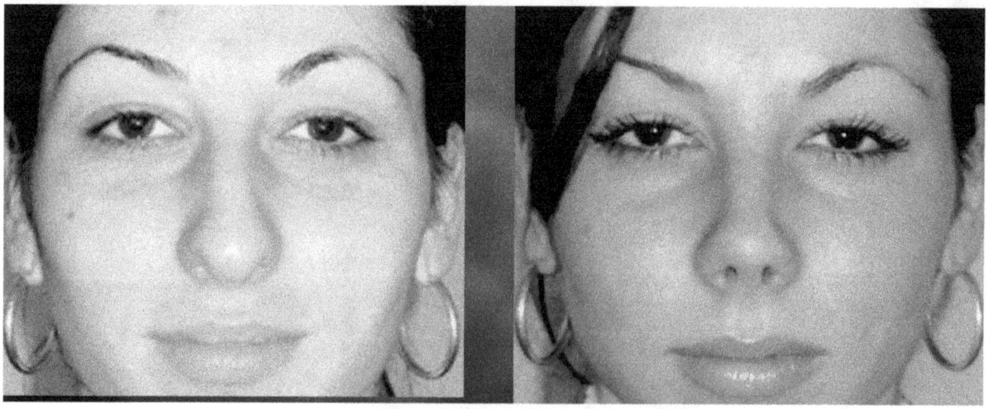

Figure 40. Nasal tip rotation, tip refinement and cheekbone lift. The nasal tip should be at the line of the cheekbones, otherwise it destroys the beauty triangle.

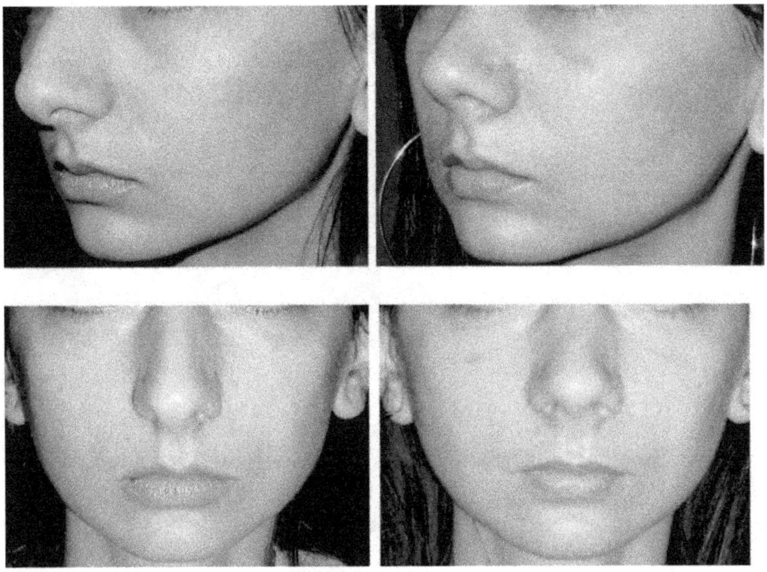

Figure 41. Nasal tip rotation for proportional beautification in a young patient. The hanging soft tissue and a shorter septum permits the tip lifting by suture.

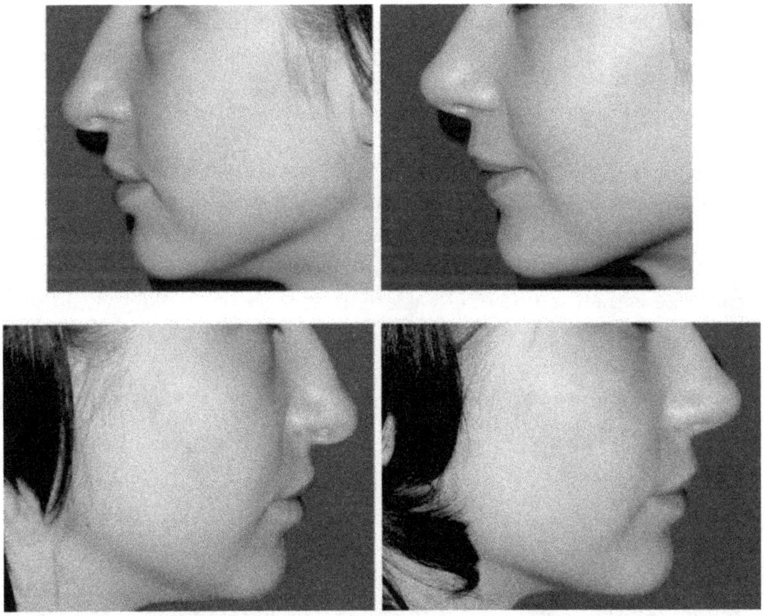

Figure 42. Nasal tip rotation for proportional beautification in a young patient. Location of the nasal tip at the line of the cheekbones.

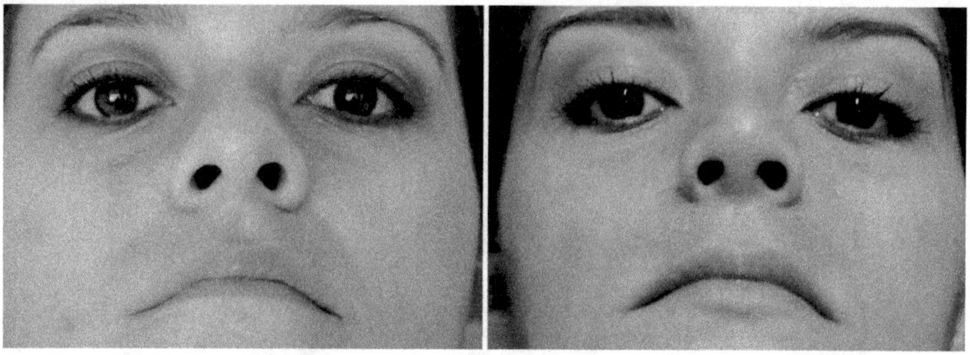

Figure 43. Before and after tip refinement and alar base narrowing in a Caucasian patient. Additional brow lift designs the brow.

Serdev Suture® techniques in rhinoplasty are time-saving, preventing trauma, with immediate results. The post-operative period is short, with no downtime, no or minimal bruising, immediate or prompt return to work and social life. No bandages are necessary.

Alar base narrowing is very important beautification in Afro-Americans and Asians. It provides refinement in Caucasian faces.

5. Scarless Serdev Suture® method in prominent ears

Various techniques have been proposed to correct prominent ears. The author presents a simplified method of auriculoplasty with sutures, by needle perforations only, without incisions. The key point of the operation is a line of sutures along the planed antihelix fold to transfix the fold at the antihelix tail, bending the scapha over the conchal cartilage to make the earlobe fall into place. The results are satisfactory, with a naturally looking antihelical fold.

This surgery is usually done to set prominent ears back, closer to the head, or to reduce the size of the visibly large ears. Prominent ears usually concern children from 4 to 14 years of age, but also adults. Non-suture techniques usually take about two to three hours, although complicated procedures may take longer. Most of the methods use incisions in the back of the ear. The cartilage is then sculpted. Occasionally, a piece of cartilage could be removed to provide a more natural-looking fold. Non-removable stitches are mostly used to help maintain the desired shape and position of the ear. Other techniques involve a similar incision in the back of the ear. Skin is removed and stitches are used to fold the cartilage back on itself to reshape the ear without removing cartilage.

Author's sutures without incisions offers a simplified method to suture cartilage on both sides from the desired fold, without the need to incise or excise skin or cartilage.

Anatomy

The most common deformity of the ear is the uni- or bilateral prominent ear. This deformity is caused by the lack of formation of the natural fold along the antihelix, a hypertrophied concha or a combination of both. The auriculo-mastoid angle is normally 20–30° from the skull. The helical rim lies about 17–20 mm from the skull. The scapho-conchal angle is 90°, and if this angle is flattened, the ear appears protruding. The size and depth of the concha affect the deformity and the surgical technique for correction.

Aim

To pin the ears closer to the head, bring the ear elements into harmony, refine ear shape and reduce large elements.

Indications

Inferiority Complex, Personal Aesthetic Requirements and Needs.

Preliminary preparations and evaluation

Surgeon and parents should never insist on surgery until the child wants the change. Pre-operative evaluation includes clinical and photographical examination. Pre-operative photographs assist in the study and evaluation of the deformities and in making appropriate decisions. Photographs demonstrate the problem from many angles. Surgery on both ears could be suggested for balance, even if only one ear appears prominent.

Anesthesia

In all cases, the author uses local anesthesia in combination with i.v. sedation

Material and method

Twenty-five patients with prominent ears (without necessity of excision of a strip of the deep concha) were included in this study: 13 patients with unilateral protruding ears and 12 cases with bilateral prominent ears. Ages ranged between 5 and 35 years (15 females and 10 males).

Ear surgery was performed as an outpatient procedure. All the cases were operated under local anesthesia with adrenaline 1/1 000 000 injection of the posterior surface of the auricle. If anterior approach is necessary, local anesthesia is used subcutaneously in the specific area.

5.1. Surgical technique

The suture method aims to suture the cartilage on both sides of the desired antihelix fold, using skin punctures only.

The sutures were performed starting from the upper part of the tail to the lower end of the antitragus in order to disrupt the strongest point where the helix, antihelix and antitragus join.

Two 0,7-0,8 cm long parallel lines are marked on both sides of the planed antihelix fold - for example: A-B and A1-B1. If necessary, a row of additional sutures is planned, such as B-C and B1-C1, C-D and C1-D1 etc. In most Asians, Afro-Americans, Latino-Americans who have soft cartilages, as well as in some Caucasian kids, less sutures could be enough, but in stronger cartilages 3 and more sutures are usually necessary to bend the cartilage and form the desired fold. The lines A-B and A1-B1, B-C and B1-C1, C-D and C1-D1 etc. mark the parallel subperihondreal transcartilagenous passes. The connecting lines between A-A1, B-B1, C-C1 and D-D1 are only subcutaneous to connect the transcartilagenous passes and bring them together. The length of the parallel transcartilagenous and connecting subdermal lines are pre-planned in respect of ear size and the desired result. Subcutaneous dissection in the area of the sutures can be done through the skin perforations, using Serdev® needles. To perform the technique, the author uses a Serdev® "mini-mini" needle, a USP 3/0 surgical suture and 4 skin perforations per suture in the posterior or anterior ear surface. The order of the passes depends on the surgeon (left or right handed), ear side, and surgeon skills. The author starts with a transcartilagenous needle pass - for example A-B, takes the suture end and positions the suture through the needle pass. After that he makes the 2 subcutaneous connecting passes to introduce both suture ends subcutaneously. Then, the second transcartilagenous pass A1-B1 is made at the other side to finalize the suture. When all sutures are done, the tightening of the knot should be done under elastic medium tension to adapt, but not to squeeze, cut or traumatize the cartilages.

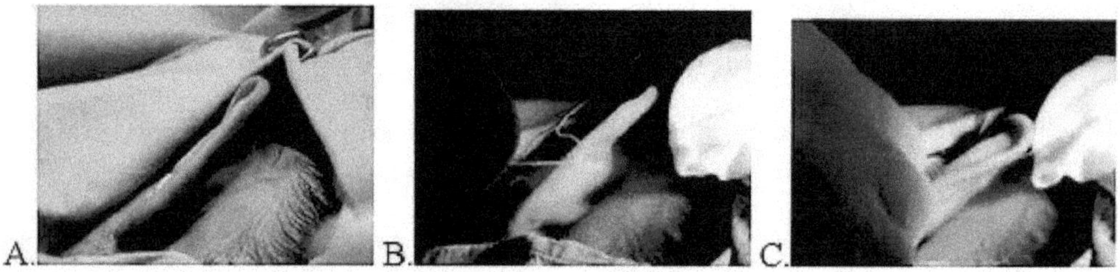

Figure 44. **A.** Before, **B.** The suture before being knotted, **C.** Knot is done under elastic tension and helix is rotated. The ear is pinned and the antihelix fold is now present.
Video: http://www.youtube.com/watch?v=P73OgGYhzDQ

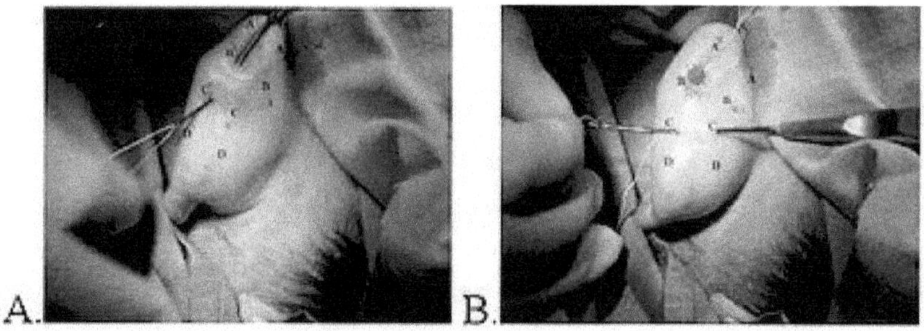

Figure 45. **A.** The first suture A-A1(subdermal) - A1-B1(transcartilagenous) - B1-B (subdermal) – B-A (transcartilagenous) is finished and the suture ends are located at point A. The knot will be done when all sutures are finalized! The needle is located intracartilagenously in B1-C1, parallel to the future antihelix fold and the suture end is in the needle eye; **B.** The suture is introduced in the B1-C1 intracartilagenous plane and the needle is in the subdermal connecting line C-C1, in order to take the suture end;

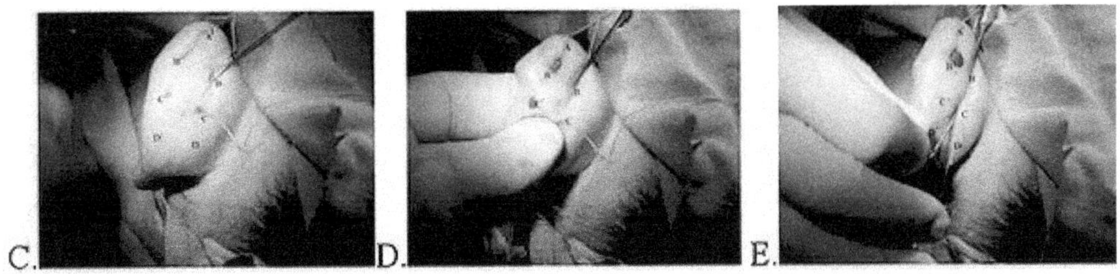

C, D, E. The suture is introduced in the connecting subdermal line C1-C, and the next transcartilagenous B-C pass is done; C-B line;

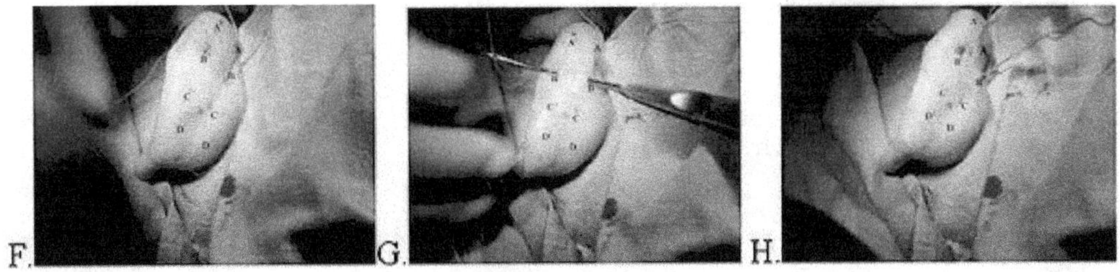

F. The suture is introduced in the intracartilagenous line B-C, **G.** The needle is introduced in the subdermal connecting line B-B1; **H.** The suture end is taken in the connecting subdermal line B-B1 and the full circle of the suture – B-B1(subdermal), B1-C1(transcartilagenous), C1-C(subdermal), C-B(transcartilagenous) – is ready. Both suture ends are at point B.

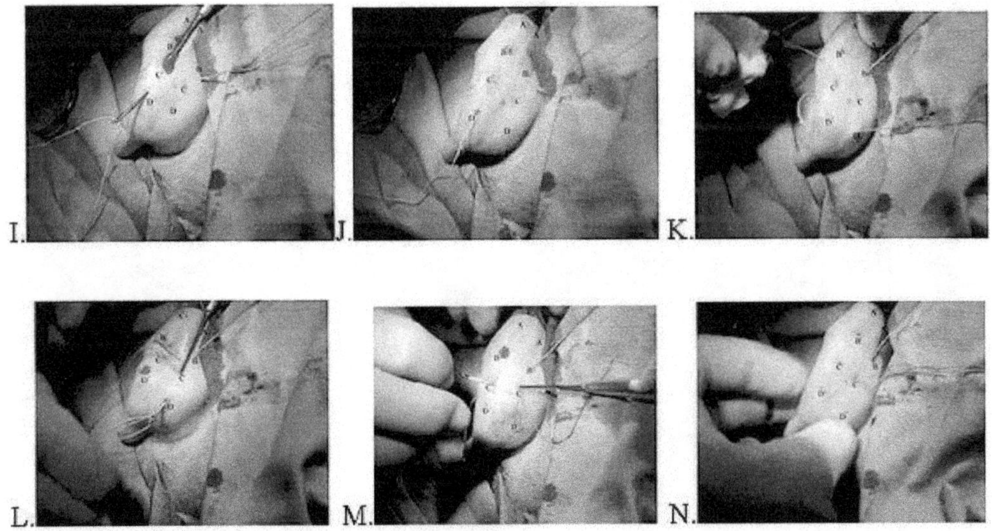

I, J, K, L, M, N. Making the 3rd suture circle C-C1 (subdermal), C1-D1 (transcartilagenous), D1-D (subdermal), D-C (transcartilagenous)

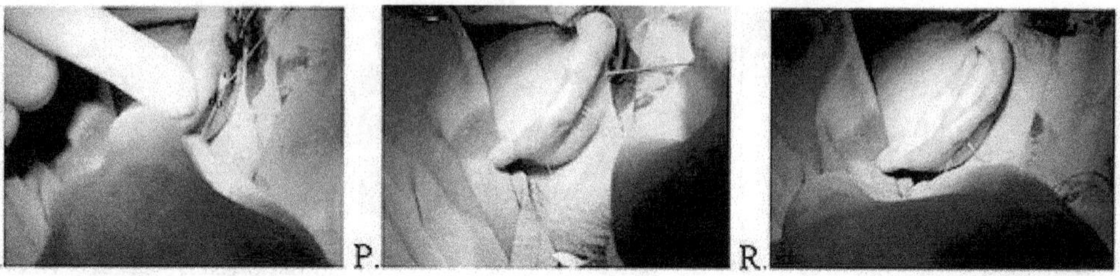

O. P. R.

O, P, R. All 3 suture circles are tightened under elastic tension, the anthelix fold is created, and the ear is pinned.

When all necessary sutures are done and tightened on both ears, symmetry is checked. Symmetry is usually obtained by the method itself. In 3 cases symmetry was perfected with additional suture on one side and in 2 cases with additional sutures on both sides. The prominent ears were corrected without incision or excision of skin from its posterior surface and without excision of cartilage. The antihelix was weakened by the line of sutures on its posterior surface and the antihelix fold was obtained successfully by the sutures only.

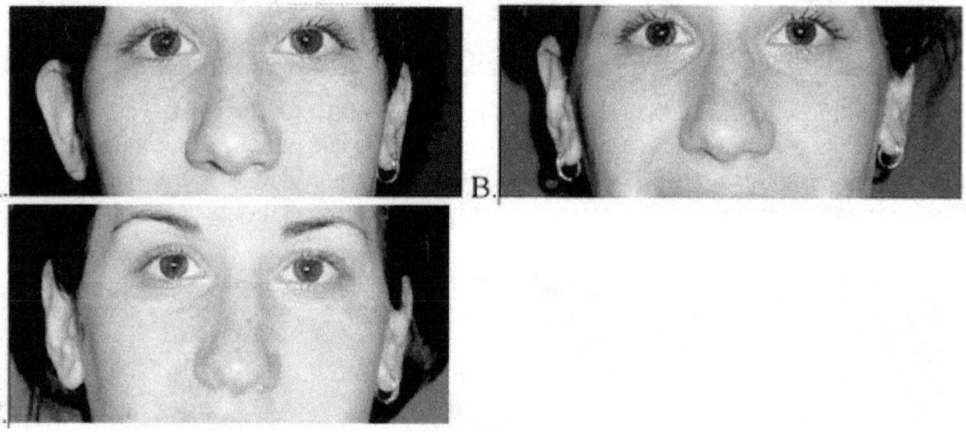

A. B. C.

Figure 46. Before, **B.** Immediate result, **C.** Result after 2 years

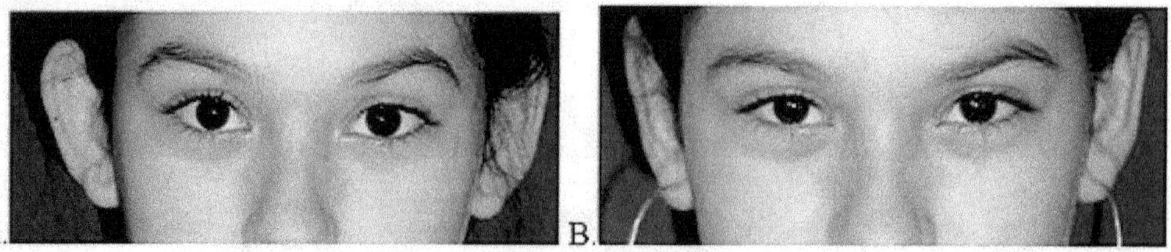

A. B.

Figure 47. Before, **B.** Result after 30 months

All patients had no need or have refused excision of the concha. In 5 cases, where lowering of the concha was necessary, the author has performed sutures of the concha cartilages to the occipital periosteum or mastoid with a good result.

Anterior surface sutures were used in 6 easier cases, when patients asked for minimal corrections, in 2 cases of difficulties with the equality and in 2 cases of secondary corrections.

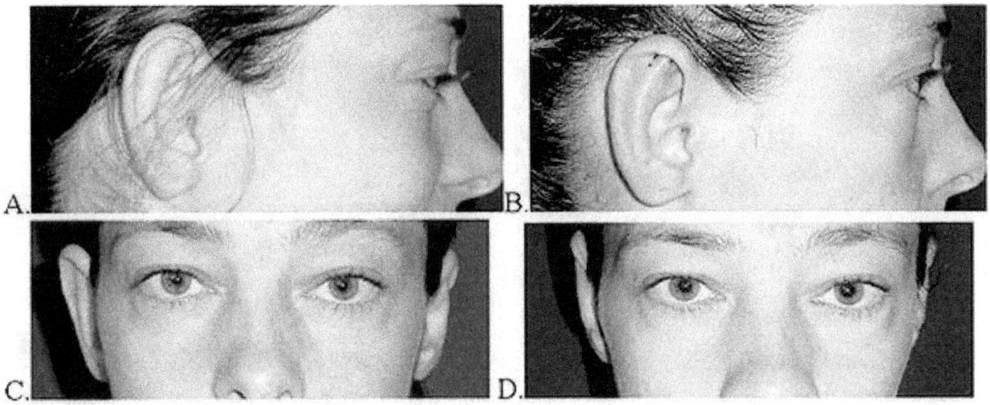

Figure 48. A suture is done on the right ear, on the anterior surface. **A., C.** Before, **B., D.** Result after 3 years.

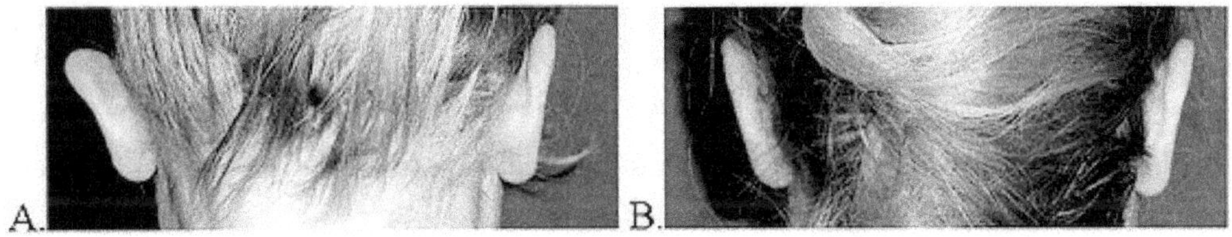

Figure 49. **A.** Before, **B.** Immediate result after suture. No wounds. Bandages can be used overnight. Patients are advised to carry an elastic band for a month.

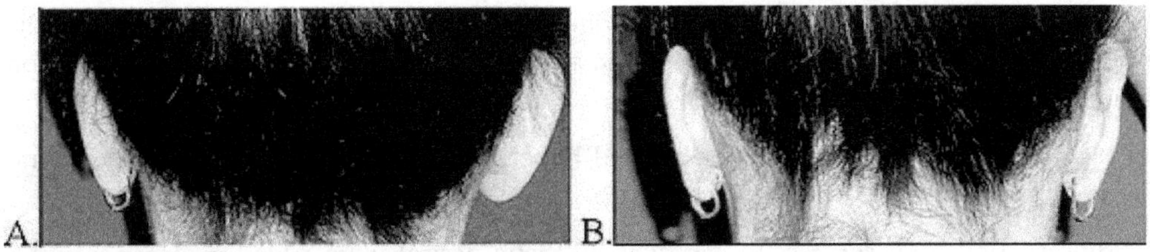

Figure 50. **A.** Before, **B.** Immediate result after suture. No wounds. Bandages can be used overnight. Patients are advised to carry an elastic band for a month.

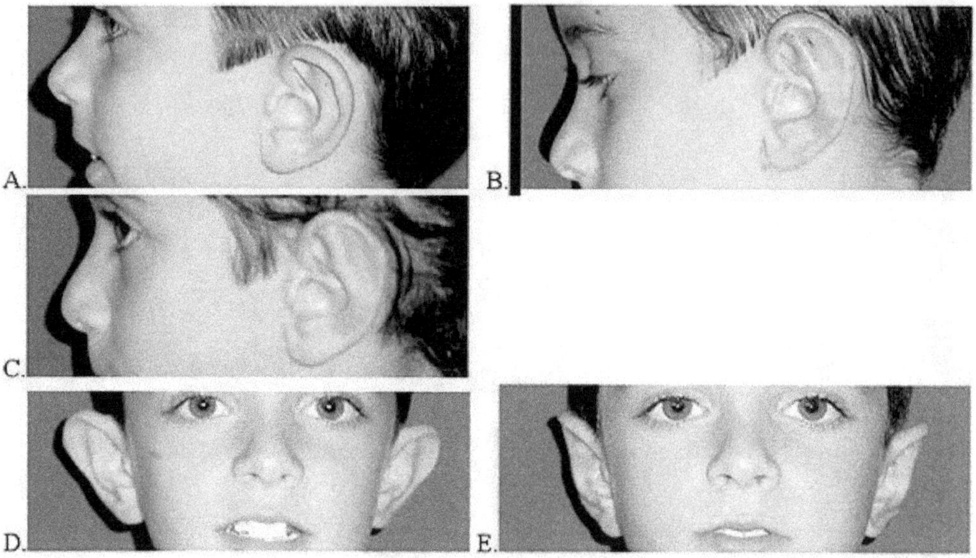

Figure 51. **A, D**. Before. **B**. Immediate result. An additional suture is done on the left ear from the anterior surface to fulfill equality of both years. **C, E**. Result after 18 months

5.2. Results

Adults and children are usually up and around within half an hour after surgery.

Any activity in which the ear might be bent should be avoided for a month or so. Most adults can go back to work on the day after surgery. Children can return to school activities 2 to 3 days after the operation, if they are motivated and careful about playground activity.

The procedture was accepted very well both by children and adults and the results were described as very satisfying.

5.3. Complications

Complications are infrequent and usually minor. Nevertheless, as with any operation, there are risks associated with surgery and specific complications associated with this procedure. Incomplete correction of prominent ears is probably the most common and undesirable outcome in otoplasty. Hematomas or seromas can complicate recovery and should be managed as soon as possible. Hypertrophic scars or keloids may form along the incision line.

In his patients, the author has not observed hypertrophic scars or keloids. There were no seromas, no infection or blood collection.

Additional unilateral sutures (to complete aesthetic desire) were added in 3 patients, 4-6 months after the primary surgery. There have been no overcorrection or chondritis.

Additional sutures can be done at any time, with no downtime or loss of social contact and work time.

5.4. Discussion

The goal of the suture technique in auriculoplasty is improvement and beautification, but not perfection. Perfect symmetry is unlikely and unnatural in human body, including the ears. Both ears never match perfectly (Fig. 52, 53). Patient and parent expectations should be discussed before the operation.

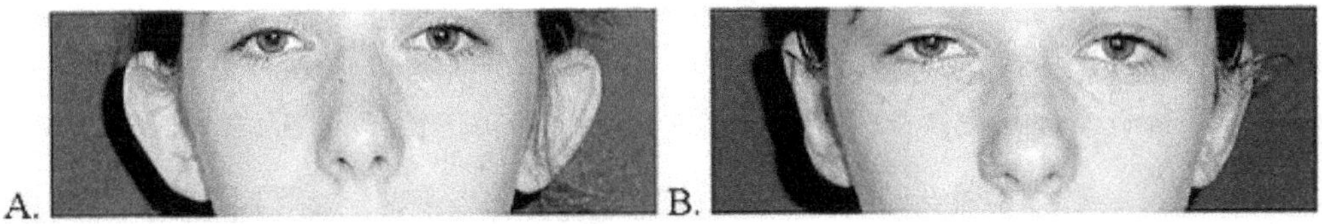

Figure 52. A. Before, B. Results after 3 years.

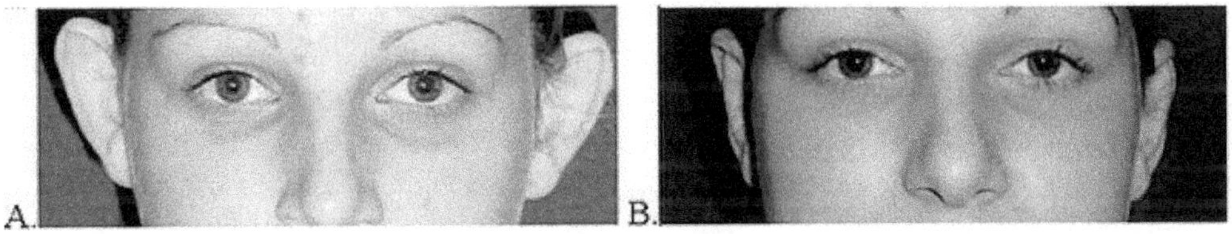

Figure 53. A. Before, B. Results after 3 years.

If the child is young, some surgeons may recommend general anesthesia, (the author uses local). For older children or adults, surgeons may prefer to use local anesthesia. Children who want the surgery and are motivated, cooperate better during the operation. The author has used local anesthesia, combined with intravenous sedation in all cases, and children do not remember the operation time.

The operation is mostly performed on children between the ages of four and fourteen. Ears are almost fully grown by age four. Ear surgery on adults is also possible and there are generally no additional risks. Discussion on state of the art techniques is always necessary like descriptions of the techniques such as Zplasty and Sandwich methods. In cases of inferiorly bulging concha an open surgery is suggested to correct the lobule and to maintain it posteriorly. In different techniques the auricle can be attached to the skull around the external meatus. Other authors use removal of cartilage where it is attached to the mastoid, with the aim of preventing the spring action of the auricle on the skull bone. The size of the concha will be taken into consideration for its correction and the proper evaluated size of cartilage to be excised.

Proper pre-operative evaluation is an essential step for satisfactory results. Not deviating from the decisions taken before the operation will avoid unnecessary excision that cannot be corrected later.

Good otoplasty makes the ears more proportional to the size and shape of the head and face.

The main function of the ear is hearing. Cosmetic ear surgery can reshape deformed or protruding ears and restore proportions.

Author details

Nikolay Serdev
New Bulgarian University, Sofia, Bulgaria

6. References

[1] Serdev, N.P. Year 1994, Suture Suspensions For Lifting Or Volume Augmentation In Face And Body (English version), 2nd Annual Meeing of the National Bulgarian Society for Aesthetic Surgery and Aesthetic Medicine, Sofia, 18 March 1994, Int J Aesth Cosm, 2001,1:1, 2561-2568

[2] Serdev, N.P. Forehead Subperiosteal Masklift in Combination with McIndoe Facelift Technique and Profile Correction. The 7th IPRAS Congress European Section, Berlin, Germany, June 2-5, 1993.

[3] Serdev N.P. Temporal SMAS lift without skin excision In: Lip Augmentation During Mask and SMAS Lift Procedure, AAARS Annual Meeting, New Orleans, USA, October 5-9, 1994

[4] Serdev, N.P. Temporal SMAS Lifting of the Face. Life Surgery Workshop. Unidad Medica Clinica Del Country, Bogota D.C., Colombia, November 8-10, 1999

[5] Serdev, N.P. SMAS Lifting of the Face by Minimal Incisions – the Serdev Technique. Life Surgery Workshop, International Academy of Cosmetic surgery and the Balkan Academy of Cosmetic Surgery, Krilig Clinic in Caracas, Venezuela, November 12-18, 1999.

[6] Serdev, N.P. Principles of Face Beautification, Ier Congresso Internacional de Cirurgia Cosmetica, Buenos Ares Argentina, 31 Octubre – 1 de Noviembre 1999
[7] Serdev, N.P. Temporal SMAS lift, Lecture and Life surgery Workshop, 1st World Congress of Cosmetic Surgery with Life Demonstrations, Edsa Shangri-La Manila and Quezon City Medical Center, February 25-27, 2000. http://www.mpint.co.jp/apacs/Congress2000/con007.htm
[8] Serdev, N.P. Temporal SMAS Lifting of the Face, Combined with Liposuction and Chin Augmentation Using Suture. Life Surgery Workshop, Tel Aviv, Israel, April 20-24, 2000.
[9] Serdev, N. P. Principles of face beautification, The 3-rd World Congress of ISAS, Tokyo, April 8-10, 2000, 9W58
[10] Serdev, N.P. Lifting del SMAS con Una Pequenna Incision Temporal, VIIIas Journadas Mediterraneas de Confrontaciones Terapeuticasen Medicina y Cirurgia Cosmetica, Sitges, Barcelona, March 16-19, 2000
[11] Serdev, N.P. Facial Rejuvenation by Minimal Skin Incisions, International Congress "Refinements in Aesthetic Surgery" Oradea, Romania, June 22-24, 2000
[12] Serdev, N.P. Ambulatory Temporal Smas Lift By Minimal Hidden Incisions, Int J. Cosm. Surg.2001;1 (2):20 - 27
[13] Mittelman H, Newman J. Smasectomy and imbrication in face lift surgery. Facial Plast Surg 2000 May; 2: 173-82.
[14] De la Fuente A, Santamaria AB Endoscopic subcutaneous and SMAS facelift without preauricular scars.Aesthetic Plast Surg1999 Mar-Apr; 23: 119-24.
[15] Maloney BP, Schiebelhoffer J. Minimal-incision endoscopic face-lift. Arch Facial Plast Surg 2000 Oct-Dec; 4: 274-8.
[16] Hagerty RC, Scioscia PJThe medial SMAS lift with aggressive temporal skin takeout. Plast Reconstr Surg 1998 May; 101 (6):1650-6
[17] Mitz, V, Peyronie M. The superficial musculoaponeurotic system (SMAS) in the parotid and cheek area. Plast. Reconstr. Surg. 1976; 58: 80.
[18] Cardoso de Castro, C. The role of the superficial musculoaponeurotic system in face lift. Ann. Plast. Surg. 1986; 16: 276.
[19] Kamer FM, Frankel SMAS rhytidectomy versus deep plane rhytidectomy: an objective comparison.ASPlast Reconstr Surg 1998 Sep; 102 (3): 878-81.
[20] Hamra ST. The tri-plane face lift dissection. Ann Plast Surg 1984 Mar; 12 (3): 268-74.
[21] Hamra ST. The deep-plane rhytidectomy. Plast Reconstr Surg 1990 Jul; 86 (1):53-61.
[22] Hamra ST, Composite rhytidectomy.Plast Reconstr Surg, 1992 Jul; 90 (1): 1-13.26.
[23] Mitz V, Use of deep planes in surgery of rejuvenation of the face Chirurgie 1991; 117 (4): 278-86.
[24] Ramirez OM, Maillard GF, Musolas A. The extended Subperiosteal Face lift: A definitive Soft-tissue Remodeling for Facial Rejuvenation. Plast Reconstr Surg 1991; 88:227-36.
[25] Bonnefon A Deep "en bloc" facial lift" Ann Chir Plast Esthet 1992 Jan; 37 (1), 85-94

[26] Bonnefon A. Deep vertical lift and its development regarding the central facial area and lower two-thirds of the neck. Our technique, Ann Chir Plast Esthet, 1999 Dec: 609-16.

[27] Teimourian B, Delia S, Wahrman A, The multiplane face lift.Plast Reconstr Surg 1994 Jan 93; 1: 78-85.

[28] Stuzin, J. M., Baker, T. J., Gordon, H. L., and Baker, T. M. Extended SMAS dissection as an approach to midface rejuvenation. Clin. Plast. Surg. 1995; 22: 295.

[29] Quatela VC, Sabini P. Techniques in deep plane face lifting. Facial Plast Surg 2000 May; 2: 193-209.

[30] Bosse, J. P., and Papillon, J. Surgical Anatomy of the SMAS at the Malar Region. In Transactions of the 9th International Congress of Plastic and Reconstructive Surgery. New York: McGraw-Hill, 1987: 348.

[31] Miura Y, Moura PD, Ramasastry S, Hochberg J. Can we simplify the nomenclature of the fascial lyers of the temporo parietal region? OnLine J Plast Reconstr Surg, Nov 1997;1: 1.

[32] Stuzin JM, Wagstrom L, Kawamoto HK, Wolfe SA. Anatomy of the frontal branch of the facial nerve: The Significance of the Temporal Fat Pad. Plast Reconstr Surg 1989; 83: 265-71.

[33] Hochberg J, Kaufman H, Ardenghy M. Saving The Frontal Branch during a Low Fronto-orbital Approach. Aesth Plast Surg 1995; 19: 161-163.

[34] Barton, F. E., Jr. The SMAS and the nasolabial fold. Plast. Reconstr. Surg. 1992; 89: 1054.

[35] Serdev N. Auriculoplasty Serdev Suture, Int J Cosm Surg 2000, Video time: 24:30 min. | Screen Size: 320 x 240 | File size: 36.2 | File Name: auriculoplasty_serdev_suture.wmv

[36] Serdev N., Auriculoplasty for beautification – a post-congress workshop, Asia Pacific Craniofacial Association. Third Conference, Shanghai, P.R. China, Oct. 30th – Nov. 1st, 2000

[37] Serdev N. Principles of Face Beautification, XIas Jornadas Mediterraneas De Confrontaciones Terapeuticas En Medicina y Cirugia Cosmetica, 21-25. 03. 2001,

[38] Serdev, N.P. Scarless Serdev Suture Method In Prominent Ears (Bulgarian), Original Papers, Int J Aesth Cosm 2009, 9:4, 1-9

[39] Barcelona 1. A.J. McDowell, Goals in otoplasty for protruding ears, Plast. Reconstr. Surg. 41 (1968) 17.

[40] Madzharov, M.M. A new method auriculoplasty for protruding ears, Br. J. Plast. Surg. 42(285) (1989) 290.

[41] Davis, J, Otoplasty: Aesthetic and Reconstructive Techniques, Springer-Verlag New York, Incorporated,1997/05

[42] Sainz Arreguil J., R. Gavirial, R. San Sebastianl, F. Ezquerral and M. Berrazuetal. Aesthetic otoplasty: the key point

[43] Hoda Saleh, Hassan Mostafa. Otoplasty for the prominent ear. Plastic and reconstructive surgery International Congress Series 1240 (2003) 603–605

[44] Ely ET: An operation for prominence of the auricles. Arch Otol 1881;10:97-99.

[45] Luckett WH: A new operation for prominent ears based on the anatomy of the deformity. Surg Gynecol Obst 1910;10:635-637.
[46] Mustarde JC: The correction of prominent ears using simple mattress sutures. Br J Plast Surg 1963 Apr; 16: 170-8[Medline].
[47] Sternstroem SJ: A "natural" technique for correction of congenitally prominent ears. Plast Reconstr Surg 1963 Nov; 32: 509-18[Medline].
[48] Wright WK: Otoplasty goals and principles. Arch Otolaryngol 1970 Dec; 92(6): 568-72[Medline].
[49] Furnas DW: Correction of prominent ears with multiple sutures. Clin Plast Surg 1978 Jul; 5(3): 491-5[Medline].
[50] Romo T 3rd, Sclafani AP, Shapiro AL: Otoplasty using the postauricular skin flap technique. Arch Otolaryngol Head Neck Surg 1994 Oct; 120(10): 1146-50[Medline]. 13. Adamson PA, Strecker HD: Otoplasty techniques. Facial Plastic Surgery 1995; 11: 284-300.
[51] Janis JE, Rohrich RJ, Gutowski KA: Otoplasty. Plastic and Reconstructive Surgery 2005; 115: 60e-72e[Medline].
[52] Serdev N. Auriculoplasty Serdev Suture, Int J Cosm Surg 2000, Video time: 24:30 min. I Screen Size: 320 x 240 I File size: 36.2 I File Name: auriculoplasty_serdev_suture.wmv
[53] Behmand RA, Ghavami A, Guyuron B. Nasal tip sutures, part I: the evolution. Plast Re cons tr Surg. 2003;112(4):1125-1129, discussion 1146-1149.
[54] Tebbetts JB. Shaping and positioning the nasal tip without structural disruption: a new, systematic approach. Plast Reconstr Surg. 1994;94(1):61 -77.
[55] Mocella S, Bianchi N. Double interdomal suture in nasal tip sculpturing. Facial Plast Surg. 1997;13(3):179-196.
[56] Baker SR. Suture contouring of the nasal tip. Arch Facial Plast Surg. 2000;2(1): 34-42.
[57] Leach JL, Athre RS. Four suture tip rhinoplasty: a powerful tool for controlling tip dynamics. Otolaryngol Head Neck Surg. 2006;135(2):227-231.
[58] Tardy ME, Cheng E. Transdomal suture refinement of the nasal tip. Facial Plast Surg. 1987;4(4):317-326.
[59] Papel ID. Interlocked transdomal suture technique for the wide interdomal space in rhinoplasty. Arch Facial Plast Surg. 2005;7(6):414-417.
[60] Daniel RK. Rhinoplasty: a simplified, three-stitch, open tip suture technique, part I: primary rhinoplasty. Plast Reconstr Surg. 1999;103(5):1491-1502.
[61] McCollough EG, English JL. A new twist in nasal tip surgery: an alternative to the Goldman tip for the wide or bulbous lobule. Arch Otolaryngol. 1985;111 (8):524-529.
[62] Daniel RK. Rhinoplasty: creating an aesthetic tip: a preliminary report. Plast Re¬constr Surg. 1987;80(6):775-783.
[63] Kridel RW, Konior FJ, Shumrick KA, Wright WK. Advances in nasal tip surgery: the lateral crural steal. Arch Otolaryngol Head Neck Surg. 1989;115(10):1206-1212.
[64] Pastorek NJ, Becker DG. Treating the caudal septal deflection. Arch Facial Plast Surg. 2000;2(3):217-220.

[65] Gruber RP, Friedman GD. Suture algorithm for the broad or bulbous nasal tip. Plast Reconstr Surg. 2002;110(7):1752-1764, discussion 1765-1768.

Chapter 3

Serdev Sutures® in Lower Face and Neck

Nikolay Serdev

Additional information is available at the end of the chapter

http://dx.doi.org/10.5772/55675

1. Introduction

The concept of lower face SMAS lift via sutures, through skin punctures alone (or by hidden incisions in the retro-lobular fold), explains how to re-structure and re-position the lower face, associated facial elements and neck, without visible pre- and retro-auricular scars. The author uses the specially designed, curved elastic Serdev® needles with lengths of 60 mm, 100 mm and 140 mm and prefers the Bulgarian semi-elastic, polycaproamide (Polycon) surgical suture USP 2, with long delayed absorption durability.

2. Lower face and neck lift by sutures, with skin perforations only or by using a hidden 2.5 cm retro-lobular incision

The first methos is a closed approach suture method of lower SMAS face and neck lift. The author uses skin punctures alone to introduce the needle and suture, in order to capture, lift and fix loose lower face and neck SMAS to stable structures like periosteum, without tissue undermining. Colli fascia, mastoid or occipital periosteum are used as anchor points to fix and elevate the lower SMAS, enabling lower face and neck lifting.

In the second method, the author uses limited undermining of 3-4 cm in front of the tragus, via retro-lobular incision. The fold behind the earlobule is the only place to hide the incision and at the same time obtain the optimal approach to cheek SMAS and platysma in front of the tragus. Usually, the retrolobular fold permits a 1.5-2.5 cm long incision. Thus, lifting the SMAS restores aesthetic angles, shape and proportions, which is the basis for beautification and rejuvenation.

2.1. The concept

Ptosis and laxity of the "subdermal facial mask" - the SMAS - in lower face and neck reflects the signs and appearance of lower face aging. The concept of using the closed approach semi-elastic sutures with delayed absorption, is to tighten and elevate the lower face and neck, without unnecessary incisions. It is a fact that soft tissue and skin are attached to the SMAS. Accordingly, lifting and fixing the SMAS into a more favourable position enables repositioning of soft tissue facial structures as well. Loose SMAS and skin laxity imparts a heavy, hanging, sad and tired facial expression. In young patients without genuine ptosis, heavy facial features, poorly expressed cheekbones and jaw lines, flawed proportions and angles, as well as sad appearance should be corrected. In many patients heavy subdermal fat and fat pad should be removed simultaneously.

Classic face lifts can not avoid some visible scars or an "operated-on" appearance, secondary to skin and SMAS rotation and pull. The concept of the suture lift of lower face and neck SMAS is to achieve immediate results and to avoid trauma, visible pre- and retro-auricular incisions, excisions and scars.

As subdermal and submental fat in the lower face is superficial to SMAS, it cannot be lifted with the SMAS lift. If necessary, it should be reduced concurrently or prior to lifting. The author uses ultrasound assisted liposculpturing in the lower face and neck since 1994 (SMEI Sculpture and later - VASER) as a best option for atraumatic fat removal and tightening of skin.

2.1.1. Definition

The two methods, described by the author, represent lower face and neck SMAS suspension, tightening or duplication, using elastic sutures durable through extended absorption delay, via needle perforations alone or via hidden retro-lobular incision, where SMAS-platysma is lifted and fixed to the mastoid, and in some selected cases - to occipital periosteum.

2.1.2. Objective

The primary goal in lower face and neck closed approach suture lifting technique is the straightening and repositioning of the subdermal facial mask - the SMAS/platysma - with the perspective of refreshing the facial appearance and obtaining rejuvenation and beautification, corresponding to aesthetic angles, proportions and anatomic position, typical for youth. It is used for sculpturing the jaw line, softening the nasolabial fold and beautification, mostly in minor and medium jowling, submental laxity. It is ideal in cases of beautification, associated with early or medium facial ptosis. In cosmetic surgery it is very important to respond to patient's requirements for immediate beautification, to avoid visible scars, as well as to give patients the chance to promptly resume work and social activities, without long recovery period.

For this objective, the author's methods were created to be minimally invasive, without trauma and scars.

2.1.3. Anatomy

Face droops with age, due to gravity, atrophy and loosening of the facial ligaments. Jowling is caused by displacement of the SMAS and skin aging. The neck is a face related area. The sagging neck is an important part of the aging face.

The SMAS is a fibro-muscular layer that connects platysma and galea and acts as a suspension for the overlying facial skin. The continuity between the facial SMAS and the platysma is an anatomical fact, useful in performing facelift surgery.

Subdermal plexus of vessels is superficial to SMAS. Motor nerves and facial muscles lie deep to SMAS. SMAS provides a suspensory sheet, which distributes the forces of facial expression. The concept that lifting this layer leads to better long-term suspension of overlying skin has become universally accepted.

SMAS continues inferiorly towards the platysma and represents aponeurotic connections between mimetic musculature and the overlying skin.

SMAS overlies the parotid gland in mandibular angle and tends to be substantial and easy to handle, because the parotid gland, zygomaticus major and minor muscles protect underlying facial nerve branches. With regard to protecting the facial nerve structures, we can accept that lower SMAS-platysma face-lift "by sutures only" or "with a retro-lobular incision" is done in a fairly secure area. The suture lift should protect the parotid gland and for this reason is performed only in the mobile superficial layers to capture the facial SMAS and platysma.

2.2. Surgical technique

The scarless lower face and neck SMAS-platysma lift by sutures takes about 10 minutes per side and is done under local anaesthesia and i.v. sedation.

2.2.1. METHOD I: using skin perforations only

1. Lower face SMAS lift by suture (A-C)

First Pass A-C

a) Perforate points A, B, and C with a No. 11 scalpel blade, only skin deep. Position the blade in direction of Langer's lines.

NB! Stay away from deep mastoid penetration (at point A), stay away from parotid gland (located deeper at point C), and submandibular gland (located more medially, could be near point B).

b) Enter the needle perpendicularly through the skin perforation at point A (without fixation of any dermal tissue), then **tangentially** through the mastoid periosteum at the anterior mastoid border.

NB! Do not push needle perpendicularly into mastoid - it is very soft and can be easily perforated (be aware of mastoid and inner ear anatomy). Do not push the needle - twist it gently forwards or backwards.

c) Proceed through fascia colli and superficial subcutaneous tissue from A to C. Proceed parallel to the skin - place the needle tip laterally. The handpiece concavity shows the needle tip position in the tissue. The pass should be superficial and below the skin. However, if too superficial - dimpling will appear above the needle. Avoid this by twisting the needle backwards and then forwards again, a little deeper (but still in a superficial plane). A deeper pass will produce a bulging effect.

NB! Stay superficial. Never introduce the needle into or below the sternocleidomastoid muscle (vascular nerve bundle, a. and v. jugularis interna). Stay away from external jugular vein as well.

d) Just before exiting at point C, SMAS (platysma) is captured. To capture SMAS, turn needle tip downwards, progress a bit and twist needle tip upwards.

NB! Stay in superficial mobile layer, away from the parotid gland (just below mobile SMAS).

e) Pass through perforation point C.

Do not push through skin perforation point C. Place skin perpendicular to needle tip, twist the needle softly and progress gently and easily. The tip should appear at perforation point C, without resistance in front. Perforation or resistance indicates engagement of dermis, resulting in a dimple that is difficult to remove. Free the needle tip and repeat the movement until the tip appears without the feeling of resistance.

f) The needle tip is threaded and is pulled out through the needle pass in line C-A.

Second Pass A-C

The second parallel needle pass goes through the same skin perforations and tissue plane, 2-3 mm away from the first one. Platysma has to be engaged again. Appearing in perforation point C, the needle is threaded with the second end of the suture that is withdrawn through the second needle pass C-A. The suture loop dives in the subdermis at point C. The knot is made under medium elastic tension. Possible skin dimples should be managed by pulling the skin away from the suture, using a mosquito instrument. Thus, the first suture of lower face SMAS fixation to mastoid (or to occipital periosteum – rare and mostly in men to hide the swelling bulging) is fulfilled (Fig. 1, 2).

PROCEDURE Video
http://www.youtube.com/watch?v=zpDvCxC9hDg

Inject local anesthesia into points A, B, and C and also into the tissue corridor to be used for the needle passes.

The points of skin perforations should be planned in advance:

Point A - fixation at mastoid periosteum

Point B - fixation of lateral border of platysma to be lifted to A. A-B direction is to cervico-mandibular angle.

Point C - fixation of check SMAS and lateral border of platysma to be lifted to A. A-C direction is to the chin.

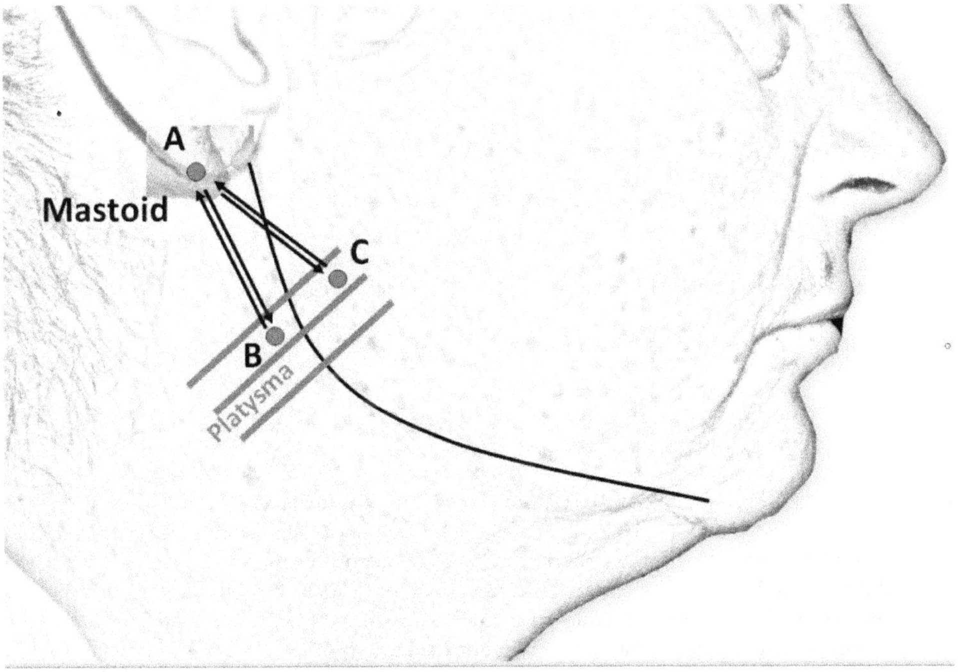

Figure 1. Lower face and neck SMAS lift, using Serdev Suture®

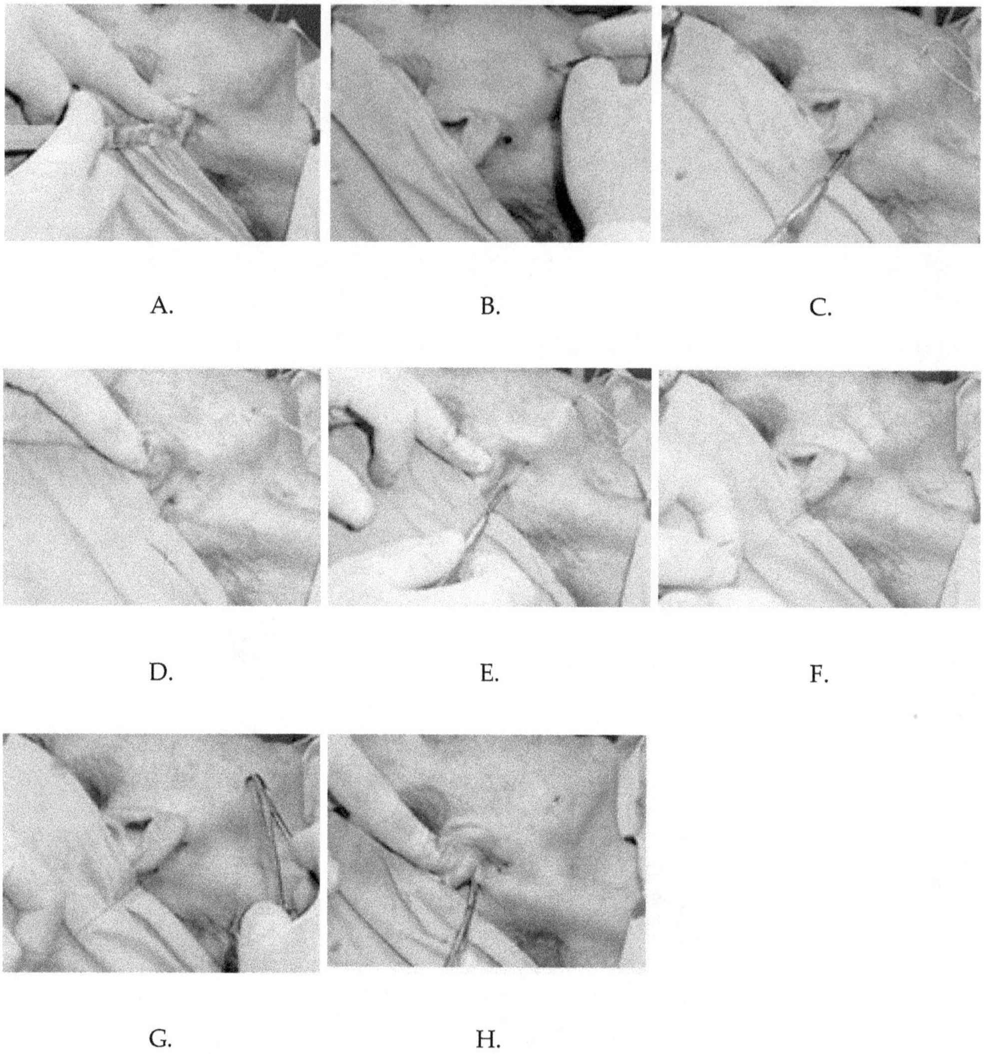

Figure 2. **A.** Lidocaine infiltration of the mastoid periosteum, colli fascia and SMAS at perforation points A, C, and along the line A-C , **B.** Scalpel blade No 11 skin perforation in the selected points, **C.** The needle is introduced through skin perforation A, then **tangentially** through the mastoid, superficial subdermal through colli fascia, SMAS/platysma and perforation point C. No dimpling should be visible above the needle., **D.** The suture is introduced through the needle pass C-A, **E.** Second pass of the needle following the same plan 2-3 mm away from the first pass, the needle eye is threaded, no dimpling is visible above the needle, **F.** The second end of the suture is introduced through the second needle pass C-A. The suture circle is fulfilled. The pull on the suture lifts the cheek SMAS, **G.** Skin dimpling has been removed by releasing the skin from attachments using a mosquito instrument., **H.** Skin is released at point A. Nice jaw line is visible.

2. Neck lift (A-B)

The second suture is done in the same manner, from point A to point B.

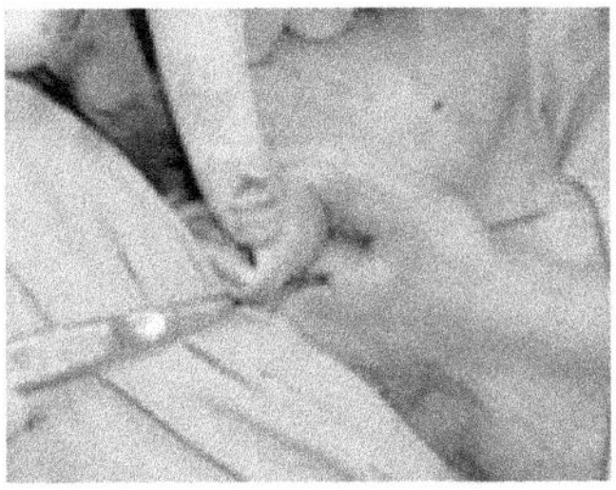
A.

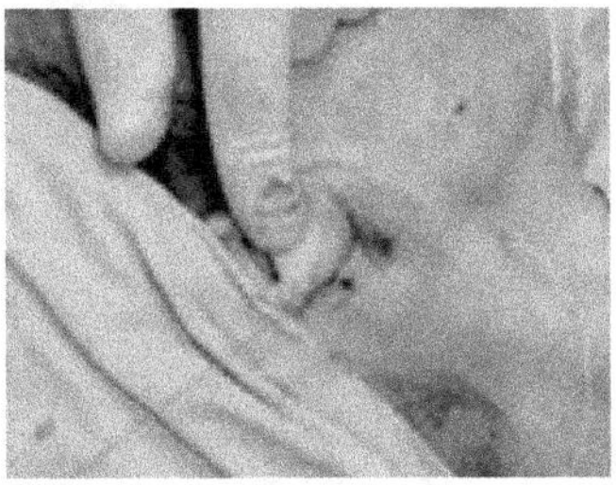
B.

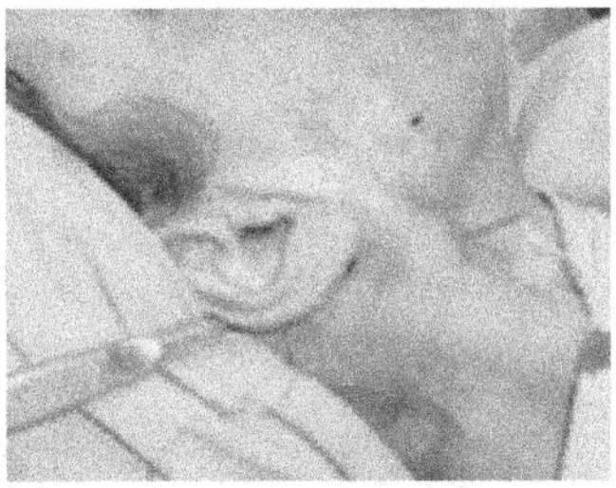
C.

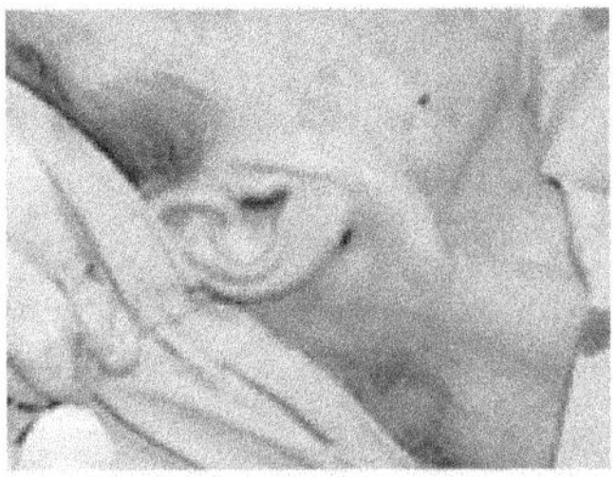
D.

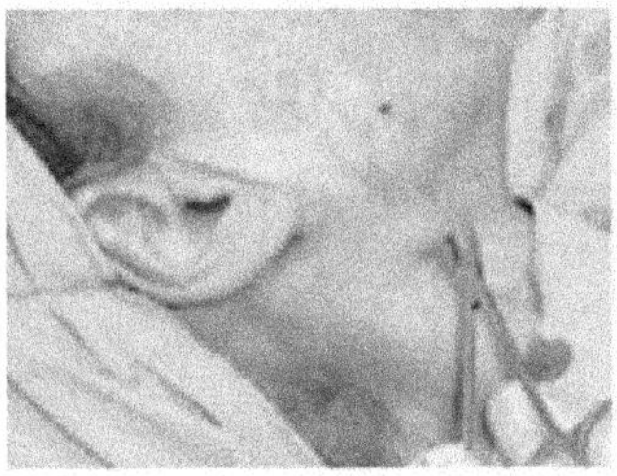
E.

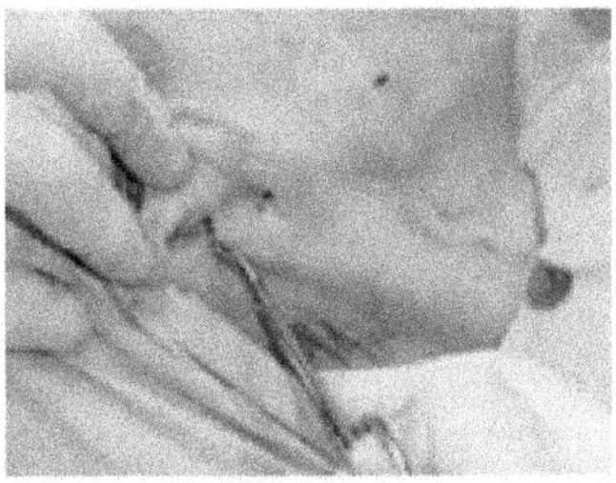
F.

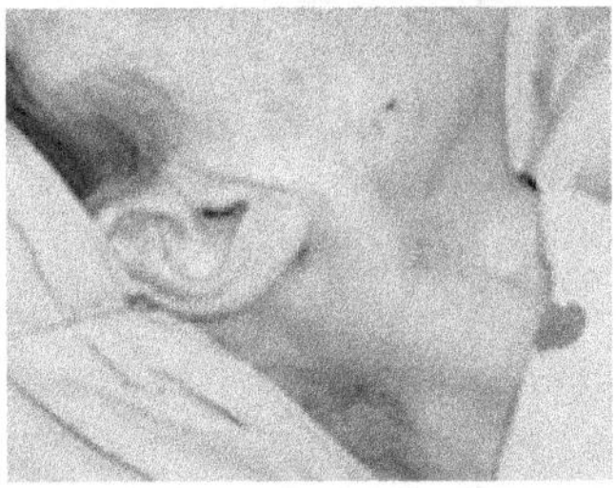
G.

Figure 3. A. The needle is introduced through the skin perforation point A, then **tangentially** through the mastoid, **superficial** subdermal through colli fascia, **above the sternocleidomastoid muscle,** through platysma and perforation point B in the direction of the cervico-mandibular angle, **B.** The suture is introduced through the needle pass B-A, **C.** Second pass of the needle following the same plan, 2-3 mm away from the first one, **D.**The second end of the suture is introduced through the second needle pass, suture loop dives into the skin perforation point B and the suture circle is fulfilled. The pull on the suture lifts the platysma, **E.** Skin dimpling at skin perforation point B is removed by releasing the skin from attachments, using a mosquito clamp, **F.** Skin dimpling at skin perforation point A is removed by releasing the skin from attachments using a mosquito clamp, **G.** The knot is made and the result of neck lift and cervico-mandibular angle is immediately visible.

At the other side, lifting is performed by suture in the same fashion.

2.2.2. METHOD II: using a 2.5 cm retro-lobular incision

The author has found that the only place to hide the incisions and at the same time have a very good approach to cheek, lower face and neck SMAS in a distance of 3-4 cm in front of the tragus, is the fold behind the ear lobule. It usually permits a 1.5 to 2.5 cm long incision, which is enough to elevate pre-auricular SMAS and retromandibular platysma into the skin incision line and to suture them to the colli fascia and mastoid.

Infiltration is done in the retro-lobular fold and 3-4 cm in front of tragus. 1.5 to 2.5 cm incision in the fold is done and a blunt subcutaneous undermining is performed through the retro-lobular opening in a radius of 3-4 cm from the earlobe in direction to: 1. oral commissure, 2. chin, and 3. cervico-mandibular angle.

After undermining there are **2 options:**

Option 1. Cheek SMAS and platysma are captured with a mosquito instrument, pulled out into the wound opening and sutured to colli fascia and mastoid. In this manner the lower face and neck SMAS lift is developed from the preauricular SMAS (at the level of the earlobule) and platysma (at the mandibular angle), and attached posteriorly to the mastoid process. Medium elastic tension is applied, providing a lower face SMAS backward & upward lift and platysma upward lift (Fig. 1). Skin is closed in one layer. Gauze dressings are not obligatory but can be used overnight or for some hours. Sutures are removed after 7 days.

Option 2. After the retrolobular incision and undermining is done, a 60 mm Serdev® needle is introduced in the undermined subdermal space and biting SMAS, arrives in perforation point C in lower face (or B in neck). After threading the needle, the surgical suture is introduced into the incision. Then, from skin perforation point A, **tangentially** through the mastoid, the needle arrives in the retrolobular incision and takes the suture end, introducing it at skin perforation point A. The suture is located in the line A-C in the lower face (or A-B in the neck area) fixing mobile SMAS (platysma) and immobile mastoid periosteum. Second pass is subdermal again taking the second suture end at point C (or B) and introducing it into skin perforation point A. Thus, the circle of the suture is fulfilled and the suture loop dives in point C (or B in neck). The knot is tied at Point A. Skin dimpling at points C and B is removed by traction of the skin perforation points C or B and the suture in opposite directions. One or two stiches are placed, in order to close the wound.

Both Serdev Suture® techniques of lower face and neck SMAS lift are quicker and safer than classic invasive face lift techniques. Mobile SMAS is lifted behind the ear lobule and sewn down to stable bone and periosteal structures. This technique gives an aesthetic and normal "non-operated on" appearance to the face, without scars and totally covers patient's expectation.

It is also possible to combine lower SMAS lift with other procedures such as fat pad removal, ultrasonic assisted liposculpturing of lower face and neck, medial platysma suturing, skin resurfacing, rhinoplasty, etc. Only a small number of patients need additional platysma sewing at the midline. In double chin cases, most important is to remove the fat collection. In authors hands, ultrasonic assisted liposuction is the best method to obtain a good cervico-mandibular angle of the neck and to tighten the skin in such cases.

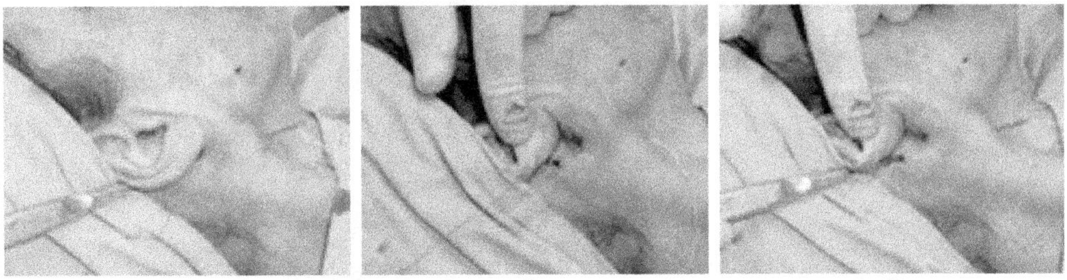

A. B. C.

Figure 4. A. After Lidocaine infiltration, retrolobular incision and about 3 cm blunt dissection of the preauricular and subauricular zones, the platysma is fixed with the needle in point B and the needle is threaded, **B.** The suture is introduced from the skin perforation point B into the opening of the retrolobular incision. A tangential bite of the mastoid from point A and suture end is introduced from the incision to point A. **C.** The needle is introduced again from skin perforation point A subdermally to perforation point B and the needle is threaded. Introduction of the suture in line B-A follows, the suture loop will dive in perforation point B and the suture circle will be finalized. The suture will be knotted, dimples removed. Closure of the retroauricular incision follows.

2.3. Results

530 patients have been operated with Method I during the period 1994-2011. Method II was performed in 386 patients. The result in these cases was immediate and optimal: there are no limitations to postoperative activities; no "operated-on" appearance, no visible scars and no real signs of operative intervention. The moderate facial tension generally imparts a pleasant sensation for the patient. Neither haematomas, nor infections have been observed. Bruising is rare.

In method I, in very loose skin cases, it is possible to obtain some swelling (bulging) effect at the sternocleidomastoid site that adapts and disappears in 2-3 weeks and could be easily covered by hair in female patients. In method II, skin undermining prevents from bulging or folding.

In method I, the skin punctures disappear in 2-3 days. In method II, the skin scar in the retrolobular fold is invisible and, additionally, there is no skin tension.

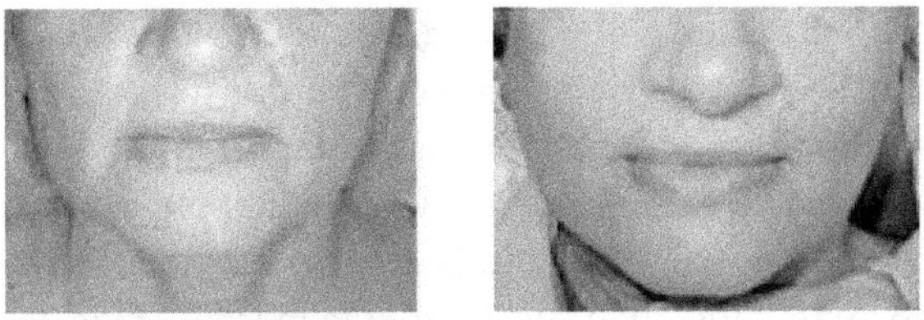

Figure 5. Visible change in the lower face appearance after lower SMAS lift by sutures with skin punctures only.

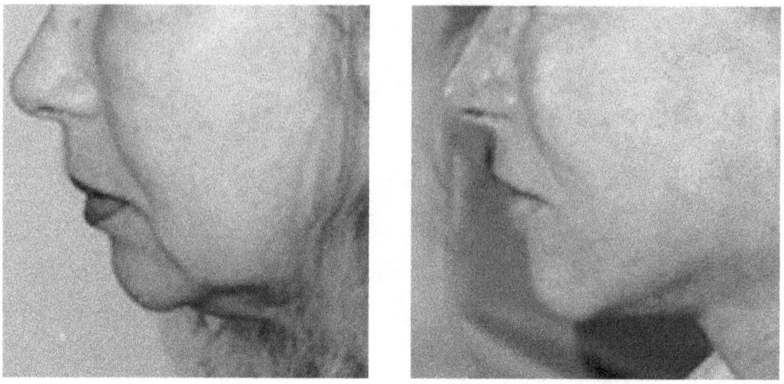

Figure 6. Result, immediately after surgery in the OP theatre. Immediate total change in the lower face after temporal, brow lift and a lower SMAS lift, using sutures with skin punctures alone.

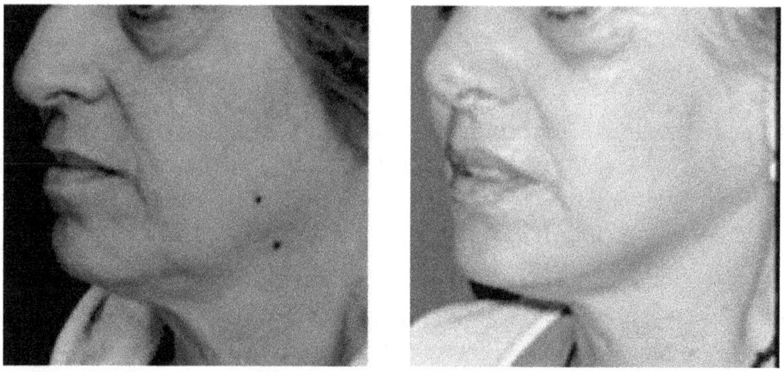

Figure 7. Before and after temporal SMAS, brow, and lower SMAS lift using sutures with skin punctures alone, combined with rhinoplasty. The change pleases the patient. Rejuvenation of the face.

In one case, when method II, option one was used, upper lid ptosis occurred during fixation of the pre-auricular SMAS. Immediate release of the suture solved this "complication" on the spot and another suture was performed without further complication. In one 63 year old patient, in line with her aesthetic requirements, an additional pre-auricular skin excision (S-lift) was performed 3 years after the suture lift. Due to the previous SMAS lift using method II, it was not possible to excise more than 2 to 3 mm skin in front of the ear.

No other complications or complaints have been observed in this period.

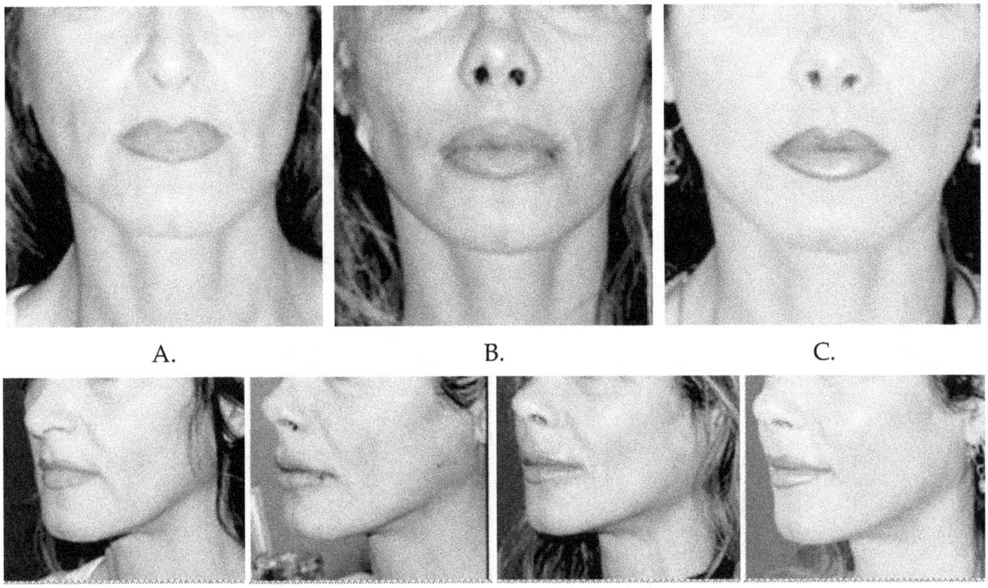

A. B. C. D. E. F. G.

Figure 8. **A, D.**Before, **B, E.** Immediately after simultaneous temporal, medial and lower SMAS face lift by sutures using skin punctures only, brow lift by sutures, rhinoplasty, and lip augmentation. The skin punctures for the lower SMAS lift by sutures are visible (E), **F.** the day after surgery.**C, G.** After 3 days with make-up.

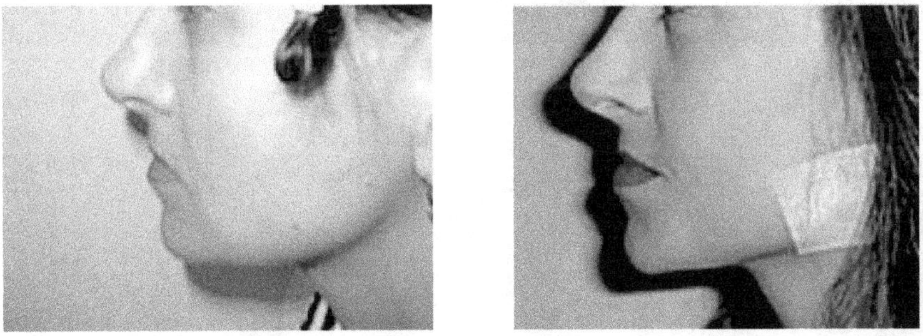

A. B.

Figure 9. **A.** Before and **B.** immediately after surgery in an 37 years old patient. A pleasant result in the lower face and jaw line. The bandage covering the skin punctures stays for overnight only. Patients usually return to work in a day or two.

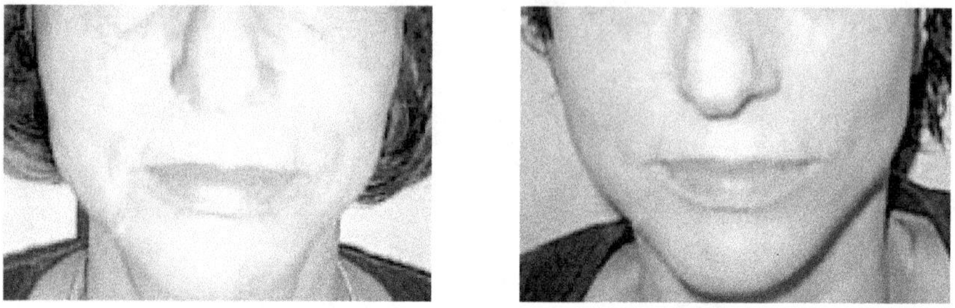

Figure 10. Rejuvenation in an elderly patient. **A.** Before and **B.** after lower face and neck SMAS lift with retro-lobular incisions. Very good result with skin beautification. The SMAS and skin attached to it is tightened.

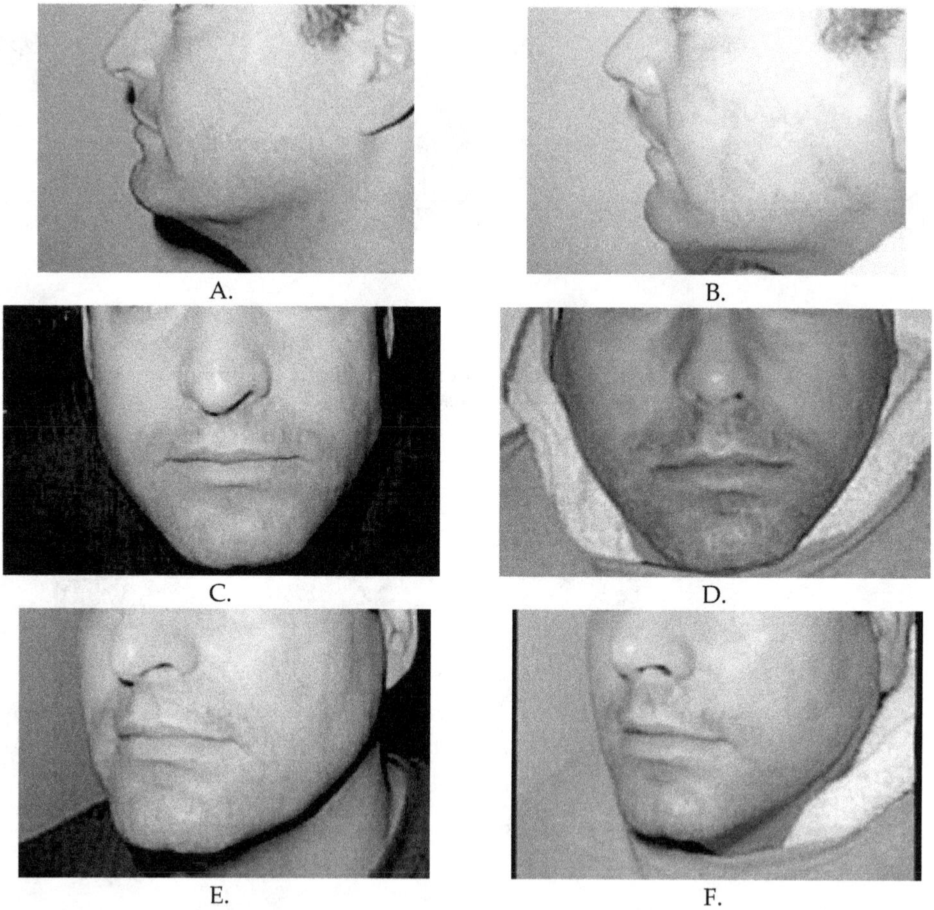

Figure 11. A, C, E. Before. **B, D, F.** After lower face SMAS lift with retro-lobular incisions in a 40 years old man, plus T-excision and columella sliding rhinoplasty. No signs of an operated-on appearance. Defined cervico-mandibular angle post op.

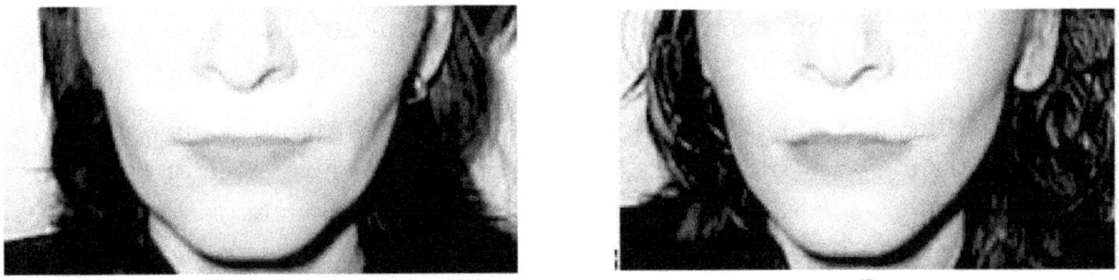

A. B.

Figure 12. **A.** Before. Thin and loose skin in the lower face. Gravity effect on the soft tissue and skin is visible in different positions. **B.** After lower SMAS-platysma lift with retro-lobular incisions in a 37 years old female patient. The SMAS, attached soft tissue and skin are tightened. No signs of gravity on the soft tissue and skin are visible in any position after surgery. Lovely tightened youthful "hungry cheeks", pleasing the patient.

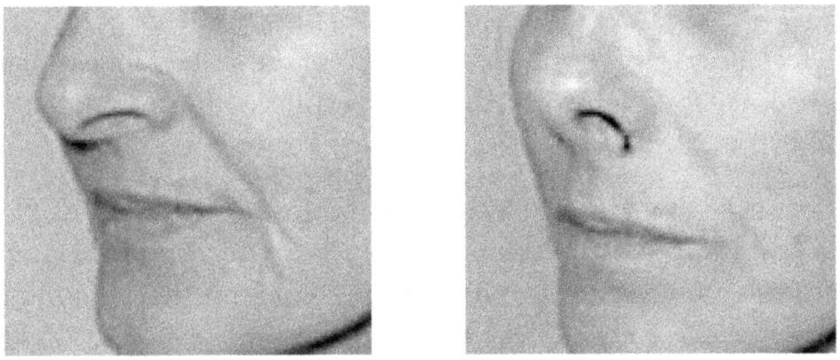

A. B.

Figure 13. **A.** Before, **B.** Effect on the nasolabial and marionette folds in a 53 years old patient after lower SMAS lift, rhinoplasty and allar base narrowing.

2.4. Complications

Minimal and very rare problems have occurred with the suture technique in some patients. As described above, one case of taking a facial nerve branch in the suture during performing method II led to ptosis of the upper lid and was solved immediately by removing of the suture. It is a rare complication, because the facial nerve runs a little higher, just below the tragus and immediately after that penetrates deep into the parotid gland. Sutures can be easily removed and placed again at any time with nearly no downtime.

In method I, the needle penetrates the tissue much lower and we have had no cases of facial nerve insertion in the suture. Three patients described some loss of sensation in the ear lobe for a couple of weeks. The trauma of involving the great auricular nerve in the suture, provoked by a lateral traction, adapts in some weeks. Swelling and bruising are rare.

2.5. Discussion

Beautification and immediate social activity are the first and most important aspect of patients' requirements. The author's experience indicates that his specific methods of lower

SMAS lift can be performed safely with minimum complications and maximum patient satisfaction.

Solely stretching the skin is an obsolete concept. Excision SMAS lifts, extended SMAS lift, deep plane, and sub-periostial face-lifts are associated with a number of complications, including haematoma, pixie ear, nerve injury, and skin sloughing. Deep-plane and composite techniques achieve a deeper suspension, but the risk of facial nerve injury is higher. Post-operative care is longer and pre- and retro-auricular incisions are not the patient's best contemporary option.

The author's suture methods are performed to obtain and preserve a youthful lower face and neck through fixing lower face and neck SMAS to mastoid (or very rarely to occipital periosteum). These techniques of "scarless lower SMAS face and neck lift" provide a safe alternative to other face lifts using preauricular skin incisions and elevation, platysmal and subplatysmal flaps, SMAS dissections, submental surgery, deep plane or composite face lifts. Injury to the facial nerve in rhytidectomy has been described in less than one percent of the cases, and a spontaneous return of function results within 6 months in more than 80 percent of these injuries.

With the introduction of the author's technique, performed without aggressive platysmal and subplatysmal flaps and SMAS dissections, the risk of injury to facial nerve branches has decreased significantly. Nevertheless, the operating surgeon must follow up the patient's reactions carefully for signs of facial palsy during operation.

The scarless lower face and neck SMAS lift by sutures, using skin needle perforations only or hidden retro-lobular incision, provides a safe and effective ambulatory method for beautification and rejuvenation of early and medium sagging face. It is an effective method that addresses problems of jowling or submental laxity. A nice and youthful shaped jaw, acute cervicomandibular angle and straightened cervical skin are the most desirable effects. The results fully correspond to patients' desires. The effect is immediate and without visible scars.

The lower SMAS lift is a bidirectional lower face and neck lift that gives a harmonious, strong lifting effect on the sub-zygomatic area and jaw and creates an acute cervicomandibular angle. It achieves partial correction of the nasolabial folds and submental area laxity.

In author's patients, the lower SMAS-platysma lift is very often combined with temporal, mid-face SMAS lift and brow lift by sutures, in order to obtain a "total SMAS lift". Generally, SMAS lifts by sutures are nice and easy ambulatory weekend procedures.

3. Chin enhancement and form correction

The primary goal of facial aesthetic (cosmetic) surgery is beautification, achieving balance and harmony. The mental area must be addressed to the complete synthesis of the face. The concept of augmenting, correcting and adjusting the chin position has evolved so significantly that it is now an important procedure in face beautification. Various autogenous implants for chin augmentation have been in use for over 100 years. The advent of synthetic materials has given rise to various types of alloplastic implants with their advantages, disadvantages and complications.

The author's technique of chin soft tissue suspension, using a simple durable suture with extended absorption delay, is indicated to correct microgenia, to obtain the necessary projection and to adjust chin symmetry. It is ideally suited for correction of most chin disproportions, such as: profile deficiencies, aging (witch) chin, asymmetries, disharmonies, and is used for beautification and rejuvenation of the entire face as a single or combined operation, with very satisfying cosmetic results.

3.1. Introduction

The importance of the chin in face beautification is determined by the fact that the chin is a part of the lower third of the face. Aesthetically it has to fit to the straight line of the noble profile, to the "beauty triangle" of the lower face, and the facial golden section rule of 3 proportionally equal parts. Chin prominence gives the essence of visage character.

Profile deficiencies are due to congenital, traumatic and aging factors with different degrees of deformity. Loss of volume or a genetically small mandible affect the aesthetics and expression of the face, mouth, chin, and neck. Disharmony between the skeletal support and the soft tissue envelope is a common cause of aesthetic concerns.

Although standards of beauty evolve over time, classical facial features such as symmetry, straight profile, good chin projection and proportions remain as rules. A comprehensive beautification (including rejuvenation of the chin) depends on accurate analysis of the lower face with attention to the contours and underlying structures.

Many surgical options are available to restore the definition of the chin region. A large variety of materials are used by surgeons for augmentation purposes, although the search for the perfect implant continues.

The author's surgical suspensory procedure, using a simple suture, has the aim to return the chin's soft tissue to a more aesthetic and youthful position and to meet patients' demands for immediate result, fast recovery and beatification without implanting foreign materials.

3.1.1. Anatomy

Although the process of facial aging is predictable, the rate of changes varies from person to person. With aging, laxity develops in the skin and subcutaneous tissues, the result of which is an aesthetically incorrect projection and contour of the anterior mandible. The soft tissues are subject to gravity and undergo progressive atrophy. Aging (Witch) chin is an unpleasant aesthetic defect, characterized by ptosis of the premental tissue and a deep submental fold. Bone resorption and soft tissue atrophy are the most important components. Loss of bone volume leads to loss of support for the soft tissues of the face.

Aesthetic cosmetic rejuvenation of the face and neck involves repositioning of poorly supported soft tissues. The effect of surgery in these cases aims to improve and restore a youthful appearance. This depends on the bone structure, amount and distribution of subcutaneous fat, as well as the interconnectedness of the superficial muscles to the overlying skin.

3.1.2. The objective of the author's specific technique is to suspend the loose and hanging soft tissue of the chin, to give natural height of the chin projection and to advance the submental skin in order to obtain a youthful jaw line. Avoidance of common problems associated with implantation of foreign materials is an additional goal.

3.1.3. Definition

Suturing and suspending the loose chin soft tissue in front of the immobile menton in order to obtain volume, projection and a straight profile. Using the suture method, the chin could be positioned forward, up or down, left or right, thus obtaining proper aesthetic proportions and facial symmetry.

3.1.4. Surgical approach

Two skin punctures to insert the needle.

3.2. Author's surgical technique

One or more Serdev Sutures® of the chin soft tissue could be used to obtain roundness and projection of the chin, where desired. The author uses only two skin perforation points (A and B) in the sub- and supra- mental folds to insert the needle and perform a suture, which, bulging the sutured fibrotic soft tissue, creates volume in front of the immobile menton. An additional option is the horizontal suture with 2 lateral skin perforation points.

Using different angles of needle positioning, the author has introduced the Serdev Suture® method for total or partial enhancement, augmentation and positioning of the chin up or down (to adapt facial aesthetic proportions), or left or right (to obtain symmetry). I.e. chin lift is created tridimentionally: up or down, forward, left or right. Creation of a dimple is another option with author's techniques.

The author prefers to start from the submental skin perforation point A. **Video**: http://www.youtube.com/watch?v=oqJreY-JsCM. If more tissue is necessary, the perforation point A is located in the submental fold. When positioning the needle in the skin perforation point, the submental perforation has to be moved forward anteriorly to the menton. **NB!** Do not perforate the muscles dorsal to the menton. If a "Witch" chin has to be lifted, the submental skin perforation point should be positioned much more anteriorly, so the projection will be higher. If the chin has to be projected downwards, the second perforation point B can be lower than the supramental fold and first point A should be maximally dorsal at the submental fold. The suture can be placed more lateral to project one side of the chin only (to equalize symmetry), or the central chin tissue can be fixed to the mental periosteum more laterally with the same result.

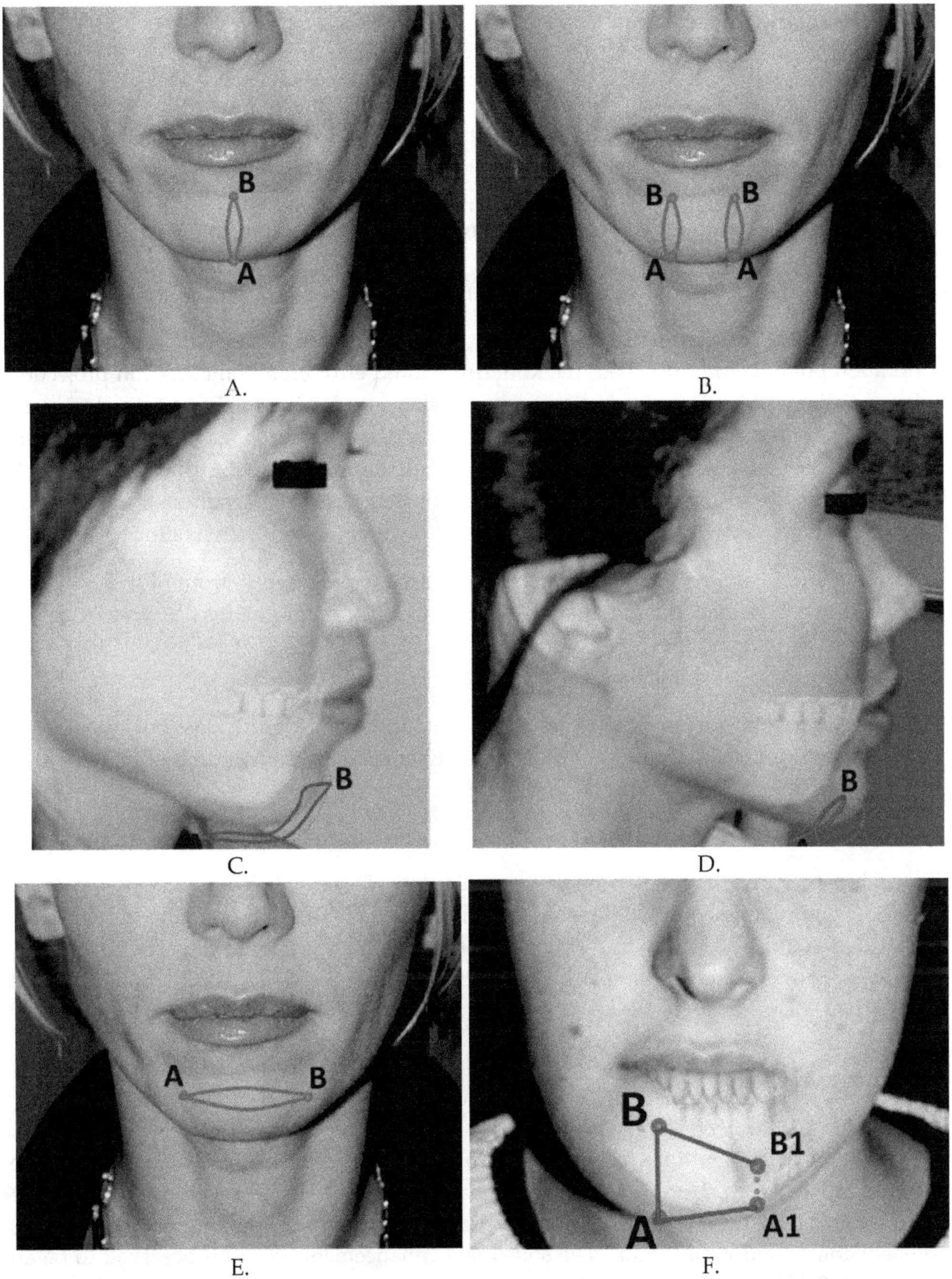

Figure 14. A, B, C, D, E, F. Different variations of fixation of the fibrotic soft tissue, with or without fixation to menton

3.3. Vertical chin suture

A 50 mm or 60 mm Serdev® needle enters through the submental skin puncture, then in front of the menton, slips along the anterior surface of the bone and exits through the other skin puncture at the supramental fold. After threading the needle with surgical suture USP 0, the suture is positioned in the deep first needle pass. Performing the second pass, the needle re-enters through point A, then medium deep through the soft tissue, and exits through point B to take the second suture end and introduce it in the second pass. **NB!** When performing the medium deep pass it should not be superficial. If skin dimpling appears above the needle, the pass is too superficial and should be repositioned deeper.

Thus, the suture circle is finalized and when pulling the suture, the suture loop dives in perforation point B. After it is tied, the knot dives into perforation point A. Chin projection is immedially visible. Then, any dimpling and skin attachment to the suture should be removed using a mosquito clamp. **NB!** If the needle pass does not engage dermis, removal of dimpling at the skin perforation points is easy. If dermis is caught, dimple removal is impossible and the suture procedure should be repeated. Twist the needle softly forward or backward to find its way through the skin perforation openings without fixation of dermis.

Performing such a suture, the available chin soft tissue is projected in front of the immobile menton and enhancement/augmentation is obtained. The angle of needle position gives direction of the enhancement - up, down, left or right. In cases of persistent deep chin dimple, 2 sutures are possible both sides.

If the projection is not sufficient, an additional horizontal suture can be added. The horizontal suture has 2 perforation points laterally and 2 passes should be done – the first one deep near the menton and the second - middle deep.

The number of sutures could be more than two, in order to obtain the necessary projection.

This ambulatory procedure takes only a few minutes. No dermal closure and no bandages are used. Facial wash should be done on the following day. The skin puncture in the supra-mental fold could be visible for 2-3 days and patients may use make up. The early post-operative period swelling is almost invisible and patients can return to their social life as soon as they wish.

3.4. Results

1095 patients underwent the above-described procedures for ambulatory suture chin augmentation in the author's clinic and abroad, between 1993 and 2012. Patients were followed up between 2 and 11 years and have reported excellent clinical success. No complications have been observed. There has been no aesthetic disappointment, no seromas, no haematomas and no infection. The soft tissue enhancement has been observed to be an average of 8.0 mm (range 4.1 to 11.8 mm). No asymmetry has been observed. On the contrary, this particular technique has been used to solve problems with asymmetry of the face. The author frequently leaves a bit of dimpling at the lower submental perforation area that defines the lower chin line better and enhances the Caucasian appearance that is very much appreciated by patients. Straight line of the profile has been obtained satisfactorily. Sometimes, additional 2-3 mm of chin prominence are required. In order to reach a straight profile line, a second suture enhancement has been done in 21 cases and in one case of pronounced retrogenia and small amount of soft tissue, the enhancement was done in 3 steps.

The obtained chin projection enhances the "beauty triangle" of the "chin and checkbone complex". The neckline becomes more slender and youthful. These visual criteria measure the degree of success in fashioning of chin aesthetics. We now believe that by using this soft tissue suture technique, with the exception of extreme cases, it is possible to satisfy the above-mentioned criteria in most patients.

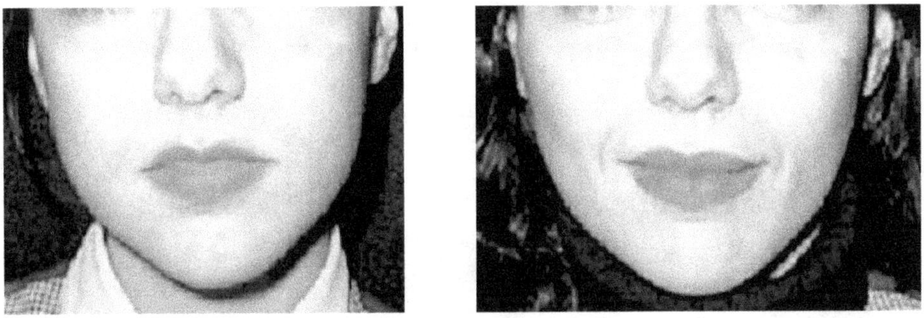

A. B.

Figure 15. **A.** Before and **B.** after chin correction and enhancement along with lower face ultrasonic liposculpture to obtain the beauty triangle of chin and cheekbones. The additional upper lip augmentation is a part of the face proportion adjustment and beautification.

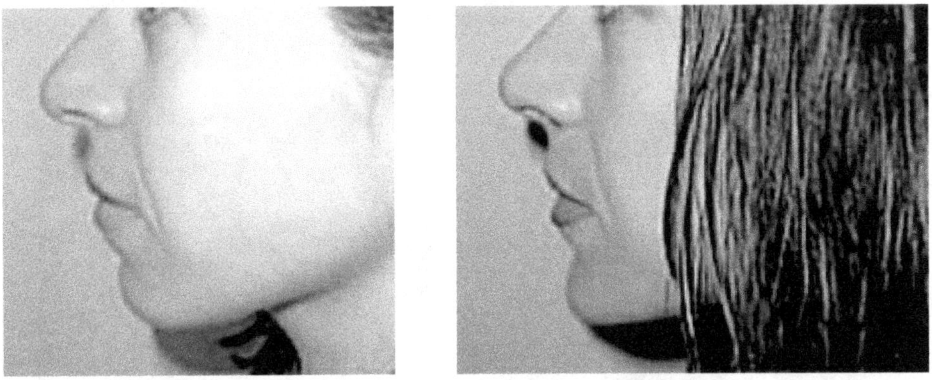

A. B.

Figure 16. **A.** Before and **B.** after chin enhancement to obtain straight line of the profile and define the jaw line, and good proportions with 3 equal parts of the face. Simultaneous rhinoplasty – T-excision and columella sliding for nasal tip rotation and projection.

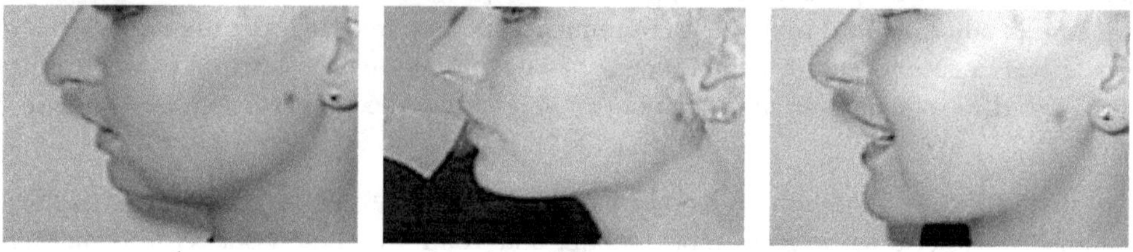

A. B. C.

Figure 17. A. Before, **B.** immediately after chin enhancement and tip rhinoplasty (T-excision and columella sliding) to obtain a straight profile and aesthetic proportions of the face (intra-op Betadine desinfection still not washed off). A slender neckline, due to skin lift forward (when moving the submental skin perforation point A in front of the menton) is obtained and is recognized as an attractive feature of youth with this method. **C.** 5 years later. It is difficult to find any change in the operated chin position during the 5 year follow up.

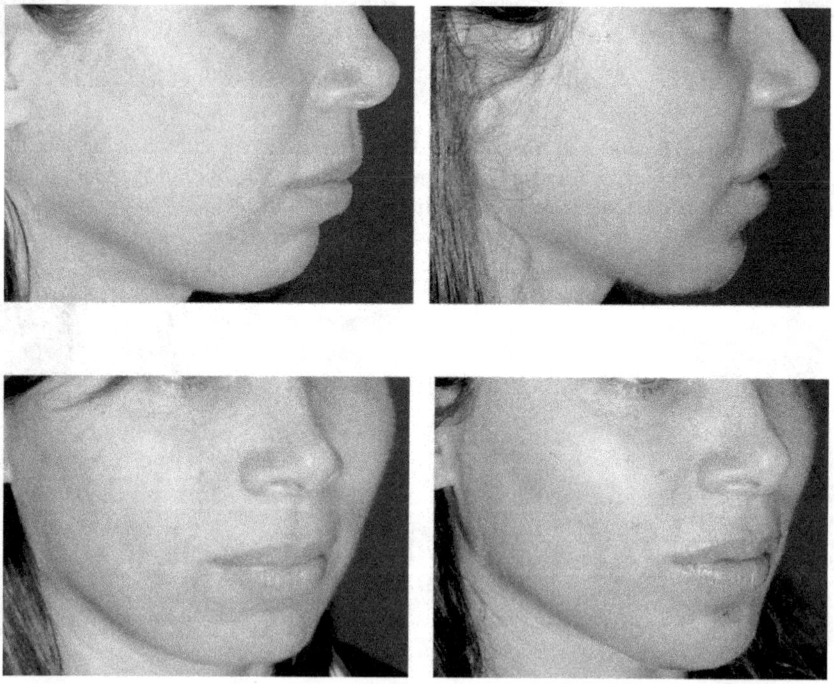

Figure 18. Better chin position is visible from all angles

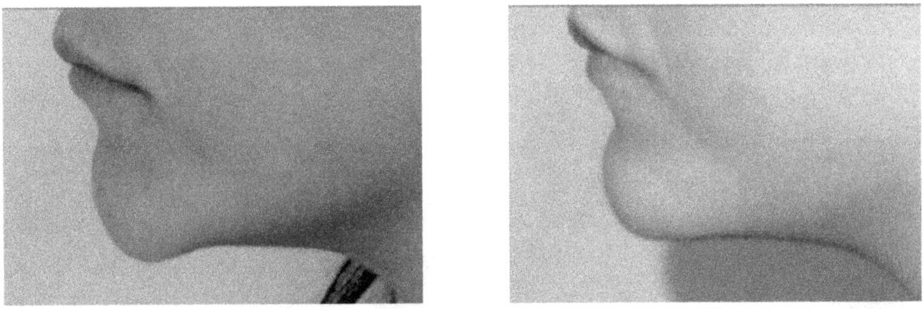

A. B.

Figure 19. **A.** Before – A witch chin in a young patient. **B.** After chin enhancement in front, suturing the tissue higher.

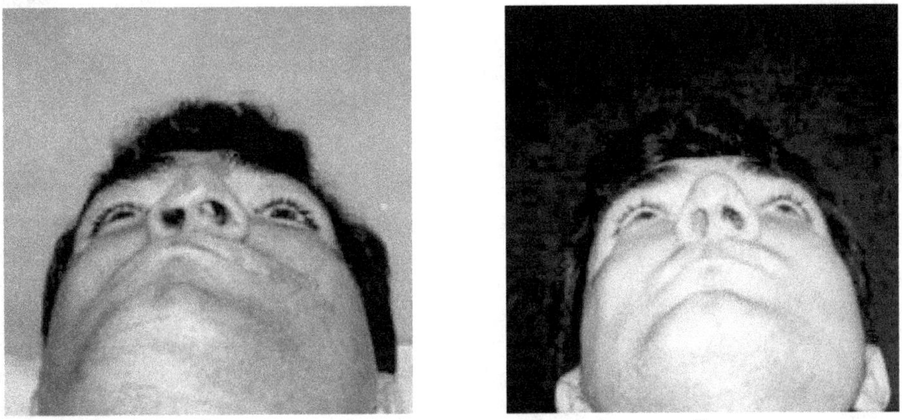

A. B.

Figure 20. **A.** Before (Betadine disinfected) and **B.** After correction of the chin position and nose deformity in one session. The chin is sutured to the left.

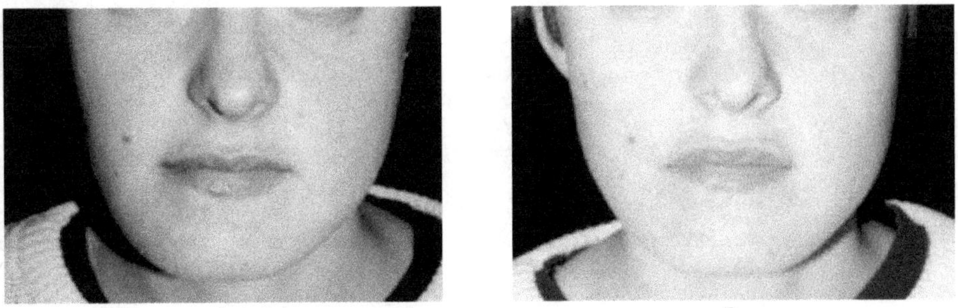

A. B.

Figure 21. **A** Before, **B.** After chin suture to the left to correct the deformity of the face.

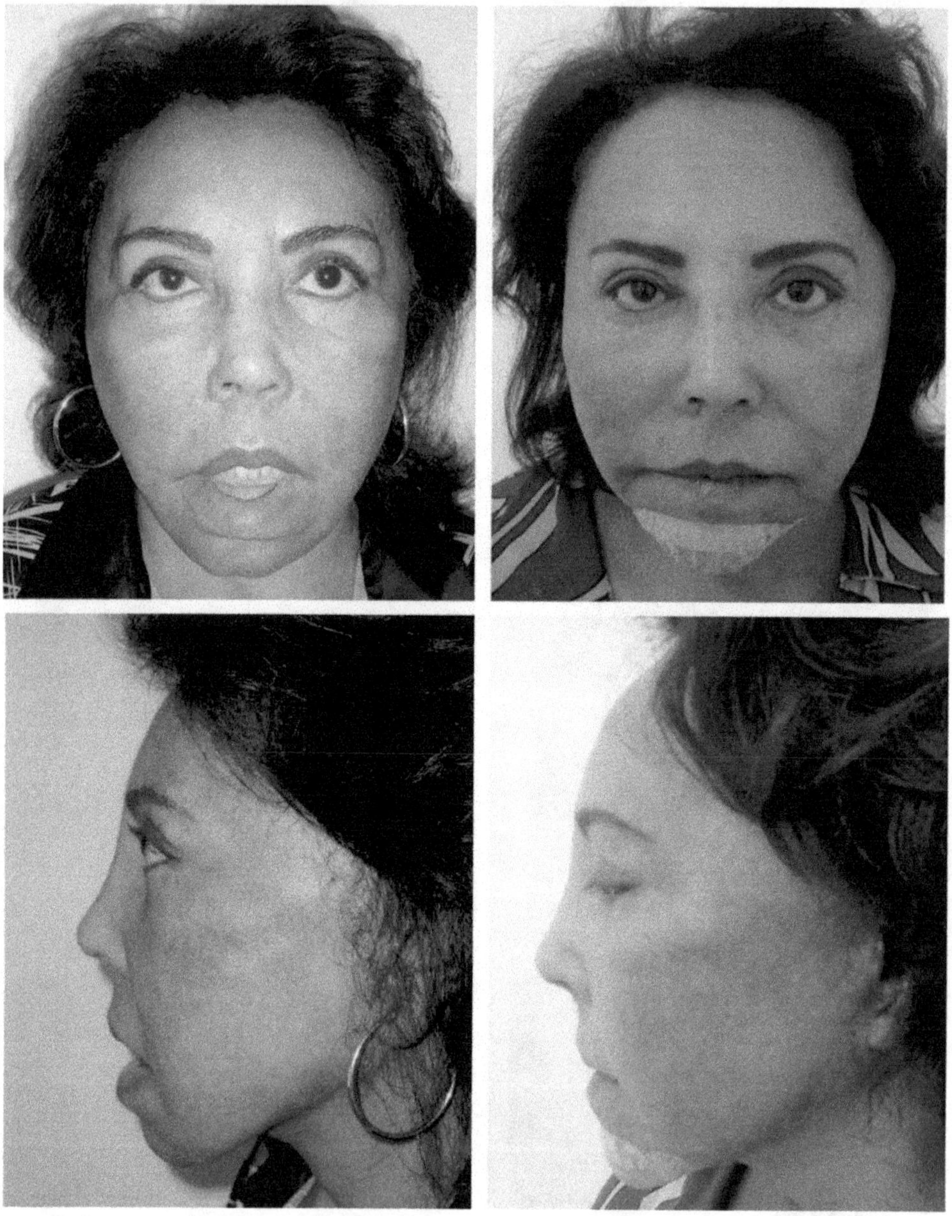

A. B.

Figure 22. **A.** Too much plastic surgery. Hanging chin/lower lip complex after removal of infected chin implant. **B.** Immediately after fixation of the chin fibrotic tissue to periosteum by suture.

The longevity of any technique depends on the stage and progression of aging, i.e. atrophy of the soft tissue and skeleton. The author has had a satisfactory longevity of results in his patients and secondary chin enhancement after years was necessary only in 5 cases. Using serial photography during the follow up period he has not noticed remarkable changes in the result.

The chin soft tissue suture technique for anterior adjustment and form correction provides a soft, natural facial appearance and it continues to be the method of choice for form correction, augmentation and beautification of the chin. All patients have rejected implantation techniques.

3.5. Chin dimple

Dimple formation is easy and consists of dermis fixation to periosteum by Serdev Suture® scarless closed approach. In such case, 2 points at the 2 ends of the dimple are used to capture the dermis between them. For this reason, the author may or may not use additional perforation points. It depends on what the patient wants – a dimple solely or with additional chin enhancement, and/or chin form correction.

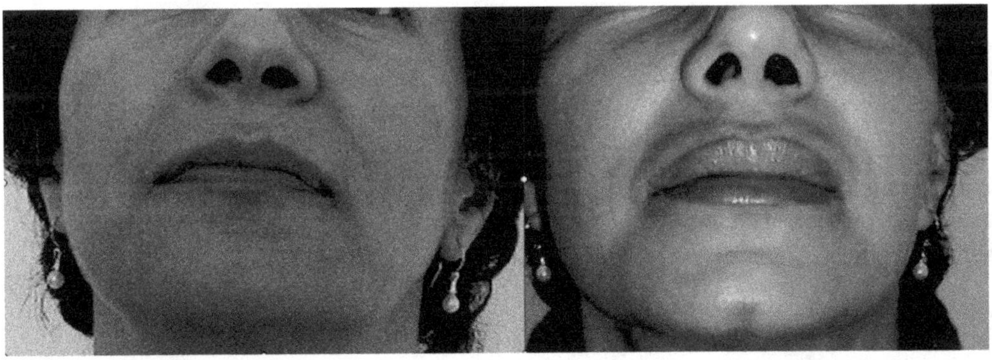

A. B.

Figure 23. Immediate result after scarless chin dimple formation by suture.

3.6. Discussion

For the past several decades, various materials have been developed to improve the appearance of the chin as one of the important subunits of the face. Initially, autogenous tissue grafts, such as: removed nasal hump, described by Aufricht in 1934, autogenous skeletal and cartilage transplants, ear cartilage grafts, rib cartilage grafts, fat, fascia, tendon, bone and dermal fat grafts have been used. Additional options became available with the development of a variety of alloplastic materials for augmentation genioplasty. Polymers are used primarily for bone deficiency substitution. Mersilene mesh introduced in 1950, silicone and silicone bag-gel inplants, Gore-Tex, Medpor, Supramid, Silastic, injectable collagen, expanded polytetrafluoroethylene (e-PTFE), high-density polyethylene (HDPE), polydimethylsiloxane (PDMS), Proplast I (PI), Proplast II (PII), porous block hydroxyapatite (PBHA) are available for correction of microgenia. Placed through an anterior oral sulcus incision or a submental incision with a screw fixation, many of these implants have good organotrophic characteristics, allowing tissue ingrowth. Available in a variety of block, sheet, and preformed shapes, they can be easily modeled and maintained. Antibiotics, irrigation, and closure of the incisions are performed. A lot of absorbable injectable materials came into the market in the last decade. Reviews of biomaterials used for mandibular implantation prove that although today's armamentarium of implant materials is vast, the search for the perfect implant continues.

Risks and complications with foreign materials: We address general considerations of toxicity relevant to all biomaterials. Investigations and overviews present data from a large number of clinical series on incidence of complications for materials used in this specific application. Although few, there are results that show infection, displacement, temporary paresthesias, incidences of absorption, rejection, or extrusion, implant migration, etc. Complications are manageable: these include implant displacement, infection has been treated with irrigation, closed system suction, etc. Most often infection requires a re-operation to remove the implant. Other complications such as internal and external soft tissue erosion, indentation, slippage, asymmetry and late bone resorption under the implant have been seen. Wound repair around implants is achieved through capsule formation. Fibrous capsule formation can be interrupted by infection, immune reaction, implant migration, or extrusion. No implant can be perfect for every face.

Due to the search of simpler techniques and based on his own experience, the author proposes an operation without implants, using only a suture of the chin soft tissue, suitable for chin enhancement, beautification and form correction. The author followed up 527 patients with chin augmentation and chin form correction for 2 and more years of whom no one had a complication. 398 of them had combined face beautification operations done.

As a single procedure or simultaneously with other facial rejuvenation operations, the chin suture of the soft tissue is ideally suited for correction of most chin aesthetic disharmonies in patients with a congenitally small mandible, patients requesting facial beautification and rejuvenation as well as correction of asymmetry. Simplicity and immediate return to social life are the major benefits of this procedure. It provides a natural, "non-operated-on" look that is largely sought after by patients today.

As implants are foreign bodies with some limits of longevity, they are mostly not accepted in the author's selection of patients and his technique became a method of choice, minimizing the tissue trauma. It appears to be an attractive alternative to other chin augmentation techniques.

4. Total face beautification using Serdev Sutures®

Beautification is the main goal in cosmetic surgery. Both words "cosmetic" in Latin and "aesthetic" in Greek language mean "beautification". Cosmetic and aesthetic surgery are wrongly understood as rejuvenation, anti aging, restoration, reconstruction etc., if no beautification is obtained.

It has been found that certain points in a face composition automatically attract the observer's attention. Many objects and scenes with certain proportions please us automatically.

4.1. Aesthetic proportions

Aesthetics as a science has been first established in ancient Greece and is based on aesthetic proportions, angles and volumes. Those aesthetic rules are intransient and are a persistent base for the understanding of beauty in all ethnic groups and cultures. It is studied in "History of Art".

In face aesthetics, the main proportion guidelines are given by **the Golden Section Rule** – the face is divided into 3 equal parts. Ancient Greeks have found that distance between columns has to be equal, to give an aesthetic perspective from different points of view. Leonardo da Vinci investigated the principle that underlies our notions of beauty and harmony and called it the Golden Section. Long before Leonardo, Babylonian, Egyptian, and ancient Greek masters also applied the Golden Section proportion in architecture and art.

Another golden rule is **the Golden Ratio** of 1.6 (1.6180339887…) that is an important rule in human body and extremity proportions. It is attracting our attention so much that credit cards have been created using the golden ratio.

4.1.1. Aesthetic angles

As face ptosis affects the lateral face, angles should be positioned higher (laterally) to create the beauty of youth, corresponding to the mask of comedy in ancient theatre, unlike the mask of tragedy. So, the lifting effect on face should be lateral.

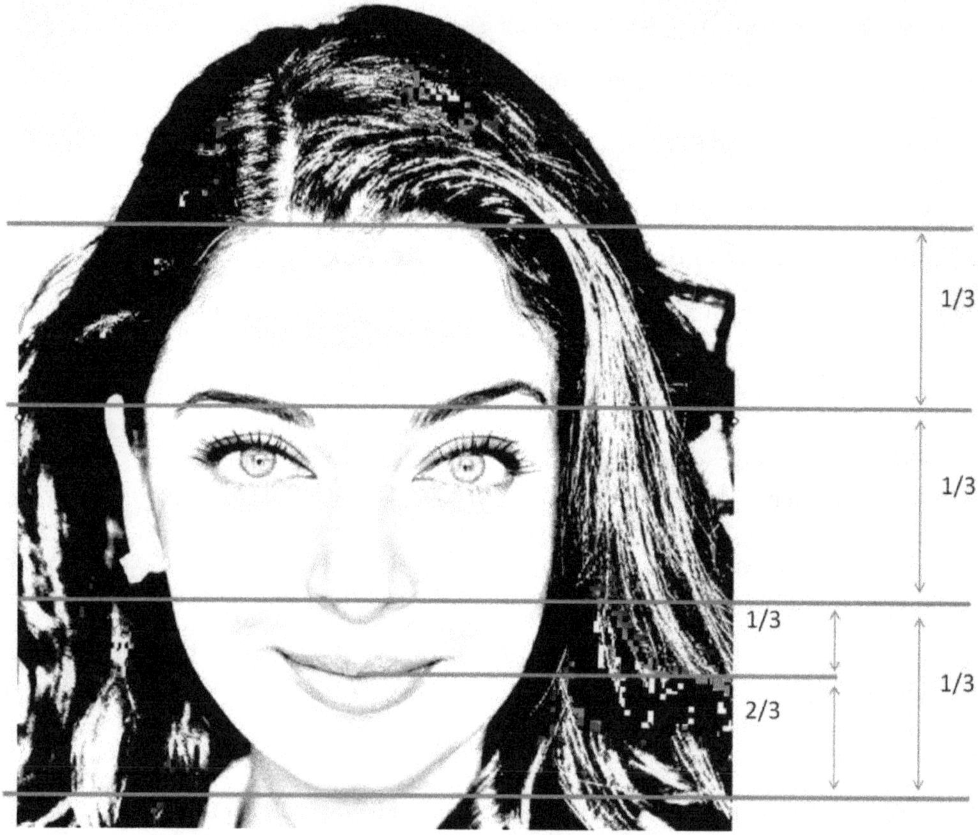

Figure 24. The Golden Section Rule permits precise examination of the face and its proportions

4.1.2. Aesthetic volumes

In the face, the "beauty triangle" visualizes apparent chin and cheekbones. Higher cheekbones represent youth.

The straight profile line is a noble sign.

As people look each other in the eyes when communicating, our first goal is to open and give light to the eyes and never modify them into an "operated-on" appearance.

Considering patient faces we can recognize unaesthetic signs. Following aesthetic rules, regardless of age, we can add beauty to a face.

The main goal of Serdev Sutures® is to create the appropriate aesthetic proportions, volumes and angles in face and body.

4.2. Some clinical cases

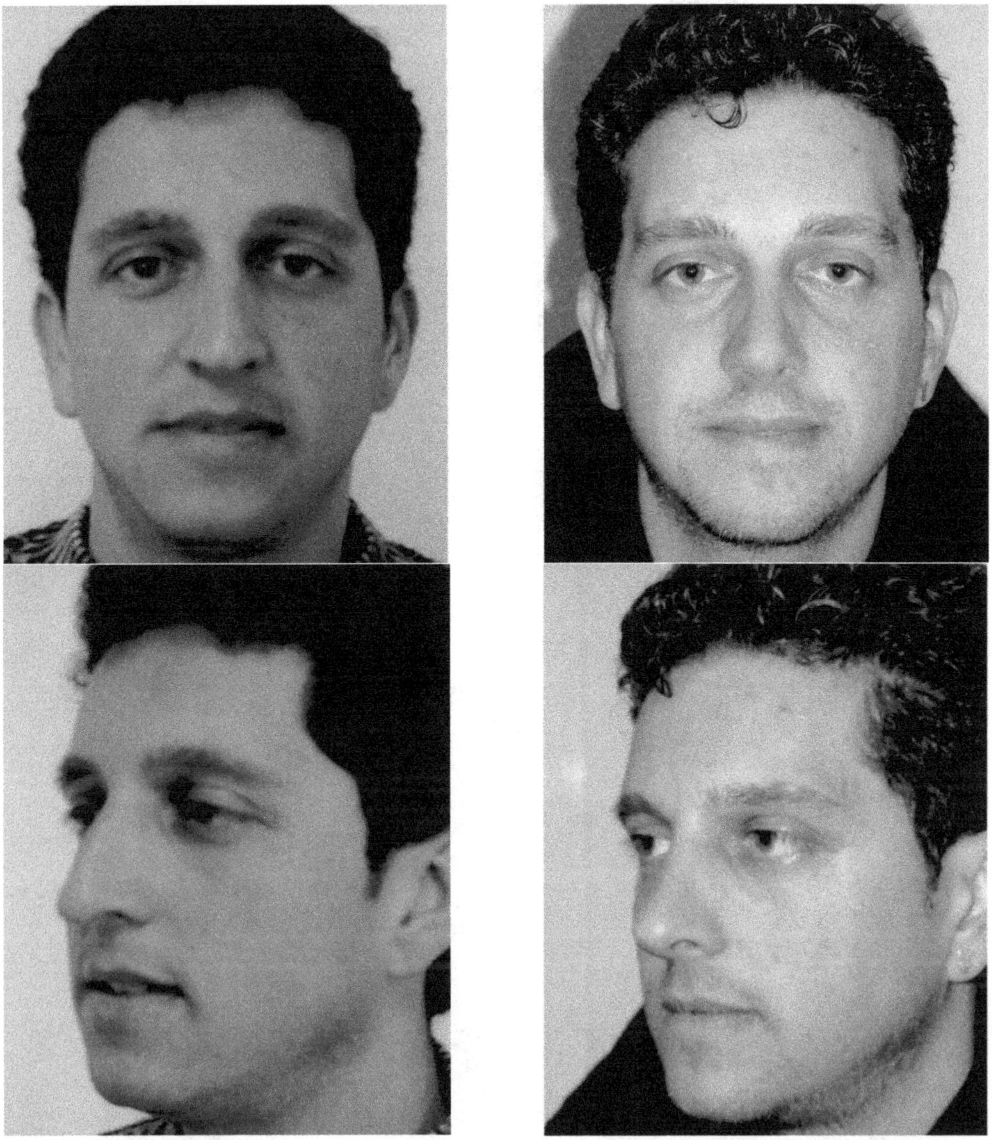

A. B.

Figure 25. A. Before: Low eyebrows give darkness to the eyes; unaesthetic proportions – the Golden Section Rule of the face is not present; nobleness is not present - retrograde chin, profile line is not straight. The proportion ratio in the lower third of the face is 1:3 instead of 1:2. **B.** After: Brow lift to open the eyes. Their color is finally visible; Rhinoplasty to create the 3 equal thirds (golden section rule), chin enhancement to create more visible beauty triangle (in men, the cheekbones should not look "sweet"), straight profile and proper lower face third ratio of 1:2. The result is **total face beautification**. "Playboy" ear pendant serves to demonstrate patient's self-confidence after surgery.

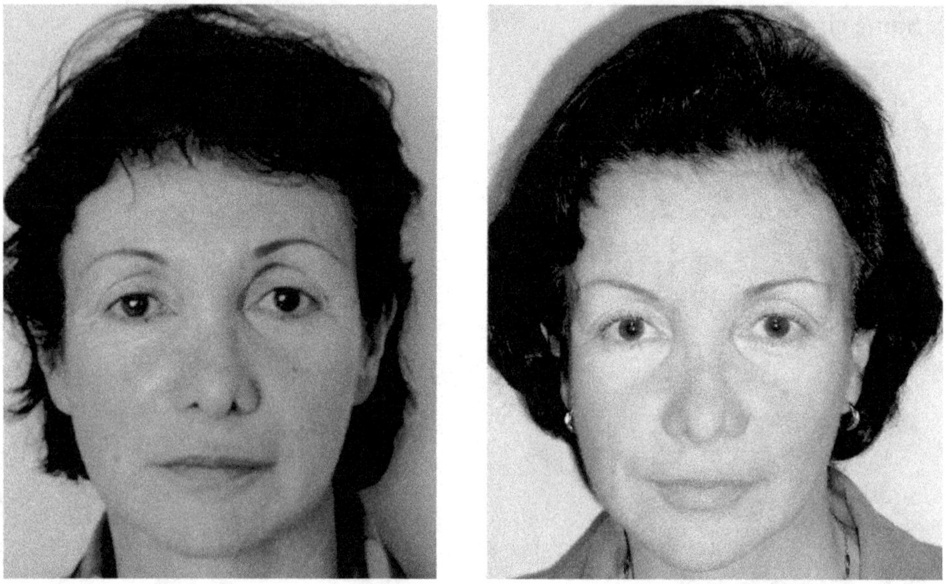

A. B.

Figure 26. **A.** Before: Brow ptosis, hollow eyes, gradual facial ptosis. Sad appearance. **B.** After Temporal and Brow Serdev Suture® lifts: eyes and face are full of light. See the color of the eyes. The Golden Section Rule is apparent. The lower face is changed from heavy and square into fresh and oval.

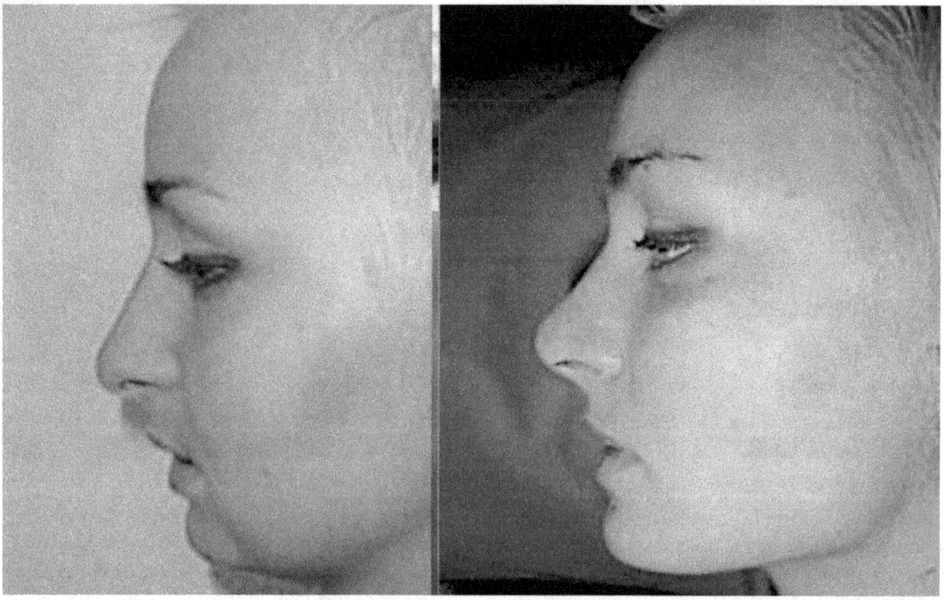

A. B.

Figure 27. **A.** Before. Nice young lady, but with longer nose, small chin; disrupted golden section rule, lower face proportion and the line of straight profile. **B.** Immediate beautification results in the operating theater after temporal lift by suture to lift the facial angles laterally and repositioning the cheekbone soft tissue; rhinoplasty to obtain the 3 equal parts of the face (golden section rule) - author's T-excision for tip rotation and columella sliding for tip projection, and chin enhancement to obtain the straight profile, beauty triangle and proper proportion ratio 1:2 in the lower third of the face. Suturing the chin in front has defined the jaw line. Skin still not cleaned from the Braunol. No operated-on appearance, immediately after 3 operations (including 2 suture lifts).

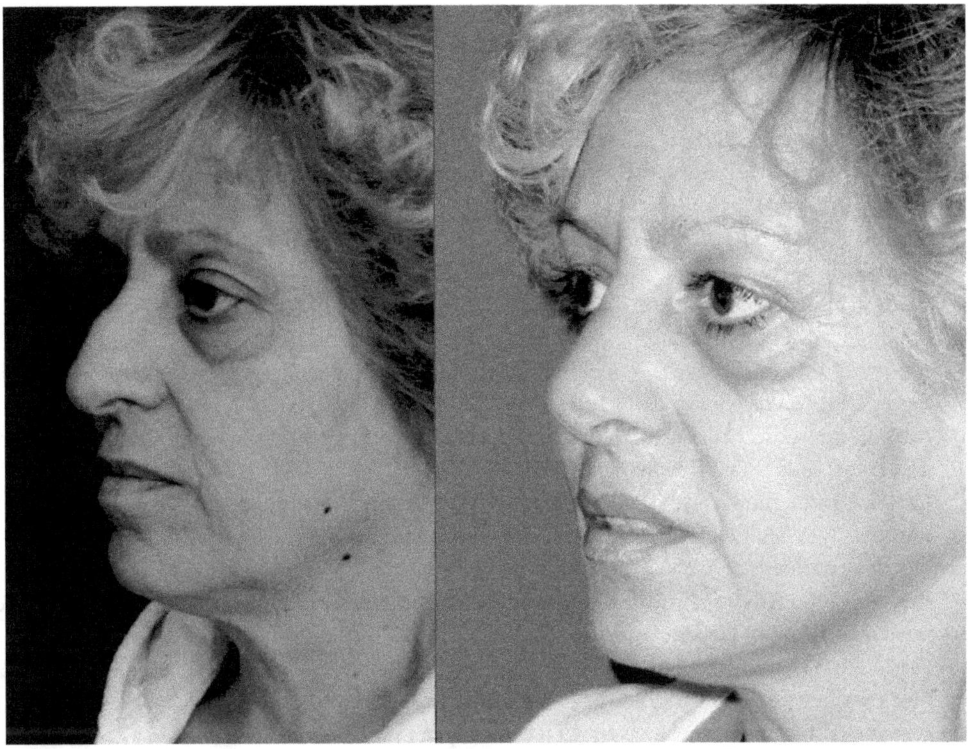

A. B.

Figure 28. **A.** Before: aging face, disproportions and lack of aesthetics in all proportions, volumes and angles. **B.** After scarless closed approach suture Brow, Temporal, Mid-face, Lower face and neck lift, Chin enhancement and Rhinoplasty. Fresh No operated-on appearance and open eye look, sparkling radiation, proper proportions are present, straight profile, angles lifted laterally, volumes, beauty triangle, defined jaw line and cervico-mandibular angle are present. Better skin texture. Blepharoplasty and cheekbone lift could be added, if and when patient decides.

5. Conclusion

In a way, cosmetic surgery as a multidisciplinary science is a fine art, inherently combining knowledge of architecture, sculpture, painting, design, fashion and even poetry. Scarless closed approach Serdev Suture® lifts, suspensions and tissue volumizing serve to create beauty on the basis of a proper understanding of anatomy, aesthetics as a science, ideal proportions, angles and volumes.

Author details

Nikolay Serdev
New Bulgarian University, Sofia, Bulgaria

6. References

[1] Serdev, N.P. Year 1994, Suture Suspensions For Lifting Or Volume Augmentation In Face And Body (English version), presented at the 2nd Annual Meeing of the National Bulgarian Society for Aesthetic Surgery and Aesthetic Medicine, Sofia, 18 March 1994, Int J Aesth Cosm, 2001,1:1, 2561-2568

[2] Serdev NP. Serdev Suture Techniques Lower SMAS Face Lift, Original Papers, Int J Cosm Surg, 2009, 9:4, 1 - 2

[3] Serdev NP.Ambulatory temporal SMAS lift using minimal hidden incisions. IJACBS, 1(2):17-24, 2001.

[4] Serdev NP. Serdev Suture Techniques Lower SMAS Face Lift (Bulgarian), Original Papers, Int J Cosm Surg, 2009, 9:4, 1-12

[5] Serdev NP. SERDEV SUTURE TECHNIQUES - Lower SMAS Face LIFT, Original Papers, Int J Cosm Surg, 2010, 10:1, 1-2

[6] Mitz V, Peyronie M. The superficial musculo-aponeurotic system (SMAS) in the parotid and cheek area. Plast Reconstr Surg 58: 80-88, 1976.

[7] Jost G, Lamouche G. SMAS in rhytidectomy. Aesthetic Plast Surg 2: 69-74, 1982

[8] Larabee WF, Makielski KH, Cupp C. Facelift anatomy. Facial Plastic Surgery Clinics of North America 1(2): 135-52, 1993.

[9] Brennan HG. Rhytidectomy: Mandibular and submandibular contouring. Facial Plastic Surgery Clinics of North America 1(2): 181-96, 1993.

[10] Kridell RWH, Covello LV. The aging face (rhytidectomy). In BJ Bailey (ed.): Head & Neck Surgery – Otolaryngology, 2nd edition. Lippincott – Raven, 1998, pp. 2693-716.

[11] Berman WE. Rhytidectomy. In CJ Krause (ed.) Aesthetic Facial Surgery. Lippincott, 1991, pp 513-31.

[12] Dedo DD. The aging neck. In BJ Bailey (ed.): Head & Neck Surgery – Otolaryngology, 2nd edition. Lippincott – Raven, 1998, pp. 2717-32.

[13] Baker DC, Conley J. Avoiding facial nerve injuries in rhytidectomy. Anatomical variations and pitfalls. Plast Reconstr Surg 6: 781-95, 1979

[14] Seckel BR. Facial Danger Zones: Avoiding Nerve Injury in Facial Plastic Surgery. Quality Medical Publishing, St. Louis, 1994.

[15] Webster RC, Smith RC, Papsidero MJ, et al. Comparison of SMAS plication with SMAS imbrication in face lifting. Laryngoscope 92: 901-12, 1982.

[16] Lewis JR. Multiple-tiered deep support of cheeks in meloplasty and rhytidectomy. Aesthetic Plast Surg 1: 21-5, 1983

[17] Owsley JQ. SMAS-platysma facelift. A bidirectional cervicofacial rhytidectomy. Clin Plast Surg 3: 429-401, 1983

[18] Randall P,Skiles MS. The "SMAS sling": an additional fixation in face lift surgery. Ann Plast Surg 1:5-9, 1984
[19] Webster RC, Smith RC, Smith KF. Face lift, Part 4: Use of superficial musculoaponeurotic system suspending sutures. Head Neck Surg 3: 780-91,1984
[20] McCoullough EG, Perkins SW, Langsdon PR. SASMAS suspension rhytidectomy. Arch Otolaryngol Head Neck Surg 115: 228-34, 1989.
[21] Hamra ST. The deep-plane rhytidectomy. Plast Reconstr Surg 86: 53-61, 1990.
[22] Hamra ST. Composite rhytidectomy. Plast Reconstr Surg 90:1-13, 1992.
[23] Ramirez OM. The subperiosteal rhytidectomy: The third-generation facelift. Ann Plast Surg 28: 218-232, 1992.
[24] Beeson WH. Extended posterior rhytidectomy. Facial Plastic Surgery Clinics of North America 1(2): 197-216, 1993.
[25] Serdev, N.P. Chin form correction and augmentation using simple suture. Int J Aesth Cosm Beauty Surg IJACBS 2001, 3 (1), 42-66
[26] Serdev, N.P. Chin Form Correction And Augmentation Using A Simple Suture, Presentations, Int J Cosm Surg, 2003, 3:3, 1-36
[27] Serdev, N.P. Chin Enhancement And Form Correction Using A Suture Of The Soft Tissue, Original Papers, Int J Cosm Surg, 2002, 2:1, 1-10
[28] Serdev, N.P. Chin augmentation using simple suture. Int J Cosm Surg 2001, 2 (1) 42-66
[29] Mottura AA. Chin augmentation with nasal osteocartilaginous graft. Plast Reconstr Surg 2002 Feb;109(2):783-7
[30] Karras SC, Wolford LM. Augmentation genioplasty with hard tissue replacement implants. J Oral Maxillofac Surg. 1998 May;56(5):549-52
[31] Cox AJ 3rd, Wang TD. Skeletal implants in aesthetic facial surgery. Facial Plast Surg 1999;15(1):3-12
[32] Hwang K. Chin augmentation with a bone graft from the mandibular region. J Craniofac Surg 2000 Nov;11(6):543-6
[33] Ramirez OM. Mandibular matrix implant system: a method to restore skeletal support to the lower face. Plast Reconstr Surg 2000 Jul;106(1):176-89
[34] Gubisch W, Kotzur A. Our experience with silicone in rhinomentoplasty. Aesthetic Plast Surg 1998 Jul-Aug;22(4):237-44
[35] Snyder GB, Courtiss EH, Kaye BM, Gradinger GP.A new chin implant for microgenia. Plast Reconstr Surg 1978 Jun;61(6):854-61
[36] Schoenrock LD, Chernoff WG. Subcutaneous implantation of Gore-Tex for facial reconstruction. Otolaryngol Clin North Am 1995 Apr;28(2):325-40
[37] Lewis RP, Schweitzer J, Odum BC, Lara WC, Edlich RF, Gampper TJ. Sheets, 3-D strands, trimensional (3-D) shapes, and sutures of either reinforced or nonreinforced expanded polytetrafluoroethylene for facial soft-tissue suspension, augmentation, and reconstruction. J Long Term Eff Med Implants 1998;8(1):19-42
[38] Singh S, Baker JL Jr. Use of expanded polytetrafluoroethylene in aesthetic surgery of the face. Clin Plast Surg 2000 Oct;27(4):579-93
[39] Gross EJ, Hamilton MM, Ackermann K, Perkins SW. Mersilene mesh chin augmentation. A 14-year experience. Arch Facial Plast Surg 1999 Jul-Sep;1(3):183-9

[40] Sclaroff A, Williams C. Augmentation genioplasty: when bone is not enough. Am J Otolaryngol 1992 Mar-Apr;13(2):105-8

[41] Kheir JN, Leslie LF, Fulmer NL, Edlich RF, Gampper TJ. Polydimethylsiloxane for augmentation of the chin, malar, and nasal bones. J Long Term Eff Med Implants 1998;8(1):55-67

[42] Yaremchuk MJ. Mandibular augmentation. Plast Reconstr Surg 2000 Sep;106(3):697-706

[43] Odum BC, Bussard GM, Lewis RP, Lara WC, Edlich RF, Gampper TJ. High-density porous polyethylene for facial bone augmentation. J Long Term Eff Med Implants 1998;8(1):3-17

[44] Dann JJ, Epker BN. Proplast genioplasty: a retrospective study with treatment recommendations. Angle Orthod 1977 Jul;47(3):173-85

[45] Qian Y, Fan Z, Yang Q. Application of MEDPOR surgical implant in the craniofacial reconstruction Zhongguo Xiu Fu Chong Jian Wai Ke Za Zhi 1998 Mar;12(2):71-3

[46] Jafar M, Younger RA. Screw fixation mentoplasty. J Otolaryngol 2000 Oct;29(5):274-8

[47] Rubin JP, Yaremchuk MJ. Complications and toxicities of implantable biomaterials used in facial reconstructive and aesthetic surgery: a comprehensive review of the literature. Plast Reconstr Surg 1997 Oct;100(5):1336-53

[48] Robinson M, Shuken R. Bone resorption under plastic chin implants. J Oral Surg 1969 Feb;27(2):116-8

[49] Maas CS, Merwin GE, Wilson J, Frey MD, Maves MD. Comparison of biomaterials for facial bone augmentation. 1: Arch Otolaryngol Head Neck Surg 1990 May;116(5):551-6

[50] Sclafani AP, Romo T 3rd. Collagen, human collagen, and fat: the search for a three-dimensional soft tissue filler. Facial Plast Surg 2001 Feb;17(1):79-85

[51] Constantinides MS, Galli SK, Miller PJ, Adamson PA. Malar, submalar, and midfacial implants. Facial Plast Surg 2000;16(1):35-44

[52] Moenning JE, Wolford LM. Chin augmentation with various alloplastic materials: a comparative study. Int J Adult Orthodon Orthognath Surg 1989;4(3):175-87

[53] Romo T 3rd, Baskin JZ, Sclafani AP. Augmentation of the cheeks, chin and pre-jowl sulcus, and nasolabial folds. Facial Plast Surg 2001 Feb;17(1):67-78

[54] Jones RH. The effects of zygomatic and chin augmentation on facial aesthetics. Ann R Australas Coll Dent Surg 1998 Oct; 14:114-8

Chapter 4

Serdev Sutures® Lifts in Body Areas

Nikolay Serdev

Additional information is available at the end of the chapter

http://dx.doi.org/10.5772/55672

1. Introduction

Excisional body lift operations are traumatic surgical procedures that result in significant scarring.

The scarless transcutaneous closed approach Serdev Suture® method in buttock lift, breast lift, abdominal flaccidity lift was first presented in 1994 as a scarless alternative to the classic excision lifts, such as circumscisional body lifts, mammoplasty, abdominoplasty (tummy tuck) and others as part of the total understanding for the scarless closed approach suture lifting method. The concept is to lift stable mobile fascias to immobile tissues such as periosteum, immobile fascia, or tendons. This is achieved by a closed approach suture lift, using special instruments – curved semi-elastic Serdev® needles and semi-elastic surgical sutures, distinguished by an extended period of delayed absorption (2-3 years).

The Serdev Suture® buttock lift presents a scarless surgical procedure for the treatment of the flaccid, flat and "unhappy buttock" form by a closed approach, without any requirement for incision and excision scars. The outcome is a visual change in buttock projection, roundness, tightness and elevation into a higher position. The buttock lift elongates the lower limbs and changes the proportions of the body. The aim is to obtain a beautification of the buttock form by creating a circumferential lifting effect on the buttock's subcutaneous tissue without scars. This is obtained by the use of a suture that takes hold of the inferiorly positioned deep fibrous tissue, elevating and fixing it to the "sacro-cutaneous" fascia (discovered by the author). This fascia fixes the overlying skin to the lateral lines of the sacrum and suspends the weight of the buttocks.

In scarless suture breast lift, the mobile breast glandular tissue and its fascia are lifted and fixed to the stable immobile anterior clavicle periosteum, or to the insertion of the pectoralis major tendon to humerus.

The Serdev Suture® method allows for an atraumatic and scarless lift of the inner thigh dermis to the tendon insertion of the gracilis muscle.

The Serdev Suture® lift can be used in selected cases of thin patients to obtain a scarless and atraumatic tightening of the abdominal skin. This suture method for abdominal flaccidity lift is achieved by a closed approach suture as well, with skin perforations alone in the abdominal skin to capture, suture and lift the mobile superficial fascias supporting the abdominal skin. To obtain outcome longevity it is important to lift and stretch the firm mobile fascias, fixing them to immobile firm tissue, such as costal periosteum and/or perichondrium, periosteum of spina iliaca superior anterior.

A stable improvement was observed in all patients. In the post-operative period, the complication rate was minimal and below 0.1%. All early comlications were resolved in the first 4-5 post-operative days. All other professional duties, social activities or obligations were possible in the next one or two days. These outpatient procedures are effective in the correction of laxity and ptosis. They also create a new form, along with improved body proportions that has been universally accepted as beautification beside rejuvenation.

2. Buttock lift

As more people seek body contour surgery, we should use our expanding knowledge and surgical experience to create new, non-scarring surgical procedures for beautification in areas like the buttocks. Former results of body contour surgery have been less than satisfying. A very small number of techniques are available for correction of the form and aesthetics of the buttocks. This is especially so for lax, ptotic and non-projected buttocks. Scarless methods are preferred and demanded by virtually all patients.

Classic methods are combinations of liposuction, lipoinjections, implants for augmentation and lipectomy. The outpatient buttock lift procedure by suture can satisfy patients' requirements for beautification of the buttock form and position without scars and foreign bodies. The post-operative period is both rapid and easily tolerated, while the outcome is durable and long lasting.

2.1. Anatomy

The well accepted gluteal position is the location of the gluteus maximus muscle. The muscle-sceletal framework is usually well formed. Unfortunately, female structure usually includes an inferiorly positioned fatty tissue deposit, elongating the female buttocks in the inferior perspective. Long and hanging buttocks are visible even from a frontal view (Fig. 1) and shorten the length of female lower limbs. The hanging buttocks soft tissue is well recognised as "unhappy buttocks" as distinct from the high gluteal position, known as "happy buttocks".

2.2. FIXATION of mobile to immobile tissue

The only useful mobile tissue for suture lift is the very fibrotic buttocks soft tissue. **NB!** Gluteus muscles and gluteus fascia cannot be lifted.

The only immobile structure to which the suture can be fixed, in order to produce buttock lifting and secure the buttock weight, is the Serdev "sacro-cutaneous" fascia (discovered by the author) which fixes the skin to the lateral edges of the sacrum, located between the "dimples of Venus" at the sacro-iliac points and the upper point of the intra-gluteal fold, located at the sacro-coccigeal point. **NB!** Sacro-coccigeal fascia is not useful for fixation. Any attempt to attach the buttocks weight to the sacro-coccigeal fascia can provoke an "ischiadic" pain.

The gluteal fatty tissue is very fibrotic. The fibrotic tissue represents a flexible support for the soft framework of the body. It forms a stable network for subdermal and deep fat layers. We use this stable fibrotic buttock soft tissue structure in order to elevate it securely by fixation to the Serdev fascia on each side.

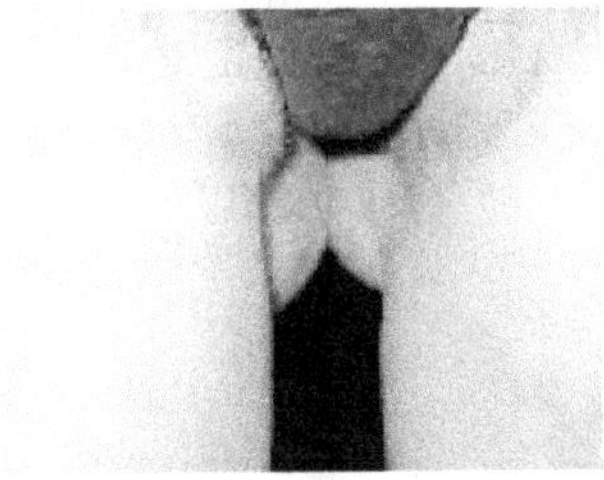

A.

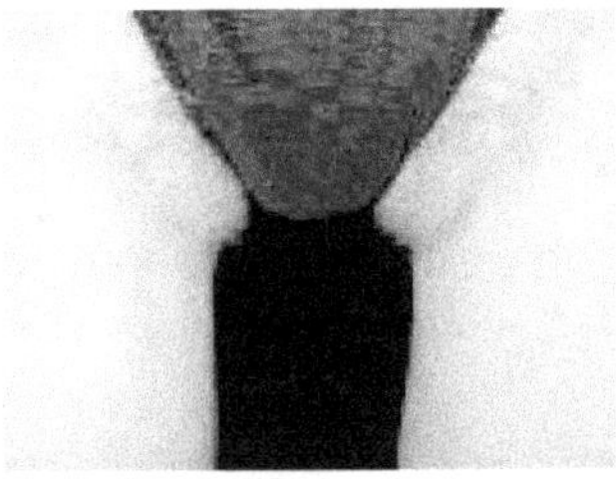

B.

Figure 1. **A.** "Unhappy", sagging, loose buttock soft tissue, drooping between the thighs, engenders disappointment in women, inclining them to request buttock lifting. **B.** "Happy buttocks" - the outcomes of lifting the hanging buttocks are visually elongated legs and more aesthetic body proportions.

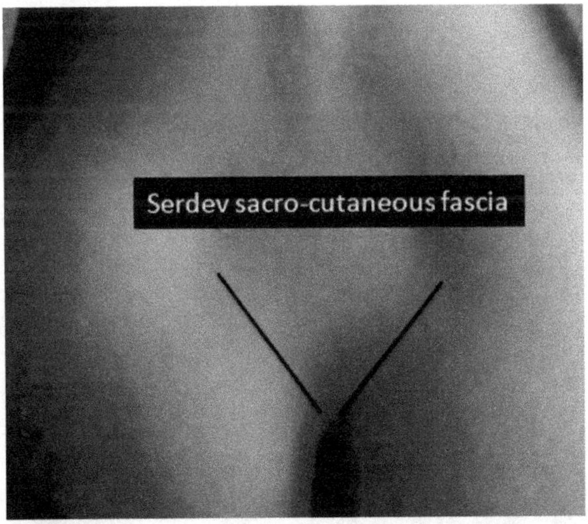

Figure 2. The Serdev "sacro-cutaneous" fascia fixes the skin to lateral edges of the sacrum in the lower part of the "rhombus of Michaelis". It is located on each side, between the "dimples of Venus" and the upper point of the intra-gluteal fold, i.e. between the sacro-iliac points and the sacro-coccigeal point.

2.3. Method

Indications: Beautification, aesthetic proportions, lifting of ptosis, elongation of the lower limbs, shortening of the body length in proportion to the legs.

The primary indication for buttock lift surgery by suture is the moderate to severe soft-tissue laxity in the lower trunk, with minimal or mild residual fat deposits. In patients with significant fat deposits, the author initially treats with UAL/VASER to reduce the volume and heaviness of the buttock fat tissue. Then, the reduced weight of the buttocks soft tissue can be lifted and fixed to the Serdev fascia in order to ensure a safe post-operative healing process.

The buttock lift by suture was created for aesthetic purposes, with the intention of creating a higher and more attractively rounded and projected buttocks, while at the same time creating a visible elongation of the legs and a change of the correlation between the body and the length of the lower limbs. True buttock sculpting demands a three-dimensional artistic appreciation of the anatomic and surgical adipose layers of the central trunk. This is essential in preventing complications from the buttock lifting, where the fixation is done without damaging neurovascular structures.

2.4. The technique

Author's surgical technique consists of a fixation of the complete buttock soft tissue fibrotic system to the Serdev sacro-cutaneous fascia on each side. The suture technique uses the specially designed Serdev® needles from 170 mm to 250 mm, and Polycon USP 4, 6 or 8, depending on the degree of tissue volume and heaviness.

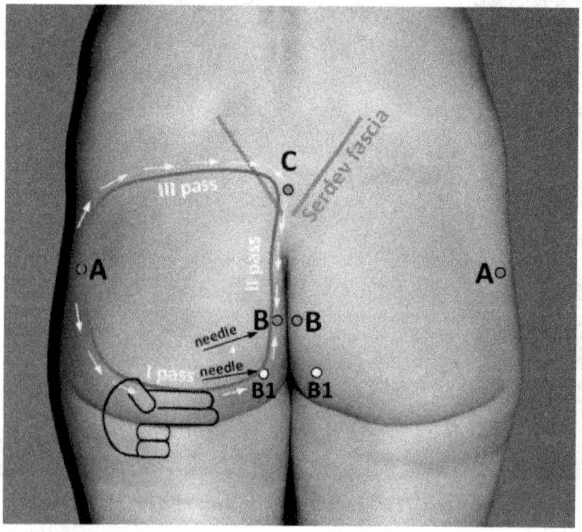

A.

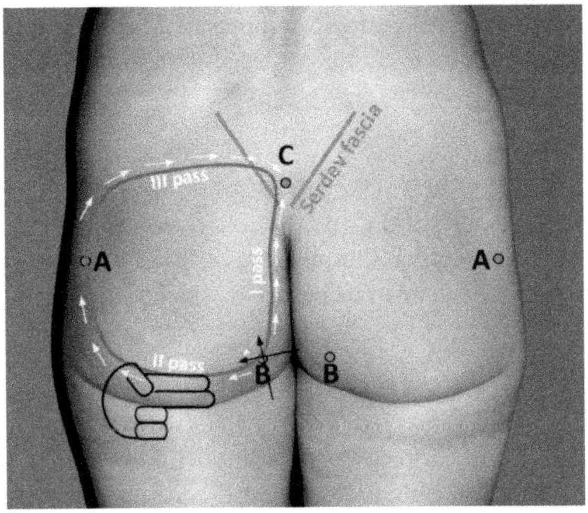

B.

Figure 3. "Serdev fascia" is marked in red color. It is perpendicular to skin and sacrum and the suture with buttocks' heaviness will hang on it. Arrows show the direction of needle passes. A minimum of three passes is necessary to complete the fixation of the buttock fibrotic soft tissue system to Serdev fascia, which realizes a lift, roundness, projection and stable fixation of the mobile lower buttock to the immobile Serdev fascia. 2 methods are presented:
A. The first pass is from A to B1, then the direction of the needle is changed toward B, but higher than the anus (B1 is only an orientation, not a skin perforation point). The suture is introduced into A-B. Then, the needle is introduced in the second pass (C-B), in order to be threaded at B. Next, the second end of the suture is taken at A and fulfills the circle of the suture at C (third pass – C-A) to be tightened and knotted on Serdev fascia. If no dermis is attached to the suture, all dimples at the perforation points are easy to remove.
B. Sometimes it is easier for beginners to perform 2 passes at once - to start from B to C and introduce the suture from C in direction to B, then change the direction of the needle tip towards A, without exiting the superficial fascia at B. This maneuver prevents beginners from dimpling at point B. After introducing the suture in lines C-B-A, the third pass C-A introduces the thread in line A-C and fulfils the suture circle at point C. The suture will be tightened and knotted at C. Dimpling at a perforation point has to be removed.

The author prefers the first step for fixation of the subdermal fibrotic tissue to be initiated from the lateral aspect of the buttock. Selection of the type of surgical suture is the surgeon's responsibility. However, the elastic tightening of the Polycon suture provides a stable support with a short elasticity, when lifting the buttock into a higher position and fixing it to the stable sacro-cutaneous fascia. The suture collects the buttock's fibroic tissue and its trabecular system into a superficially convex "bouquet". This roundness is moved superiorly and fixed to the Serdev sacro-cutaneous fascia. The fixation of the suture to the stable inelastic fascia maximally ensures the longevity of the aesthetic effect. The semi-elastic quality of the antimicrobial polycaproamide suture Polycon (as preferred by the author) reduces the possibility of trauma and decubiti of the fibrotic tissue and reduces complications.

The buttock lift by suture requires 10 to 15 minutes of operating time per side, no blood transfusions, no stay at the clinic, no nursing care and no more than a day or two absence from work.

2.5. Directions

Mark skin perforation points A, B and C (B1 should be only marked, not perforated, it is an orientation point). Point A should be located laterally, at the midpoint of each buttock, near the place where the trochanter can be palpated. This ensures equal distance to points B and C.

2.6. Tips and tricks

- Perforation point B could be located above the anus (preferable because of hygienic reasons) or below, and somewhat lateral from anus, in order to secure point B from contamination.
- If skin perforation point B is planned higher than the anus, an imaginary point B1 should be taken into consideration and when arriving from point A, deep under point B1, the needle direction should be changed to B as shown in Fig. 3.A.
- If perforation point B is planned below the anus, the superficial fascia at that point B should be perforated very well and the perforation must be widened to avoid fixation with the needle and introduction into the suture. Otherwise, its attachment to the suture will produce dimpling.
- Point C should be between both Serdev fascias, inside of the triangle of the sacral region. This will ensure that the passes C-B and C-A on both sides will cross the Serdev fascia from below and above, and the suture will be fixed to the Serdev fascia. Serdev fascia is perpendicular to the skin and sacral edges and the weight of the suture will be suspended on it.
- Perforation of sacrococcigeal fascia and fixation of the suture on it produces ischiadic pain and should be avoided!
- Do not fix the gluteus fascia or gluteus muscle to the suture. Both are immobile and will not permit lifting.
- Perform an oval, circular suture, in order to place equal tension to all points. Do not perform triangles or Z sutures. Higher tension in the angles will cut through the tissue and will not permit longevity of the lift.

After anesthetic infiltration intradermally and deep in points A, (B1), B and C, and deep in the soft tissue along the marked suture circle, make small perforation at points A, B and C. Then, open the perforations and deep subdermal fat in perpendicular fashion with a mosquito clamp. Take sterile needle caps from 18-guage needle, cut part of the closed needle cap tip. Insert these plastic cannulas in twisting perpendicular fashion, maximum deep into perforation points A, B and C, in order for the suture to stay deep in the fat fibrotic tissue (near but above the gluteus fascia) and away from dermis and subdermal fibrotic tissue. This maneuver prevents dimpling.

2.7. Technique

Video: http://www.youtube.com/watch?v=mn0O2bNkG7o

First Pass - A-B: It should be deep in the soft tissue, 2 fingers higher than the infragluteal fold (see Fig. 3) in order to stretch and flatten it when the buttock is lifted:

Variant A (Fig. 3. A)

- **First pass - A-B:** Introduce a long Serdev® needle 170mm or 230mm from point A to point B1, deep in the soft fibrotic fat tissue. **NB!** The Serdev Suture® circle should be located deep, just above the gluteus maximus fascia. Be sure not to be too superficial as it will cause skin/tissue dimpling on the path of the needle. If so, twist the needle backwards to free the superficial tissue and proceed deeper. Stay near, but above the gluteus fascia, which will block your needle if perforated. Arriving deep at B1, turn the needle toward B, as shown in Fig. 3A. Find the deeply positioned opening of the plastic cannula and go out through the plastic hub. Load the needle at point B with a thread USP 4, 6 or 8 (depending on buttocks size) and pull through. The surgical sutures will be located deep in the soft tissue, in the mobile line B-A. **NB!** The deeply introduced plastic cannulas prevent from engaging dermis and fibrotic tissue in the suture (prevent from dimple formation).
- **Second pass - C-B:** Proceed from point C to B, deep in the fat tissue, 1-2cm away from the intra-gluteal fold (without superficial skin/tissue dimpling). **NB!** If dimpling appears, the needle is too superficially located. Proceed deeper, without perforating the sacrococcigeal fascia (pain!). Find and exit through the plastic hub at point B and load the needle. Pull through from B to C. In this way, the suture has crossed the Serdev fascia medially.
- **Third pass has two options: A-C or C-A:**
  - **Pass A-C:** Load the needle at point A. From A, proceed to C - deep subdermally (without superficial dimpling), and cross laterally through the upper part of Serdev fascia. Perforate the Serdev fascia near the upper pole and exit at point C through the plastic hub. Unload the needle at C and pull back the empty needle through point A. The suture circle is finalized and both ends of the suture are located at C. Remove cannulae, tighten and knot. Remove dimpling at perforation points. **NB!** If you want to tie the knot at point A, proceed with empty needle from A to C and load needle at C. Introduce the suture at C-A. Then you will have both ends at A. Tightening and knotting the suture at A is somehow difficult for beginners. Most doctors prefer to knot at C.
  - **If pass C-A is selected:** From C, proceed to A, load the needle at A and unload it at C. Both ends of the suture will be located at C. Remove cannulas, tighten and knot at C. Remove dimpling.

Tie the suture as closely as possible to medium tension. In this way, the whole buttock tissue will be collected and projected like a "bouquet" by the suture and fixed higher to the Serdev fascia. Pull out all dimpling at points A, B and C, using a mosquito clamp.

NB! Do not perform suture triangles ABC. The higher pressure in the angles will cut the tissue and the suture will become loose. The circle of the suture should be round to apply equal pressure at each point and minimize trauma of the tissue.

The close proximity of the wounds to the anus area makes antibiotic prophylaxis and strict hygiene obligatory.

2.8. Warnings

1. Do not perforate gluteal fascia or muscle. They cannot be lifted.
2. Do not perforate the sacrococcigeal fascia or periosteum at point C – this causes ischiadic pain.
3. Make a circular suture to obtain equal pressure around all points. Do not perform triangle sutures - tension on the angles will cut the tissue and produce pain.

2.9. Author's experience

More than a thousand buttock lifts have been performed by the author in the last 19 years, both in his clinic and during live surgery workshops around the world. Patients ranged in age from 18 to 62 years. The author reports his experience with patients followed up for up to 10 years.

2.10. Combined methods

63% of the patients had moderate lower trunk and lower limb cellulite and fat deposits, which required additional ultrasonic liposculpture of the lower body and limbs. In patients who have had buttock lift in combination with ultrasonic assisted liposculpture, UAL was performed to reduce the volume and to sculpture the buttocks and other areas for total leg or body beautification. Additional positive qualities of UAL are skin tightening and weight loss. When using UAL for buttock sculpturing, the goal is to minimize fat deposits, buttock's weight and to obtain a nicely rounded and higher positioned buttocks (over the gluteus maximus muscle).

2.11. Results

The buttock lift by suture requires 10 to 15 minutes of operating time per side, there is no blood loss or transfusions, no stay at the clinic, no nursing care and not more than a day or two absence from work.

The cosmetic results were evaluated with pre-operative and post-operative photographs and by patient satisfaction. No patient was dissatisfied with the results and all of them considered their results as excellent or very good.

2.12. Risks and complications

Risks are: higher pressure on one tissue being different from the tension in other areas and points; contamination - skin perforation point B near the anus area.

- Higher pressure should be prevented, by performing a circle – a round form suture that equalizes pressure in all points and prevents from tension and trauma of the tissue.
- Infection can be prevented with better selection of point B and antibiotic prophylaxis. The Bulgarian surgical sutures are antimicrobial, semi-elastic and are preferred by the author.

In all his cases, the author has observed only one patient with a painful hardness in point B, near the infra-gluteal fold and four other cases with a local infection in one of the wounds. The cause for the first complication was the rigid nylon suture that was used in this first patient. Rigidity, hardness and inelasticity caused a tissue decubitus in the point of tension on the soft tissue. This complication has since then been avoided by changing the suture material to the semi-elastic Bulgarian antimicrobial Polycon suture. In all other cases, the local infection was easily treated in a matter of days. Infections are very rare, occurring mainly at the skin perforation points and are easily treated. No hematoma or nerve damage have been observed. Pain is limited to the first 1-2 weeks in sitting position. In limited cases, when the pain goes away, patients forget the advices to gradually commence physical activities. In these few cases, abnormal friction and trauma can cause pain that is usually on one side. Palpation along the suture gives information about presence or absence of infiltration and location of the pain. It is usually near a perforation point.

In very rare cases, the skin perforation point was opened and some seroma or blood drops have been evacuated with the disappearance of the pain. If there is no infiltration around the suture, slowing down activities, non-steroid anti-inflammatory drugs and pain killers are enough. Antibiotic can be added if considered necessary.

2.13. Clinical cases

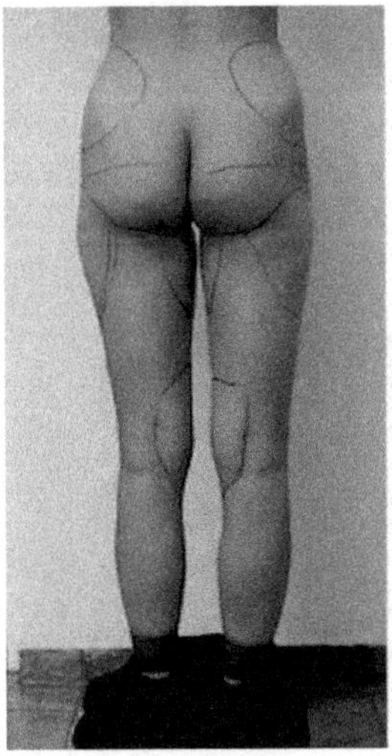

A.

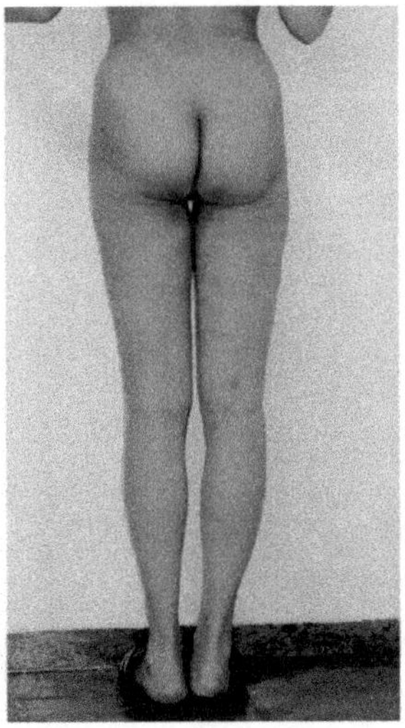

B.

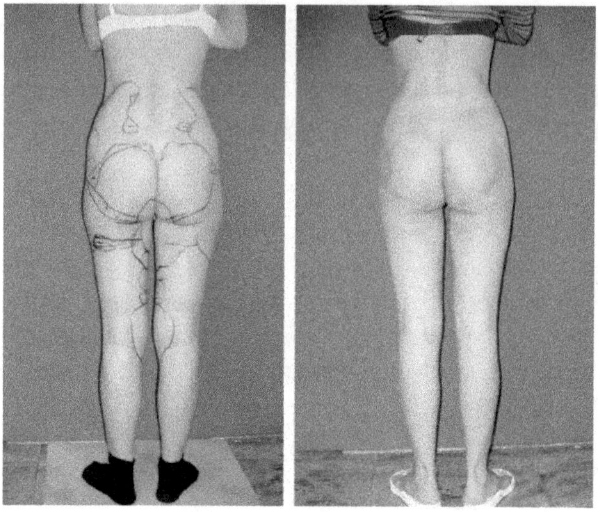

C. D.

Figure 4. **A., C.** Before UAL and Buttock lift. **B., D.** Day one after ultrasonic liposculpturing of lower extremities, buttocks and flanks and simultaneous Buttock lift by Serdev Suture®. Pre-operative drawings are still visible. Very rare bruising verifies that surgery has been atraumatic. Tight, higher buttocks, straight and elongated legs, correct proportions.

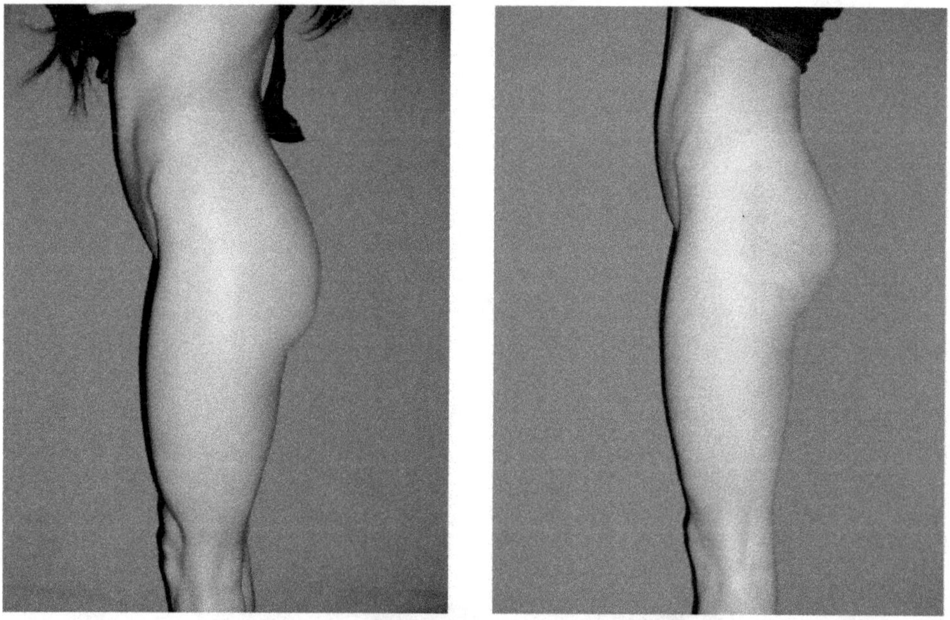

A. B.

Figure 5. **A.** Before, **B.** Result after a buttock lift by suture in a dancer. Elongation of the legs. Better projection and higher buttocks are visible even in anterior half-profile position. No incision scars.

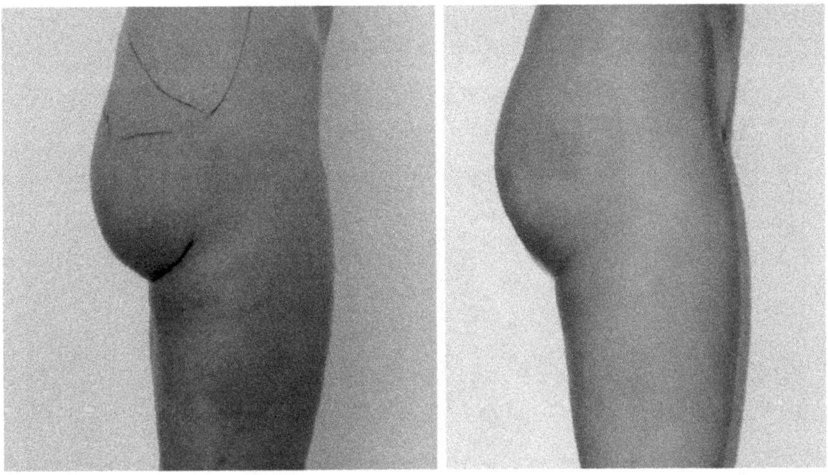

A. B.

Figure 6. **A.** Before, **B.** Result after a buttock lift by suture. Elongation of the legs. Better projection and higher buttocks.

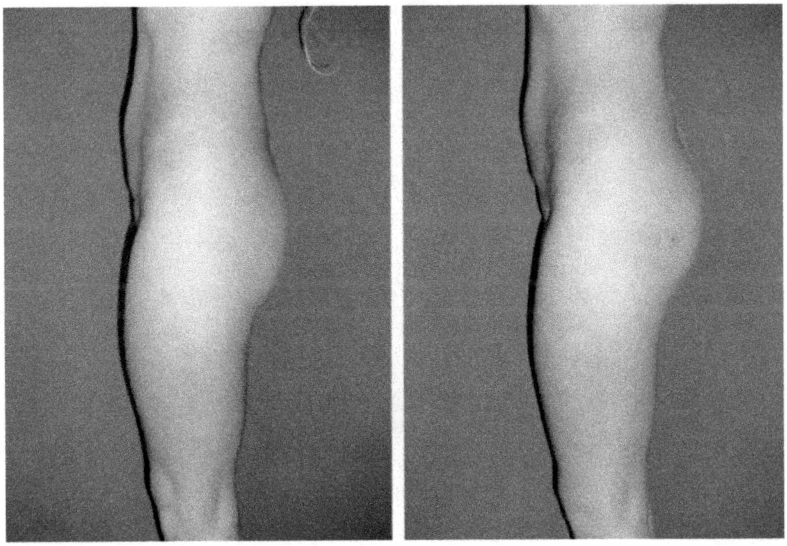

A. B.

Figure 7. **A.** Before and **B.** After buttock lift by Serdev Suture®. Visible elongation of the lower extremities and shortening of the trunk after buttock lift.

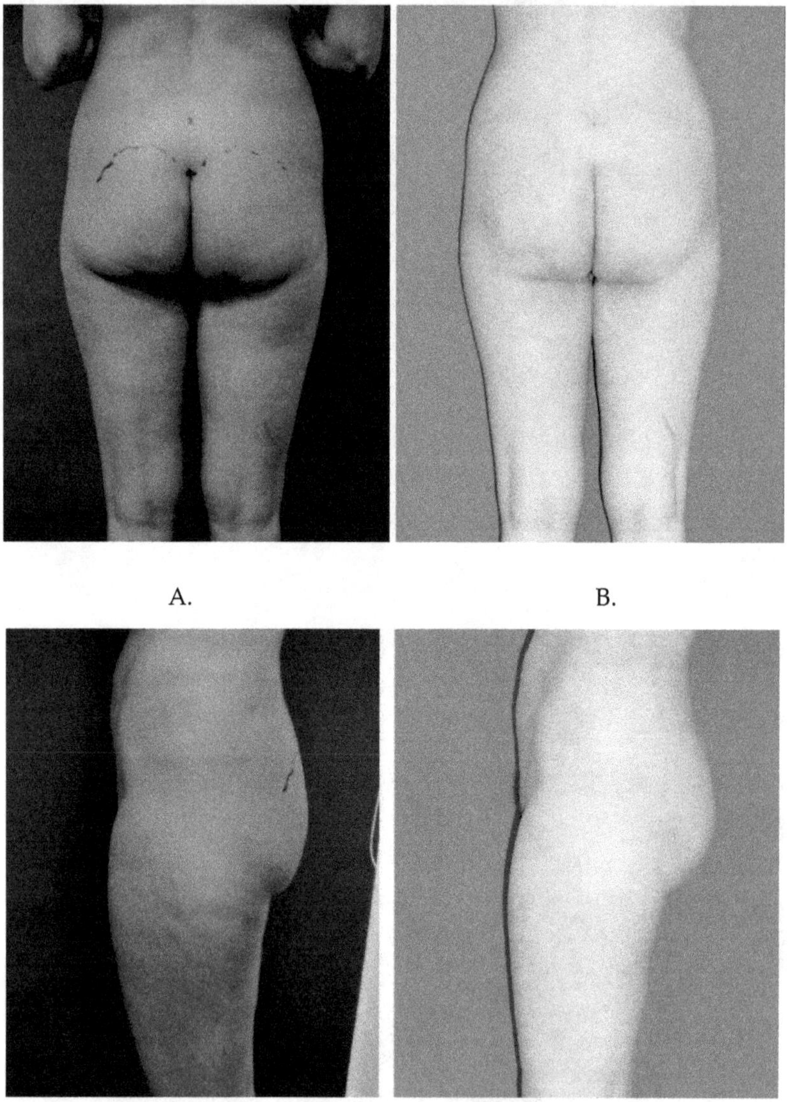

A. B.

C. D.

Figure 8. **A., C.** Before, **B., D.** Result after buttock lift by suture in a 62 y.o. patient. The buttocks are visibly lifted and a better-rounded form is obtained. There is improvement of the whole body shape.

2.14. Discussion

There is an increasing demand for surgical correction of the body contour in modern society. There is a limited number of operations that aim to correct non-aesthetic buttocks form as part of the total body contouring and proportions. The hips, thighs and the lower back frame the buttock contours. Ethnic differences in the shape and proportions of the buttocks create a variety of aesthetic perceptions in size and shape. However, high positioned "happy" buttocks and elongated legs have always been fashionable.

Flat and sagging buttocks are a common clinical condition. However, before the introduction of the suture butt lift, there was no proven aesthetic and effective therapeutic option at hand. Sole excision of skin cannot obtain a true lift of the heavy buttocks. Subcision is a surgical technique that has been used in treating advanced degree of cellulite. To treat excesses of fat and skin tissue in that area, liposuction and/or dermolipectomy have been mostly used. The indication for liposuction has been restricted to the conditions in which the overlying skin is capable to retract and adapt itself to the new contour. If excess skin is the cause of the deformity, a dermolipectomy has been mostly indicated.

2.15. Buttock augmentation, wrongly named "lifting"

Liposuction of the buttock area is infrequently mentioned in the literature and for some authors it is a forbidden zone. Two additional approaches in suction lipectomy of the buttock region are described: liposuction of the "banana" and liposuction of the "sensuous triangle". A common complication of liposuction of this area is ptosis of the buttocks. To improve buttock roundness, fat transplantation and different implants, including mammary ones, have been introduced. These procedures do not lift, but only augment buttocks. Free fat graft has been used to avoid the most common complications of doing a buttock augmentation with silicone prostheses and to find a better surgical procedure that is simpler, complementary with liposuction while better able to deal with body irregularities. Lately, excessive augmentations can be observed in Brazil and Latin America, which are not acceptable in Caucasian communities, where aesthetic proportions are important.

Furthermore, the suture lift is the best option for Afro-Americans and Asians, where there is a tendency to hypertrophic scarring.

3. Breast lift

3.1. Clavicular fixation

Video: http://www.youtube.com/watch?v=bHKA5HaiZs0

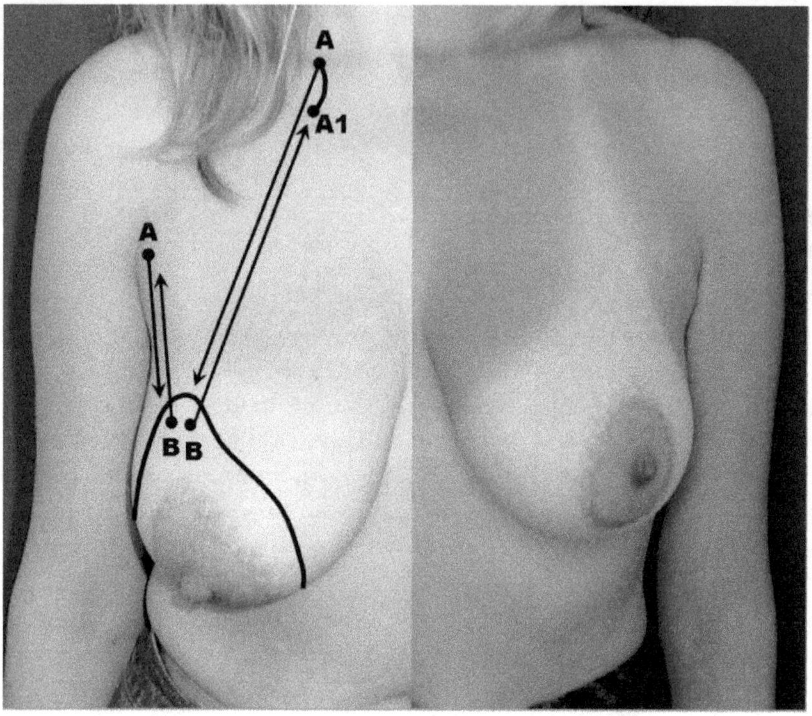

A B

Figure 9. **A.** Before breast lift to clavicle and to pectoralis tendon. **B.** Result – 14 cm lift of the nipple

NOTES:

- The circular line indicates the glandular tissue edges,
- Points A and A1 in clavicular fixation are at the upper and lower borders of the clavicle. Take anterior clavicular periosteum and never posterior.
- Arrows show the direction of the needle pass.
- In larger breasts a longer needle could be necessary and 2 sutures may be required.
- Using "Clavicular fixation", nipples can be raised as much as 14 cm or more. Due to the shorter distance between the pectoralis tendon A point and the upper glandular breast tissue B point, "Pectoralis tendon fixation" can be used for small lifts (suspensions) or for additional support to clavicular fixation in larger breasts.

DIRECTIONS:

a) Mark the borders of the breast glandular tissue. Select the breast fixation point B depending on the breast heaviness in the upper part of the glandular tissue.

b) Select the position for the clavicular fixation. It could be:

Central position

Place a plastic tape measure around the neck directed to the nipples and mark the lines. Measure and mark the distance "nipple to clavicle" on both sides.

Medial or Lateral – for medial or lateral nipple position

If requirements for more central or more lateral nipple position, select a more central or more lateral clavicular fixation point.

c) Local anesthesia in points A, A1, subperiosteally in A-A1, intradermally in point B and perpendicularly into the breast fascia, upper breast tissue and below, on the A-B line in deep subdermal fat layer.

d) Perforate points A, A1 and B using a No. 11 scalpel blade. Perforate the blunt subdermal fascia in points A, A1 and the breast glandular tissue fascia in point B using mosquito clamp.

Warning: If not perforated, the superficial fascias will be engaged in the suture, forming a dimpling effect on the surface

e) Clavicular Fixaction A-A1:

Pass an unloaded "mini mini" (50 mm) or "mini" (60 mm) Serdev® needle from point A to A1 under the anterior clavicle periosteum. Load the needle with a USP 4 or 6 surgical suture (depending on breast size) and introduce it under the anterior clavicle periosteum A-A1.

Warning: Do not pass dorsal to the clavicle (danger: subclavian a. and v., brachial plexus)

f) Take the upper breast glandular fascia and tissue at point B, using "medium" (140 mm) Serdev® needle. Proceed to point A1 in the deep subdermal fat. Feed the suture end into the Serdev® needle at point A1 and introduce it toward B.

Warning: Unwanted superficial needle pass forms dimpling on the skin surface. Try again a deeper pass to obtain a smooth surface over the needle.

Stay above the pectoralis fascia. If engaged, the pectoralis fascia will block the needle and the suture and then it will produce immobility of the suture.

g) Proceed with the needle from point A in deep subdermal tissue and then over the breast tissue to point B. Feed the second suture end into the needle from point B passing it into point A to accomplish the circle of the suture.

Warning: Do not perforate through dermis at the skin perforations, as this will result in a dimple. In the skin perforation points, pass the needle perpendicularly to the skin surface, without catching dermis (without resistance in front), by gently twisting the needle. Do not push - twist the needle gently forwards or backwards.

h) Tie at point A. Check for equality. After securing the knot, release any dimpling at points A, A1 and B with a hemostat.

Warning: Serdev Sutures® should not engage skin. Skin cannot hold or support the suspended tissue.

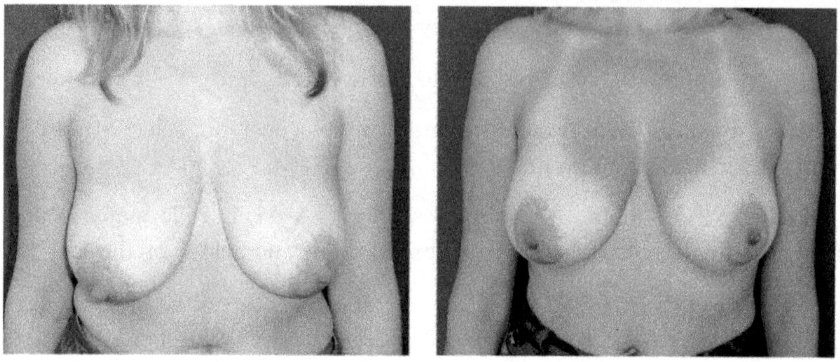

A B

Figure 10. **A.** Before, **B.** After a 14 cm breast lift by clavicular suture in large ptotic breasts. A second "step-by-step" breast lift by suture can be performed after months.

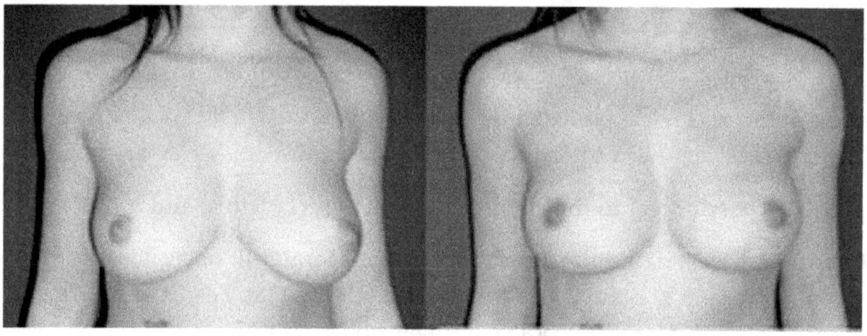

A B

Figure 11. Breast lift by suture to the clavicle in a young patient.

3.2. Pectoralis tendon fixation

DIRECTIONS:

a) Select the place of fixation to the pectoralis major tendon at its insertion to the axilla - Point A.

Note: In point A, the needle pass through the tendon should start from the dorsal side of the tendon to the front of it - Point A1. In other words - Point A should be posterior to the pectoralis tendon, near its insertion to the brachium.

b) Local anesthesia in point A1, through the tendon to Point A, intradermally in point B and perpendicularly into the breast fascia, upper breast tissue and below, and in the deep subdermal fat layer on the A-A1-B line.

c) Perforate points A and B, using a No. 11 scalpel blade. Perforate the subdermal fascia and breast fascia bluntly in point B, using a mosquito clamp.

Warning: If not perforated, the fascias will be engaged in the suture, forming a dimpling effect on the surface.

d) Using an unloaded "medium" (140 mm) Serdev® needle, pass from point A, through pectoralis major tendon to A1. Point A1 can be a skin perforation or not. If no skin perforation point A1 is selected, change the needle direction, passing deep in the subdermal fat layer. then under the upper breast tissue, then perpendicular up through breast tissue and skin perforation at point B. Thread needle with USP 4, or 6 suture. Pull through point A.

Note: If easier, perforate A1 and introduce a threaded "mini" or "mini mini" Serdev® needle in line A-A1. Then, using an unloaded "medium" needle proceed from point B through the upper breast fascia, upper breast tissue, and in the deep subdermal fat to point A1. Next, thread the needle at A1 and pull it through at point B.

e) With the unloaded needle, take a different plane in the subdermal fat in line A-B, exiting at point B **(do not grab the tendon and the glandular breast fascia with the second pass, but stay in deep subdermal fat tissue)** Load needle at point B and pull through at point A.

f) While pulling both suture ends at point A, release any dimpling seen at point A1 and B. Tie with medium tension at point A. After tying and securing the knot, release any dimpling with a hemostat at **point A, A1 and B.**

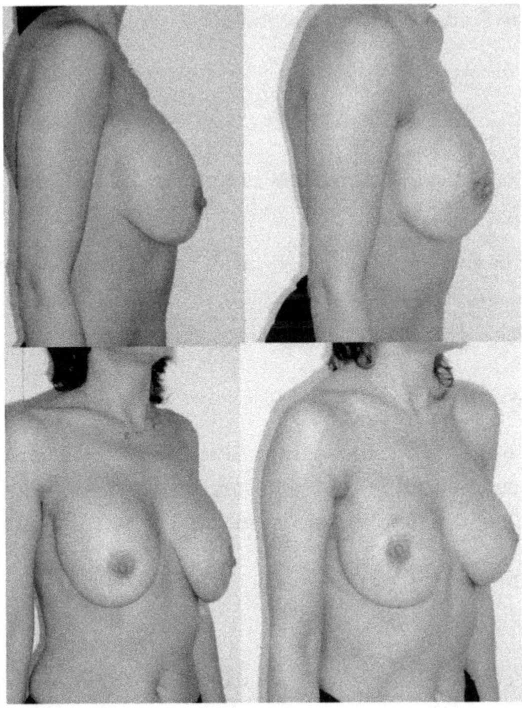

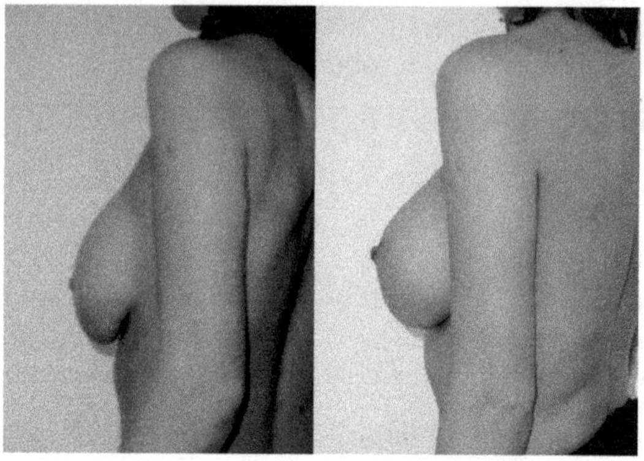

Figure 12. Before and after a breast lift with fixation to the pectoralis tendon. After subpectoral implants placement, the patient has given two births and after breast-feeding the breasts have dropped. Breast lift by suture solves the problem without additional surgery for bigger implant placement or excisional mastopexy.

4. Inner thigh lift

4.1. Introduction

Excisional thigh and buttock operations are traumatic surgical procedures that result in significant scarring. The Serdev Suture® method allows for an atraumatic and scarless lift of the inner thigh.

4.2. Anatomy

Inner thigh fat is attached to skin that loosens with time and descends with age, obesity and weight loss.

Between the major labia and the inner thigh fat deposit, there is about 3-5 cm skin that is free from any attached fat. The length of the fat-free skin depends on age, fat weight and skin laxity.

4.3. Surgical concept

The Serdev Suture® method is a stable suture fixation of movable to non-movable fibrous structures. The use of semi-elastic, absorbable surgical sutures is crucial, as they do not cut the target mobile tissue and when fibrosis is finalized (6 to 18 months) the sutures will be absorbed (in 2-3 years).

4.4. The procedure

The Dermis layer, precisely adjacent to the fat deposit, has to be sutured to the Gracilis tendon, near its insertion point at the Pubis (Fig. 13).

Position the patient so that the upper inner thigh is exposed (leg externally rotated). In this position the Gracilis muscle is the only visibly prominent muscle and tendon under the skin of the upper inner thigh. To identify the Gracilis tendon, palpate along the Gracilis muscle. The Gracilis tendon will be located immediately below the Pubic Tubercle.

Administer local anaesthetic injection to the dermis to be sutured (exactly over the upper fat border), surrounding soft tissues and in the proximal Gracilis tendon.

Make a stab incision with a No. 11 blade into the free-from-fat skin (in the lowest point possible) on both sides of the Gracilis Tendon. Incisions will be 1-1.5cm apart.

Perforate skin opening **A** with the Serdev® needle (mini-mini, or mini), elevate the skin with the needle to the Gracilis tendon insertion and securely pass through the tendon insertion. Lift the skin perforation on the other side to the level of the needle tip (needle is fixed in the tendon). Pass the needle through opening **B**. Load a USP 2 Bulgarian (Polycon) suture into the needle eye at point B and retrogradely withdraw the needle through point **A**. With this pass, the suture is fixed to the immobile Gracilis Tendon insertion. Allow the skin to relax back to its original position. Now make the second pass precisely through the firm dermis from **A** to **B** (very difficult – gently twisting forward (not pushing) the Serdev® needle) and passing through the skin opening at point **B**. Now load the free end of the suture into the eye of the needle. Retrogradely withdraw the needle from point **B** through the dermis pass and point **A**. With this pass, the movable firm dermis is attached to the suture and the circle of the suture is finalized with the 2 free suture ends at point **A**.

Tie a secure surgical knot under medium elastic tension. Cut the suture just short of the knot and let it dive into the opening. At this point is very important to release the skin at points **A** and **B** with a mosquito clamp to remove any dimpling of the skin.

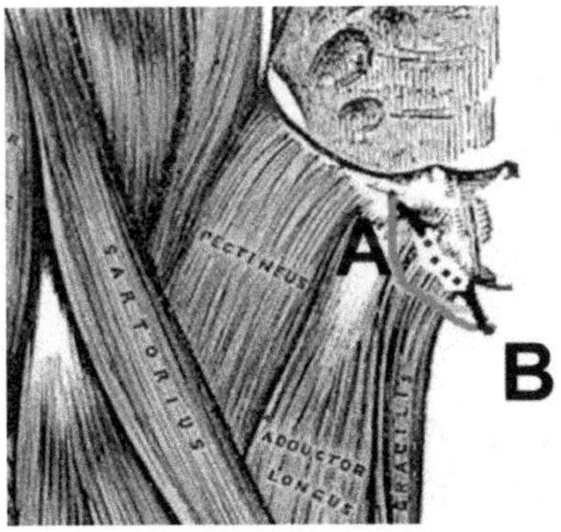

Figure 13. Inner thigh lift by suture is fixed to the incertion of the gracilis tendon

The medial thigh will now be lifted and the inner thigh skin will be stretched.

Skin folding will be placed high in the fold, laterally from the major labia. The initial skin folding due to skin lifting, anesthesia and swelling will adapt to the very wrinkled skin in this area and will disappear in 2-4 weeks.

5. Abdominal flaccidity lift

5.1. Introduction

This suture method for abdominal flaccidity was first presented in 1994 as a scarless alternative to the classic abdominoplasty (tummy tuck) and a part of the total understanding for the scarless closed approach suture lifting method all over face and body. The concept is the lift of abdominal skin without engaging it in the suture. This is achieved by a closed approach suture lift, using special instruments – curved semi-elastic needles and semi-elastic surgical sutures, distinguished by an extended period of delayed absorption (2-3 years).

The author uses skin perforations alone in the abdominal skin to capture, suture and lift the superficial fascias and linea alba supporting the abdominal skin. To obtain outcome longevity, it is important to lift and stretch these firm mobile fascias, fixing them to immobile firm tissue, such as xiphoid periosteum, costal and spina iliaca anterior superior periosteum.

The Serdev Suture® lift can be used in selected cases of thin patients to obtain a scarless and atraumatic tightening of the abdominal skin.

5.2. Anatomy

Anatomy landmarks are linea alba, superficial fascia, bone periosteum around the abdomen.

Firm mobile fascias fixing the abdominal skin are linea alba and superficial fascia. Firm immobile structures utilized in turn for fixation of the mobile fascias are the xiphoid process, the costal line, spina iliaca anterior superior.

Linea alba runs from the xiphoid process to the pubic symphysis and is mostly composed of collagen connective tissue. It fixes the abdominal skin longitudinally to the mid-line and consisting only of connective tissue, does not contain important nerves or blood vessels.

The superficial fascia of the abdomen fixes the anterior abdominal skin by a trabecular system. The superficial fascia consists of one thicker fatty superficial layer (Camper's fascia). There is also a membranous deep layer (Scarpa's fascia). The superficial vessels and nerves run between these two layers. It is important to preserve the a.and v. epigastrica inf.

The Procedure – see video http://youtu.be/oXU_80OqtOg

"sad navel", "sad abdomen" = flaccidity

The aim of the transcutaneous, scarless, closed approach Serdev Sutures® for abdominal flaccidity lift is:

1. Cephalic lift - to produce a "happy navel" when shortening the length of linea alba.

Two skin perforation points are used: Point A at the xiphoid and point B at a selected length of the linea alba in the upper abdomen. After anesthetic infiltration in the points A and B and along the length of linea alba, introduce the "medium" 140 mm Serdev® needle into point A, without capturing the dermis. In abdomen lifts the author uses a set of Serdev® needles with different lengths.

Take periosteum of the xiphoid and, by gently twisting the needle forward through the linea alba, exit at B. Load the needle and pull through. Second pass A-B is without catching periosteum. Load the second end of the suture and pull it through line B-A. The circle of the suture is fulfilled. Tie at A using medium elastic tension to lift the mobile linea alba in the direction of the xiphoid periosteum fixation. **NB!** Shortening of the linea alba length can be produced as well, without fixation to the periosteum, but only by shortening the lengths between 2 selected points of the linea alba, above the navel.

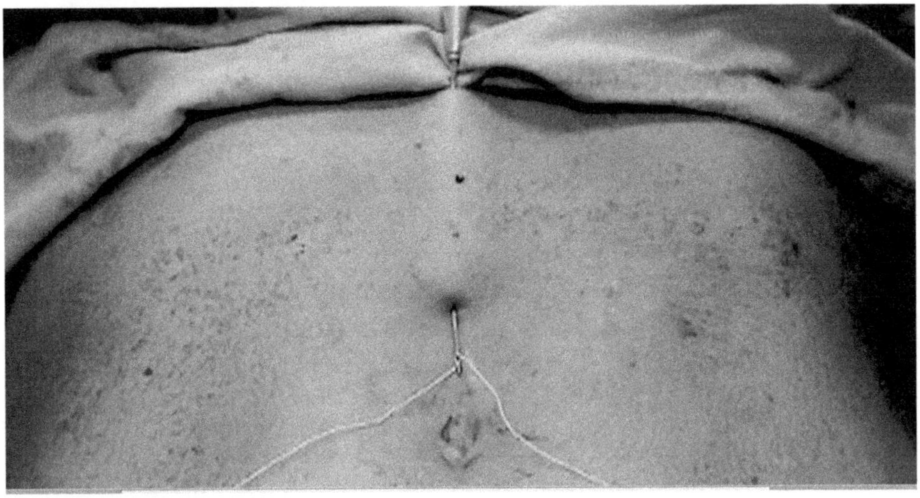

Figure 14. The needle is fixed to the xiphoid periosteum at A. Then, with soft, twisting zigzag motions through the length of linea alba it exits through point B, without catching dermis. The tip is loaded and the thread will be pulled through the line B-A. The second A-B pass will be more superficial, without producing dimpling on the surface (dimpling indicates an overly superficial pass), in order to load the second suture end and pull it through. The knot will be tied at A. Both passes could be located at both sides of the linea alba.

2. Cephalic, lateral and distal lifting - to stretch the flaccid abdominal skin in cephalic, lateral and distal direction is performed by a fixation of the mobile superficial fascia to immobile structures, such as:

a) the costal line periosteum/perichondrium,

b) the spiina iliaca anterior superior

5.3. Surgical procedure

Mark point A at costal periosteum/perichondrium level, or at spina iliaca anterior superior. Check the flaccidity level and mark point B (medial to A) at a selected distance. After anesthetic infiltration in points A and B and along the length of line A-B, introduce "medium" (140 mm), "small" (100 mm) or "mini" (60 mm) Serdev® needle into point A, without capturing the dermis. Take periosteum and proceed a little deeper to capture the superficial fascia and exit at B. **NB!** Be careful not to perforate through the anterior abdominal wall. Superficial fascia is just below the abdominal skin. Move the needle laterally to check fascia fixation. Load the needle and pull it through. The second pass A-B is more superficial, without catching superficial fascia or periosteum. Load the second end of the surgical suture and pull it through line B-A. The circle of the suture is fulfilled. Tie at point A, using medium elastic tension, to stretch the mobile superficial fascia in direction to the immobile periosteum, perichondrium or linea alba at A, which reflects in stretching of the attached abdominal skin.

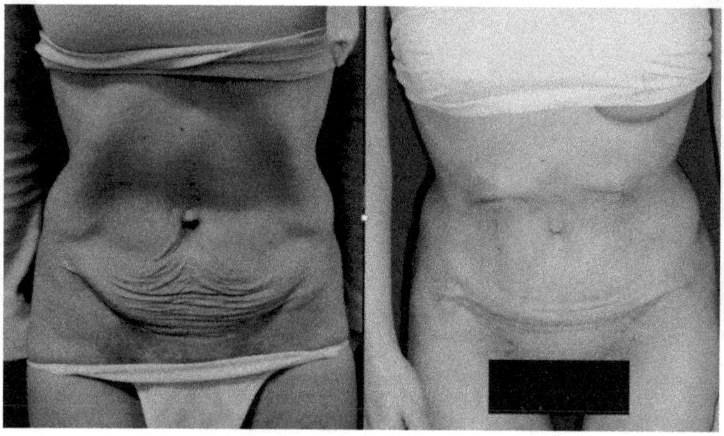

A

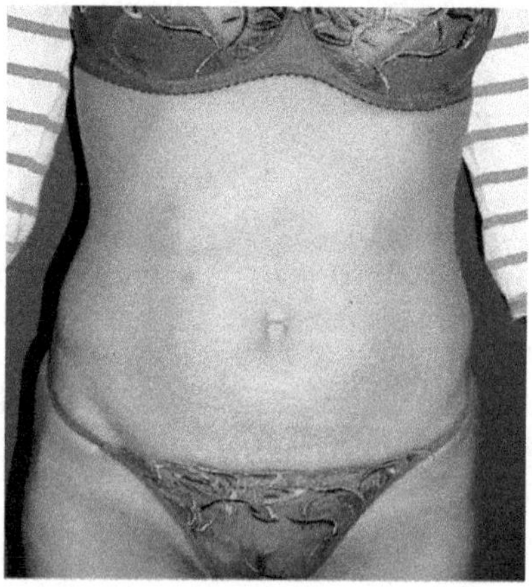

B

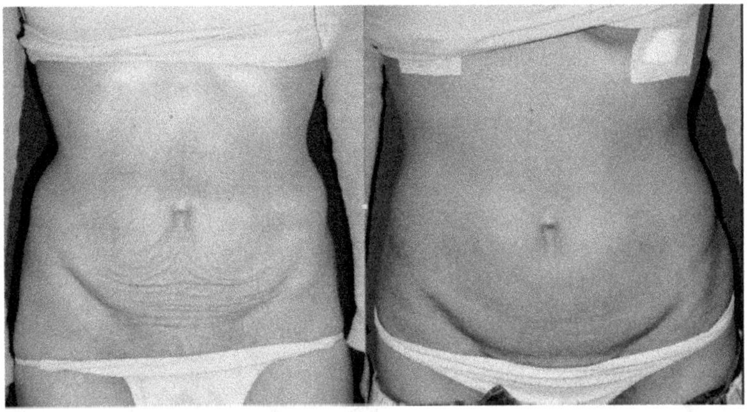

C D

Figure 15. A. Before and immediately after linea alba lift, superficial fascia lift to costal periosteum and to spina iliaca anterior superior, **B.** Edema absorption after 20 days, **C.** before and **D.** final result. Bandages in the thorax area are connected with early post op secondary breast augmentation period.

Edema absorption in the fixation locations takes about a month.

Results are more than satisfactory. Selection of patients is important.

5.4. Conclusion

Buttock lifts: Redundant tissue in sagging buttocks can be corrected by excision lifts. However, these are seldom used procedures because of post-operative problems, such as unacceptable inferiorly displacement, wide scars, early recurrence of ptosis, large trauma, blood loss and a prolonged post-operative period.

In order to limit these complications in flat and sagging buttocks without remarkable fat deposits, the author has developed a surgical technique, using a circumferential suture of the soft tissue to the sacro-cutaneous fascia discovered by the author. The circumferential suspension gives strong vertical support with minimal tension in each point and reduces the complications, which are traditionally associated with other procedures. The author's suture lift offers fewer complications than any others described. It is an efficient and safe procedure to correct or enhance buttock contour. It has virtually eliminated most complications of liposuction and dermolipectomies under general anaesthesia.

In patients, whose problem was excessive fat in conjunction with flabbiness, UAL of the buttocks combined with the buttock suture lifting method completed the main goals of the procedure in one or more different stages. The combination of UAL and buttock lift by the suture technique described in this chapter is a minimally invasive procedure that can be used to reduce and lift the buttocks at the same time.

The Serdev Suture® buttock lifting technique is simple and low in cost, with minimal morbidity and very good results. It is important to note that a good result does not depend on great surgery but rather on more simple and acceptable procedures for the patients. Outcomes incorporate harmonious structuring and positioning of the form, lifting of the lower portion of the buttocks, augmentation in the upper gluteus part and better projection. Complications with suture lift of the buttocks are few and patient satisfaction is high. The result is a visual change in the buttock projection, roundness, tightness and higher positioning. The buttock lift elongates the lower limbs and visibly changes the proportions of the body. Patients of regular weight seeking higher, rounded and projected buttocks with better proportions are indicated. Heavy buttocks and obesity are contraindicated.

Breast Lifts: Redundant tissue in ptotic and giant breasts can be corrected by excision lifts. However, these are procedures with wide scars, early recurrence of ptosis, large trauma, blood loss and a prolonged post-operative period, post-operative problems, such as unacceptable displacement etc.

The Serdev Suture® breast lifting technique is simple, with minimal morbidity and very good results. Complications with suture lift are few and patient satisfaction is high. The result is a visual change in the projection, tightness and higher positioning, as well as position of the nipple at the middle of the humerus. Heavy breasts and large ptosis are contraindicated.

Inner Thigh lift by suture is indicated mostly in skinny patients.

Abdominal Flacidity: Serdev Suture® for abdominal flaccidity lift is a satisfactory procedure that can be done in several steps. It is scarless and atraumatic. No complications have been observed. Selection of patients and their acceptance of a time interval for the adaptation of some bulging/edema in areas of fixation to the costal periosteum is crucial for patients' satisfaction. It is a good alternative to abdominoplasty in thin and selected patients.

Author details

Nikolay Serdev
New Bulgarian University, Sofia, Bulgaria

6. References

[1] Serdev, N.P. Year 1994, Suture Suspensions For Lifting Or Volume Augmentation In Face And Body (English version), presented at the 2nd Annual Meeing of the National Bulgarian Society for Aesthetic Surgery and Aesthetic Medicine, Sofia, 18 March 1994, Int J Aesth Cosm, 2001,1:1, 2561-2568

[2] Serdev, NP. Buttock lift. Two own methods. 3rd International Congress of the South-American Academy of Cosmetic Surgery, Buenos Aires, Argentina, October 19-21, 2001

[3] Serdev, NP. Buttocks lift by ultrasonic assisted liposuction - My technique International Journal of Aesthetic Cosmetic Beauty Surgery Volume 1, Number 3, 1991, 130-54

[4] Serdev, NP. Buttocks lifting without implants - Serdev technique no visible scars" Aesthetic Surgery Course In Sofia, Bulgaria, Medical Center "Aesthetic Surgery, Aesthetic Medicine, November 26, 2001
[5] Anikina TI. Soft framework of the human body, Arkh Anat Gistol Embriol 1980 Mar;78(3):5-15
[6] Hexsel DM, Mazzuco R., Subcision: a treatment for cellulite. Int J Dermatol 2000 Jul;39(7):539-44
[7] Gargan TJ, Courtiss EH., The risks of suction lipectomy. Their prevention and treatment. Clin Plast Surg 1984 Jul;11(3):457-63
[8] Schlesinger SL. Two arcane areas in liposuction: the banana and the sensuous triangle. Aesthetic Plast Surg 1991 Spring;15(2):175-80
[9] Gasparotti M. Superficial liposuction: a new application of the technique for aged and flaccid skin. Aesthetic Plast Surg 1992 Spring;16(2):141-53
[10] Pitanguy I. Surgical reduction of the abdomen, thigh, and buttocks. Surg Clin North Am 1971 Apr;51(2):479-89
[11] Delerm A, Cirotteau Y. Cruro-femoro-gluteal or circumgluteal plasty. Ann Chir Plast 1973;18(1):31-6
[12] Agris J. Use of dermal-fat suspension flaps for thigh and buttock lifts. Plast Reconstr Surg 1977 Jun;59(6):817- 22
[13] Gasperoni C, Salgarello M. MALL liposuction: the natural evolution of subdermal superficial liposuction. Aesthetic Plast Surg 1994 Summer;18(3):253-7
[14] Shaer WD. Gluteal and thigh reduction: reclassification, critical review, and improved technique for primary correction. Aesthetic Plast Surg 1984;8(3):165-72
[15] Chajchir A., Fat injection: long-term follow-Up. Aesthetic Plast Surg 1996 Jul-Aug;20(4):291-6
[16] Cardenas-Camarena L, Lacouture AM, Tobar-Losada A., Combined gluteoplasty: liposuction and lipoinjection. Plast Reconstr Surg 1999 Oct;104(5):1524-31;
[17] Lack EB. Contouring the female buttocks. Liposculpting the buttocks. Dermatol Clin 1999 Oct;17(4):815-22
[18] Lewis JR Jr. Body contouring. South Med J 1980 Aug;73(8):1006-11
[19] Pereira LH, Radwanski HN., Fat grafting of the buttocks and lower limbs. Aesthetic Plast Surg 1996 Sep-Oct;20(5):409-16
[20] Hanke CW, Bullock S, Bernstein G., Current status of tumescent liposuction in the United States. National survey results. Dermatol Surg 1996 Jul;22(7):595-8
[21] De Pedroza LV., Fat transplantation to the buttocks and legs for aesthetic enhancement or correction of deformities: long-term results of large volumes of fat transplant. Dermatol Surg 2000 Dec;26(12):1145-9
[22] Teimourian B, Adham MN. Anterior periosteal dermal suspension with suction curettage for lateral thigh lipectomy. Aesthetic Plast Surg 1982;6(4):207-9
[23] Guerrerosantos J. Secondary hip-buttock-thigh plasty. Clin Plast Surg 1984 Jul;11(3):491-503Lewis JR Jr. Body contouring. South Med J 1980 Aug;73(8):1006-11
[24] Lockwood T. Lower body lift with superficial fascial system suspension. Plast Reconstr Surg 1993 Nov;92(6):1112-22

[25] Regnault P, Daniel R. Secondary thigh-buttock deformities after classical techniques. Prevention and treatment. Clin Plast Surg 1984 Jul;11(3):505-16
[26] Gonzalez M, Guerrerosantos J. Deep planed torso-abdominoplasty combined with buttocks pexy. Aesthetic Plast Surg 1997 Jul-Aug;21(4):245-53
[27] Carwell GR, Horton CE Sr. Circumferential torsoplasty. Ann Plast Surg 1997 Mar;38(3):213-6
[28] Heddens CJ. Belt lipectomy: procedure and outcomes. Plast Surg Nurs 2001 Winter;21(4):185-9, 199
[29] Pascal JF, Le Louarn C. Remodeling bodylift with high lateral tension. Aesthetic Plast Surg 2002 May-Jun;26(3):223-30
[30] Lavigne P, Loriot de Rouvray TH. The superior gluteal nerve. Anatomical study of its extrapelvic portion and surgical resolution by trans-gluteal approach Rev Chir Orthop Reparatrice Appar Mot 1994;80(3):188-95
[31] Karnes J, Salisbury M, Schaeferle M, Beckham P, Ersek RA. Hip lift. Aesthetic Plast Surg 2002 Mar-Apr;26(2):126-9
[32] Hagen K, Sorhagen O, Harms-Ringdahl K., Influence of weight and frequency on thigh and lower-trunk motion during repetitive lifting employing stoop and squat techniques. Clin Biomech (Bristol, Avon) 1995 Apr;10(3):122-127
[33] Niechajev I, Sevcuk O., Long-term results of fat transplantation: clinical and histologic studies. Plast Reconstr Surg 1994 Sep;94(3):496-506
[34] Guerrerosantos J., Autologous fat grafting for body contouring. Clin Plast Surg 1996 Oct;23(4):619-31
[35] Peren PA, Gomez JB, Guerrerosantos J, Salazar CA. Gluteus augmentation with fat grafting. Aesthetic Plast Surg 2000 Nov-Dec;24(6):412-7
[36] Ichida M, Kamiishi H, Shioya N., Aesthetic surgery of the trunk and extremities in the Japanese. Ann Plast Surg 1980 Jul;5(1):31-9
[37] Lawrence N, Coleman WP 3rd., The biologic basis of ultrasonic liposuction. Dermatol Surg 1997 Dec;23(12):1197-200
[38] Serdev, N.P. Breast Lift: My Methods Presentations from the Congress "VI Sharing with the Experts" - San Salvador, Int J Cosm Surg 2009, 9, 2, 1 – 39
[39] Serdev, N.P. Serdev Suture Techniques Breast Lift Original Papers, Int J Cosm Surg, 2009, 9, 4, 1 – 3
[40] Serdev, N.P. Minimally Invasive Author Technique For Breast Lift Without Scars Using Sutures Abstracts - The First World Multidisciplinary Congress on Cosmetic Surgery and Medicine Int J Cosm Surg, 2010, 10, 3, 1 – 1
[41] Serdev, N.P. Tratamento De Flacides Cutanea Abdominal Com Filos Elasticos Serdev / Scarless Serdev Suture Methods For Abdominal Skin Flaccidity, 12 Congresso Brasiliero Medicina Estetica - 15 - 18 June 2005, Salvador, Int J Cosm Surg, 2006, 6, 1, 1 - 25

Chapter 5

Percutaneous Suspension Sutures to Change the Nasal Tip

M. B. Des Fernandes

Additional information is available at the end of the chapter

http://dx.doi.org/10.5772/56249

1. Introduction

Although a number of procedures have been described for placement of "shaping sutures" during open and closed rhinoplasty, scant attention is given to the possibility of percutaneous placement of sutures without dissection of the skin envelop. Periodically patients will present who want minimal changes to their nose because the tip is too bulky, not well defined and the nose is longer than ideal. Many of these patients have no concerns about the bridge width and do not have a dorsal hump. This is the perfect patient to consider using the operation that will be described.

Many other patients have had an attractive straight nose when they were young and as they have aged, the nose has become coarser, broader and tends to lengthen and lose support from the septum and then droops into becoming a hooked nose. The operation that will be described specifically addresses these changes and with this surprisingly simple operation, the nose can be restored to much closer to the original.

Other patients who have had a corrective rhinoplasty develop a typical "polly-beak" deformity. By elevating and rotating the nasal cartilages one can restore a normal nasal tip projection and a straight bridge.

2. Methods and instruments

The following instruments and materials are required:

1. 11 or 15 blade scalpel
2. 18 gauge (green) needle or a 22 (yellow) spinal needle.
3. Sharp pointed fine scissors
4. Fine dissector (optional)

5. Toothed Adson's forceps.
6. Fine needle holder to tie the knot.
7. Skin hook to free the skin from the buried thread
8. 4/0 or 5/0 non-absorbable suture. This could be an elasticised suture as described by Serdev.

The procedure is usually done in an office setting on an ambulatory patient under simple local anaesthetic usually without the need for any sedation.

The guide-line markings are made on the nose with the patient sitting up to assess the degree of droop of the nose and get an impression of the amount of lift and rotation of the tip of the alar cartilages that will be required to get the ideal result and then to feel how much more the nose may comfortably be lifted to exaggerate the immediate result.

3. Standard markings

1. A dot is placed to the right side of the dorsum of the nose immediately below the osteo-cartilagenous junction of the bridge of the nose, about 4 mm from the midline. This point is chosen so that when the anchoring transfixion suture goes through the cartilaginous septum, the tract will be anterior to the anterior nasal mucosal recess inside the nose.
2. Then a line is drawn on the side of the nose directed towards the lowest part of the columella (see Fig 1).

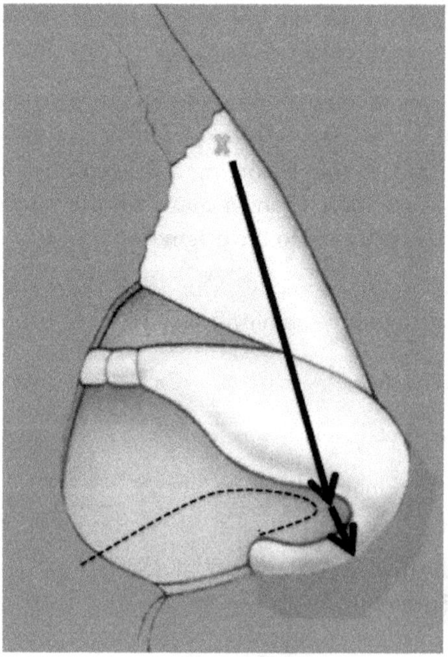

Figure 1. Showing the markins on the lateral side of the nose for the standard nose.

3. The line will traverse the soft triangle of the nostril as it courses towards the lowest part of the columella. Usually this is at the position where the columella changes angle in the "ideal" nose.
4. As one draws this line one has to take into account the shape of the lower lateral alar cartilages. (See Fig 2). Normally as seen from the front in figure 2, the line is straight downwards.

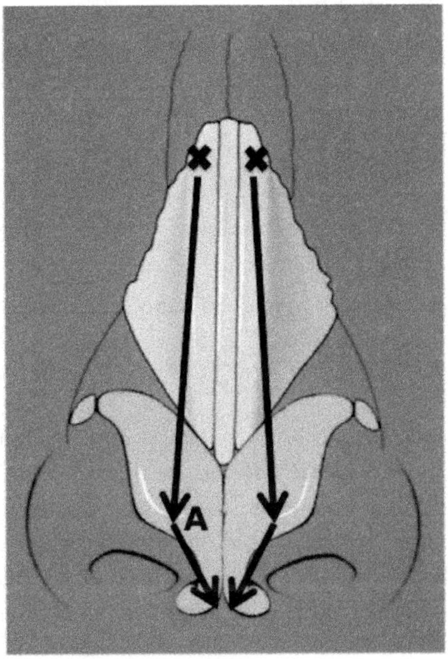

Figure 2. Showing the skin markings for the standard nose

5. However, if the cartilages are bulging and wide then one should deviate the line laterally towards the maximum width as seen from the frontal view. (See Fig 3) Generally if one presses on the lateral alar wings one can determine where this essential point is to apply medial pressure in order to narrow the nose tip. Its worth spending time familiarising yourself with these little details.
6. Then mark the midline of the columella with a vertical 3-4 mm line where the incision will be made. This incision is also dependant on where the columella will be lifted.
7. Similar markings are made on the opposite side.

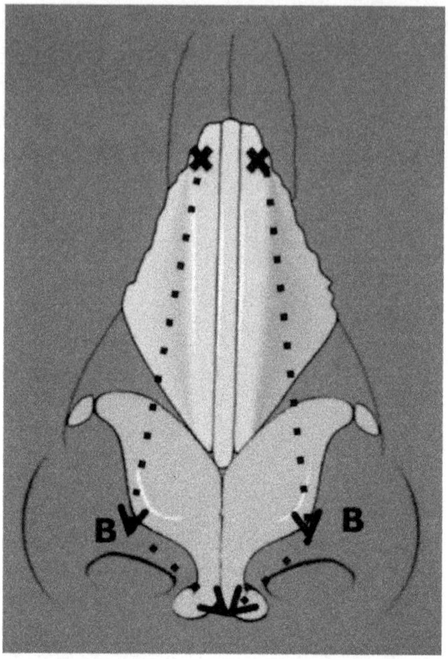

Figure 3. Showing the markings for a nose with broad alar dome cartilages.

4. Anaesthesia

An inferior orbital nerve block should be done first and in some people this gives excellent anaesthesia of the whole nose especially if the local anaesthetic is placed in the inferior orbital foramen. In other people it may be necessary to add specific block to the lateral nasal nerves as well as the nerves at the nasal spine to the columella. By blocking these nerves, anaesthesia is achieved easily and painlessly. It is advisable to check that the septal cartilage is numb by infiltrating across to the other side where the anchors will be placed.

5. Placement of the suspension sutures

1. Two stab incisions need to be made at the points marked X in figures 1 and 2 and then use the sharp pointed scissors to make sure to dissect the skin away from the cartilage that the skin is entirely free of the surrounding deep tissues. These holes should be as small as possible.
2. Make the incision on the columella and then dissect the skin away from the vertical alar cartilages in the area and extend the dissection area across into the "soft triangle" and even to the inferior edge of the lateral lower alar cartilages. By doing this one reduces the possibility of the needle passing into the nose as it is pushed across the "soft triangle" down towards the incision in the columella.
3. Insert the chosen needle perpendicularly through the incision on the right side of the nose

4. Once one reaches the layer just outside the upper lateral cartilage, change direction of the needle and point it down under the guidelines previously marked.
5. One has to distort the nose by pushing it medially and at the same time it is useful to put the Adson's forceps into the columella incision in order to retrieve the needlepoint. Make sure that the needle does not catch any tissue of the columella.
6. The needle is now positioned outside of the nasal cartilages and the non-absorbable thread (4/0 or 5/0) is passed up the needle until it protrudes through the hub at the end of the needle.
7. Pull back the needle until one reaches the entry point on the side of the nose, change direction to be perpendicular again and then push the needle through the septal cartilage to emerge through the opposite incision without catching any of the tissues attached to skin. This is the anchor so one has to be sure that the thread is not too close to the edge of the cartilage. It is easy to avoid the anterior nasal mucosal recess because it does not come into the sharp angle between the nasal septum and the upper lateral cartilages
8. Hold on to the thread and remove the needle. Most people expect that the bevel of the needle will cut the suture as it goes through the septum, but it generally never does. In doing this type of procedure for several thousands of times, the thread has been cut only twice. By this stage we have constructed more than half of the important loop that will eventually narrow, rotate and lift the alar cartilages.
9. The final stage is approached differently. The needle is now carefully inserted into the columella incision taking care not to catch any of the outer skin layer in the soft triangle of the left nostril and then pushed up to the stab incision on the left side of the nose.
10. By using the Adson's forceps one can guide the needle tip out through the stab incision without catching the surrounding soft tissue.
11. The thread is passed through the needle until it emerges from the needle hub before the needle is pulled out.
12. The suspension loop has now been created outside the upper and lower lateral alar cartilages and one can check what the nose looks like as one tightens the threads. The nose tip is lifted and the lower lateral alar cartilages are compressed towards each other medially and narrowed.
13. Examine the inside of the nostrils to be certain that the thread has not been accidentally placed medial to the alar cartilages. If this has been done and has not been detected, then it might cause a chronic infection and pain.
14. It is advisable to make two throws in the same direction so that the knot can be adjusted before the third throw which seals the knot. A double throw is recommended and altogether I recommend about six throws to ensure that the knot never slips. The knot is cut exactly on the knot so that the ends do not later protrude through the skin.
15. Always over-correct. In general it is unlikely that one over-corrects even though the nose tip is rather exaggeratedly lifted. Of course one should not over-correct too excessively. One major advantage of this operation is that it is easy to do and should one not over-correct sufficiently then the procedure is easy to repeat. The same is true should one over-correct.

16. Should you feel that the nose has not been adequately lifted a second suture can be inserted. I do not try and remove the first suture.
17. I suggest taping the nose with micropore for about two days to limit swelling and also to ensure immobility. The nose tip can be rather sensitive for the first few days.
18. Over the next three to six weeks the nose tip will drop down into a stable position. By 8 to 10 weeks one reaches a stable position.

6. Further modifications

In some patients the described procedure makes a difference but one does not achieve the refinement of the nose tip that is desired. In these cases one needs to add extra sutures. Experience has shown that generally these sutures need to be shorter.

1. If the suture designed above will not narrow the nose sufficiently then one needs to add a suture lower down on the nose with more direct pressure on the upper edges of the lower lateral cartilages. (See Figs. 5 and 6)

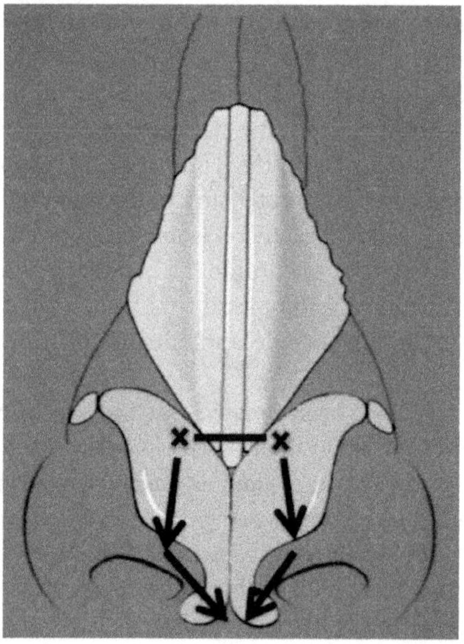

Figure 4. Showing the frontal view of the skin markings where one needs more pressure on the alar wings.

As one creates this suture in much the same way as described above, take care to ensure that the alar cartilages are not lifted anteriorly which will create a ridge on the lower nose instead of maintaining a straight bridge to the tip, or supra-tip bump. This suture is often important for creating a really fine nose tip.. A variant that can be done, depending on the anatomy, is the pass above the lower lateral alar cartilages through the septum and then around them to make a more defined cinched tip (See Fig 6 and 7).

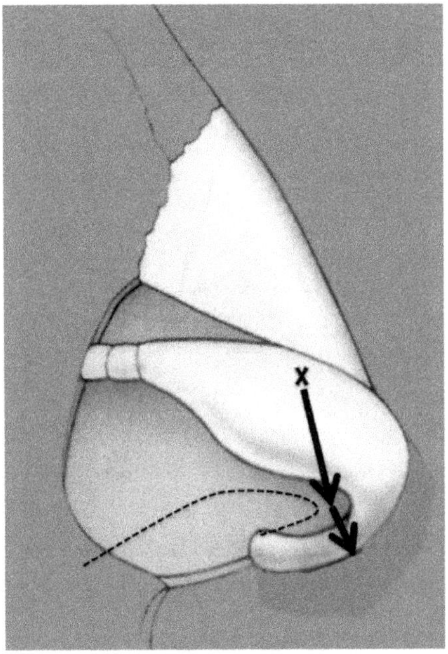

Figure 5. Showing the lateral marking for the shorter suture to compress the alar cartilages more directly.

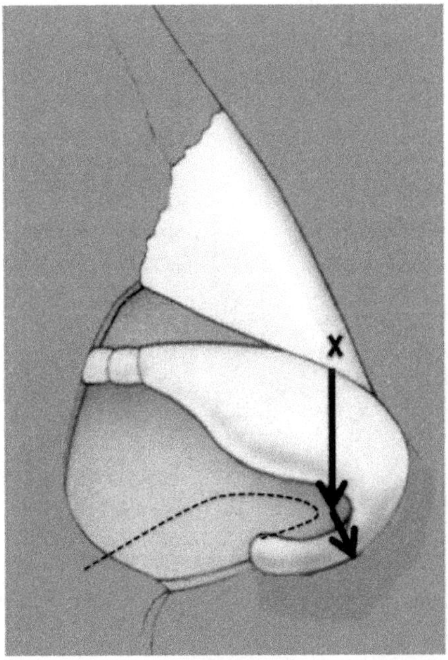

Figure 6. Showing the markings for a more pinched tip with the suture going through the septum only.

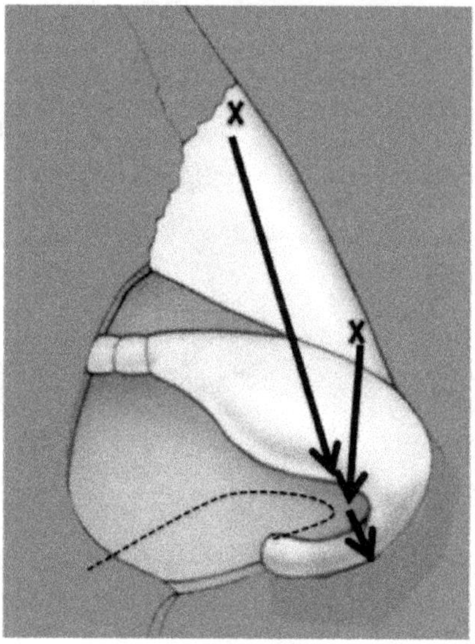

Figure 7. Showing the composite view of both longer and then a shorter cinching suture to the nasal tip.

2. In some cases with very bulky lateral alar wings we need to do a slightly different suture to get better compression. Here it is necessary to make four stab incisions on the alar cartilage in a design that allows more compression on the alar cartilage and compresses the tip as well. (See Fig. 8)

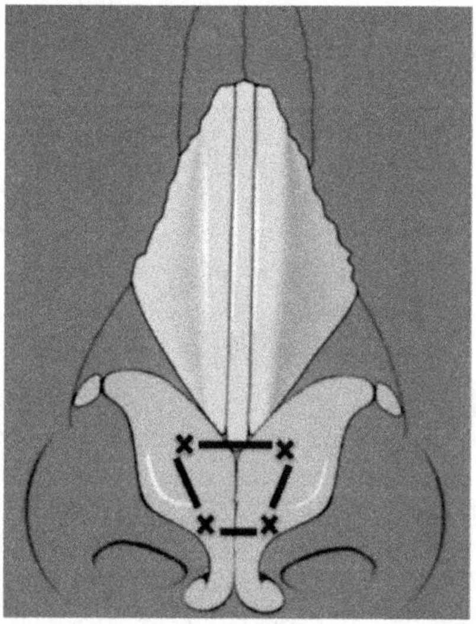

Figure 8. Showing the square suture combination in the upper edge of the medial wing of the lower alar cartilage.

Here we have to be cautious about not entering the nasal cavity. These sutures do not need to be anchored to the septum. I rarely use this suture.

3. In some cases the alar cartilages are not positioned evenly and one cartilage may be lower than the other. In this case the displaced cartilage can be lifted by a loop created in the same fashion as described above but one goes medial to the "normal cartilage so that the one thread of the suspension loop lies in between the alar cartilages and the other part lies exterior to the lower cartilage as shown in figure 9.

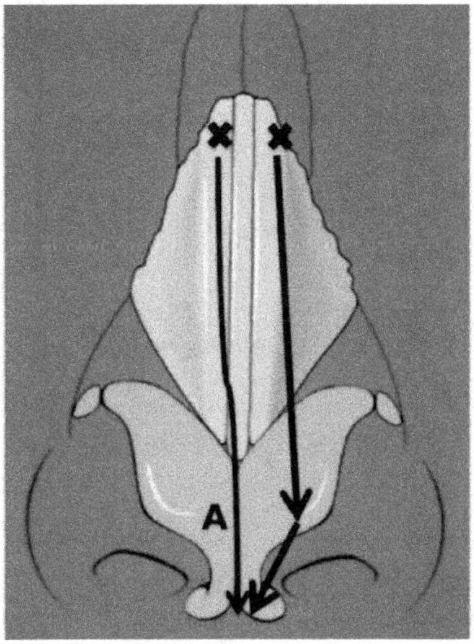

Figure 9. Showing the surface markings of the suture used to pull up the left alar cartilage. It would be the mirror image for the right side.

Tightening the loop will lift the alar cartilage to a matching position and then the suspension suture for both alar cartilages can be positioned. Do not expect that a simple loop will correct this type of asymmetry.

4. In cases of excessive bulk of the columella that hangs very low, then one should consider an elliptical excision of mucosa to lift the columella. Suspension sutures alone cannot remedy this situation.

7. Postoperative phase

Initially patients may worry that the tip of the nose has been lifted too much but if sensible exaggeration has been done, the nose takes up a pleasing position very quickly. (see Figures 10 through 1)

For the first four five days the nose looks over-corrected but rapidly changes as the swelling disappears and within a week the patient feels much more confident. By ten weeks. Weeks the nose has settled to very close to the final appearance.

The nose can be rather sensitive to minor trauma and even to kissing but that also settles quite soon. The patients may be aware of the suture for up to six months.

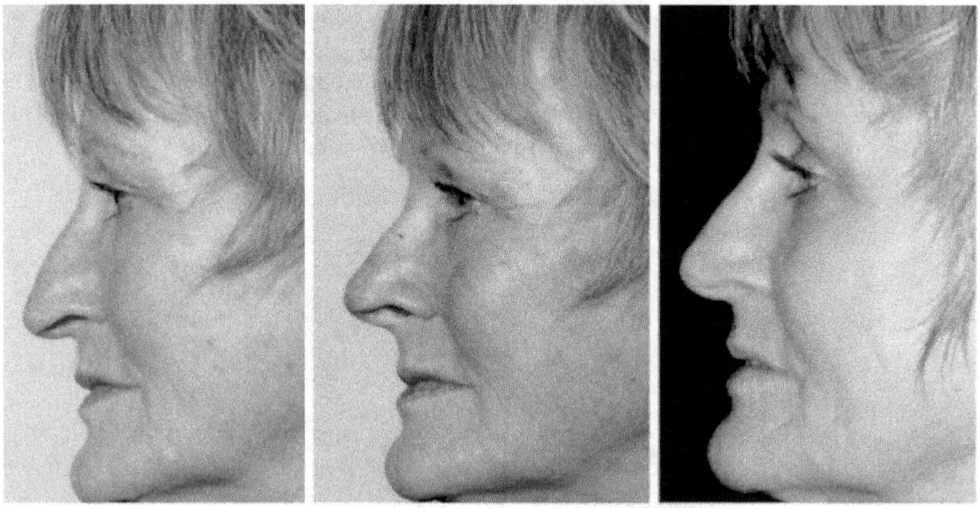

One realises quite quickly if the nose has not been over-corrected sufficiently. Patients should be warned that this is a possibility and that they might need a second minor procedure.

8. The advantages

This is a simple low cost procedure easily done in the office that does not disrupt the alar cartilages and yet shapes them easily. It is rapidly done with little morbidity and the patient can rapidly return to normal social activity. The worst luck is that the nose might need some modification with some extra sutures.

One of the greatest advantages for older people is the improvement in breathing through their nose when the tip has been lifted. Another major advantage for people who have had previous surgery is how easily their nose can be re-fashioned into the nose they hoped for.

9. Summary

A simple technique is always a benefit and this technique of lifting and compressing the nasal tip combines a very simple surgical procedure with rapid results and minimal discomfort. It can be used in old people whose nose tips have dropped and also in patients who have had a previous rhinoplasty. Its simplicity also makes it an inexpensive minimally invasive procedure that is also suitable for many minor nasal deformities.

Author details

M. B. Des Fernandes
The Renaissance Body Science Institute, Cape Town, South Africa.
Department of Plastic Surgery, Groote Schuur Hospital, University of Cape Town, Cape Town, South Africa

Chapter 6

Chin Enhancement Using Serdev Suture: Five Case Reports

Meity Hidayani, Syarief Hidayat and Dali Amiruddin

Additional information is available at the end of the chapter

http://dx.doi.org/10.5772/56711

1. Introduction

The main goal of aesthetic facial cosmetic surgery is to achieve balance and harmony to the facial features. Chin augmentation and correction are the most important procedures to obtain overall facial beauty. Chin augmentation has been conducted since 100 years ago. Some synthetic implant alloplastic materials have been used including the observation of benefits, loss, and complication accompanied with it. The beauty of the chin is one of the important factors to enhance aesthetic facial features, where the chin is the lower most from 3 facial parts. Aesthetically, protrusion of the chin should be parallel to the line of facial profile. Protrusion of the chin gives character to the face. However imperfection and protrusion of the chin as a result of trauma, congenital or aging may hinder an individual's appearance. Inconsistency between the bone and soft tissue is a common cause of impaired aesthetic beauty. [1,2]

Aging causes the skin to wrinkle and an increase in subcutaneous tissue causes change in projection and facial contour. This is caused by the laxity of the skin and facial muscles that support the gravity force. The area of the face that creases due to age includes cheeks and chin, which causes face disproportion in some individuals. [1,3,4]

There are many techniques/methods used to correct and tighten sagging facial skin, one of them by employing Serdev suture. This method involves lifting part of the face to correct the volume and position of the soft tissue with fixation of the fascia/muscle percutaneous without conventional incision. This method is preferably chosen because it is relatively safe (with minimal side effects), easy, and quick with satisfactory results. This method was invented by Dr. Nikolay P. Serdev. Besides chin lift, the method can also be applied to lift other facial parts, buttocks and abdominal area. [2,5]

Serdev suture involves passing sutures by needle into the soft tissue under the skin and stitched according to the desired purpose. This action can be performed in an outpatient unit because it is relatively safe and complications are relatively mild, such as edema, hematoma, infection and scar (rare). Patients must be selected, amongst others, patients must not have a history of heart disease, hypertension, uncontrolled diabetes mellitus, blood clotting disorders, and not taking any anti-coagulant medications; also the surgery is suggested not to be performed to patients who are under 20 years old due tothe mandible bone has not yet fully grown. [2,3,5,6]

Five cases of chin enhancementis reported on women ages between 40-53 years old using Serdev suture and without any complication.

2. Case reports

2.1. First case

A 34-year old woman came to aesthetic clinic of Mintohardjo hospital for chin enhancement. From anamnesis, no chronic medical history is found like diabetes mellitus, hypertension, heart disease, or bleeding disturbances. In terms of physical examination, no abnormality to the chin is found. Routine laboratory blood test is within normal limits. With a clean medical

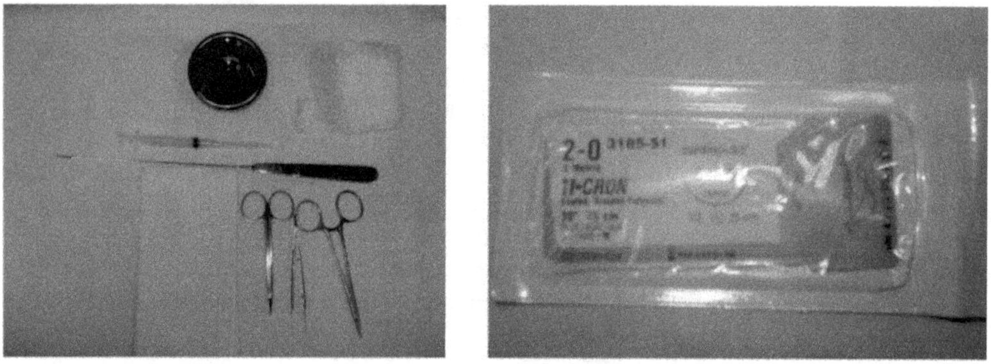

Figure 1. (A) and (B) Surgical instruments and materials prepared

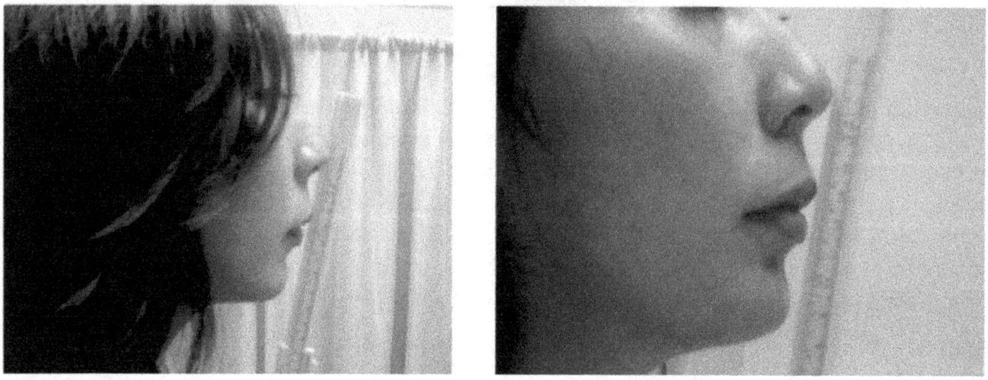

Figure 2. (A) Pre-Operation (B) Post-operation

record, chin lift can be performed using Serdev suture and after the patient read, understand, and agree to sign a medical consent.

SurgeryReport:

1. Document chin from different angle.
2. Chin position is measured by drawing a line between the lower lip and chin, then place a mark under the chin for needle insertion and exit point. .
3. The patient is laid on the operating bed.
4. Surgical instruments are disinfected using Betadine/povidone-iodine.
5. Sterile drapes are placed around the field to delineate sterile areas.
6. Local anesthesia is given by injecting 2% lidocaine on the lowermost of the chin, under inferior lip.
7. Chin skin that has been marked is punctured using a special needle by following the internal chin muscle until it penetrates the mark below inferior lip.
8. Serdev thread is inserted in the hole at the tip of the needle, and then pulled down, thus appearing under the chin.
9. Needle is inserted back to the lowermost chin following the outer chin muscle until it penetrates to the same mark below the inferior lip.
10. Thread is inserted to the needle tip then pulled again until the thread appears in the lowermost of the chin.
11. The tip of the thread is stitched to the first thread until reaching the desired chin lift.
12. The thread is cut just above the knot.
13. The skin around the knot is freed.
14. The wound is given betadine and covered with bandage as needed.
15. Document the results after operation is finished.

After the operation is completed, patient can perform activities as normal, however, the patient should take amioxcilin-clavulanic acid 3x500 mg for 5 days and administer mefenamic acid 3 times in one day if in pain.

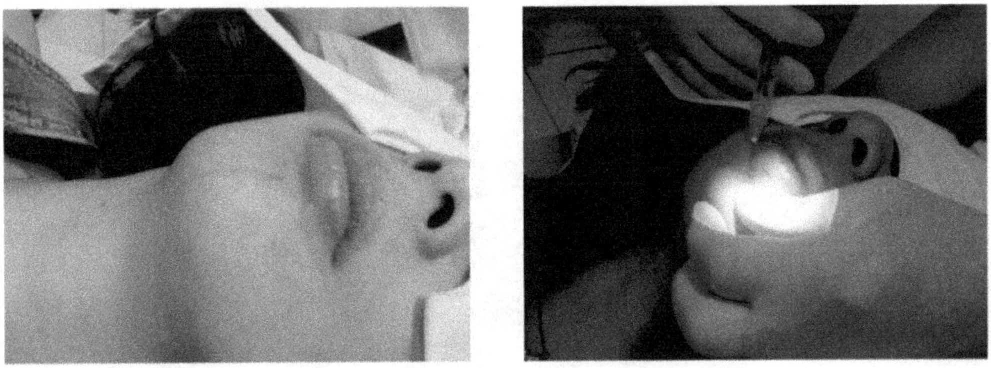

Figure 3. (A) marking for insertion and exit point (B) Anasthetic lidocaine 2%

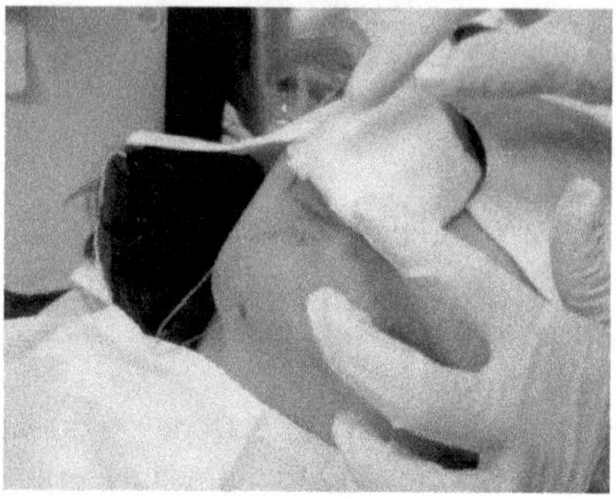

Figure 4. Thread is inserted to the tip of the needle and pulled until thread is seen in the lowermost of the chin.

2.2. Second case

A 42 year old woman came to aesthetic clinic of Mintohardjo Hospital to enhance the chin which she felt was slightly flabby. From anamnesis, no chronic medical history is found like diabetes mellitus, hypertension, heart disease, or bleeding disturbances. In terms of physical examination, no abnormality to the chin is found. Routine laboratory blood test is within normal limits. Thereby, chin lift can be performed using Serdev method after the patient read, understand, and agree to sign a medical consent.

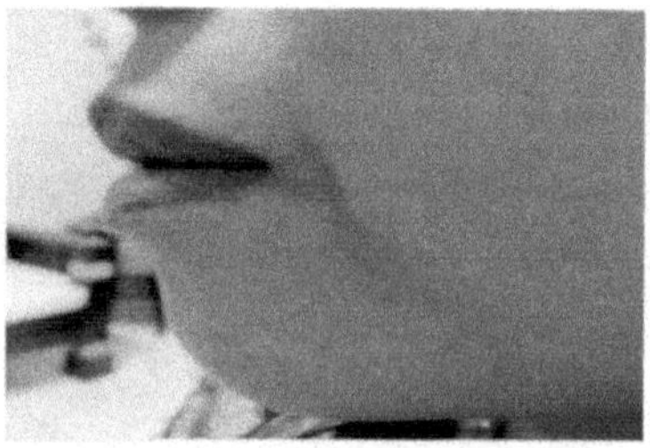

(A). Side view

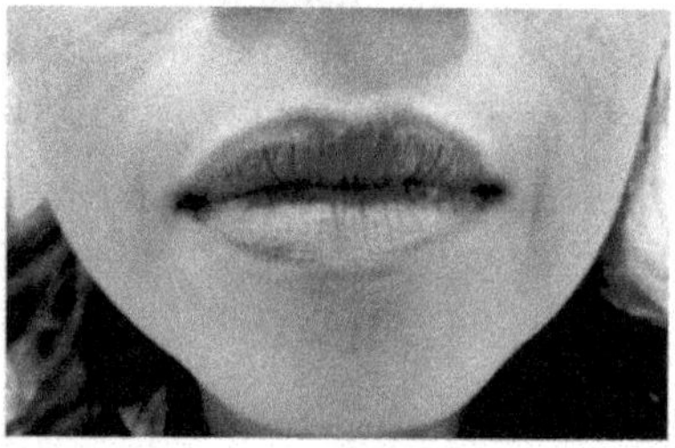

(B). Front view

Figure 5. Before procedure

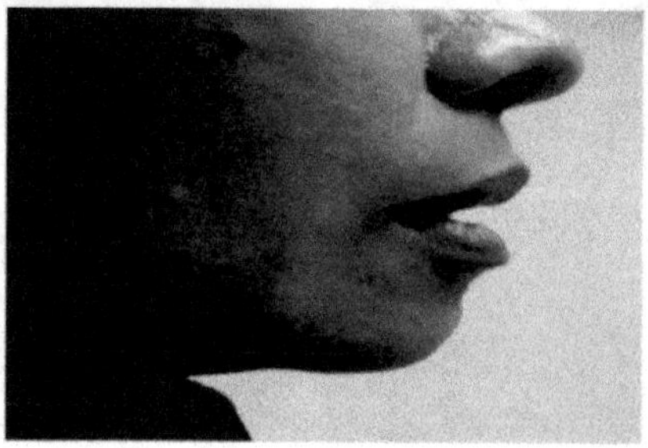

Figure 6. After procedure

Surgery report:

1. Document chin from different angle.
2. Chin position is measured by drawing a line between the lower lip and chin, then place a mark under the chin for needle insertion and exit point. .
3. The patient is laid on the operating bed.
4. Surgical instruments are disinfected using Betadine/povidone-iodine.
5. Sterile drapes are placed around the field to delineate sterile areas.
6. Local anesthesia is given by injecting 2% lidocaine on the lowermost of the chin, under inferior lip.
7. Chin skin that has been marked is punctured using a special needle by following the internal chin muscle until it penetrates the mark below inferior lip.
8. Serdev thread is inserted in the hole at the tip of the needle, and then pulled down, thus appearing under the chin.
9. Needle is inserted back to the lowermost chin following the outer chin muscle until it penetrates to the same mark below the inferior lip.
10. Thread is inserted to the needle tip then pulled again until the thread appears in the lowermost of the chin.
11. The tip of the thread is stitched to the first thread until reaching the desired chin lift.
12. The thread is cut just above the knot.
13. The skin around the knot is freed.
14. The wounds is given betadine and covered with bandage as needed.
15. Document the results after operation is finished.

After the operation is completed, patient can conduct activities as normal, however, the patient is advised to minimize the use of the lower jaw, like chewing hard foods. Patient is given amioxcilin-calvulanic acid 3x500 mg for 5 days and administer mefenamic acid 3 times in one day if in pain.

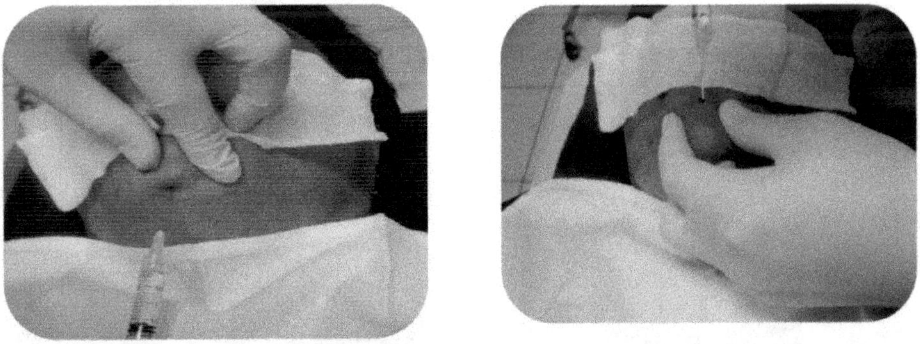

Figure 7. (A) and (B) Anesthetic lidocaine 2%

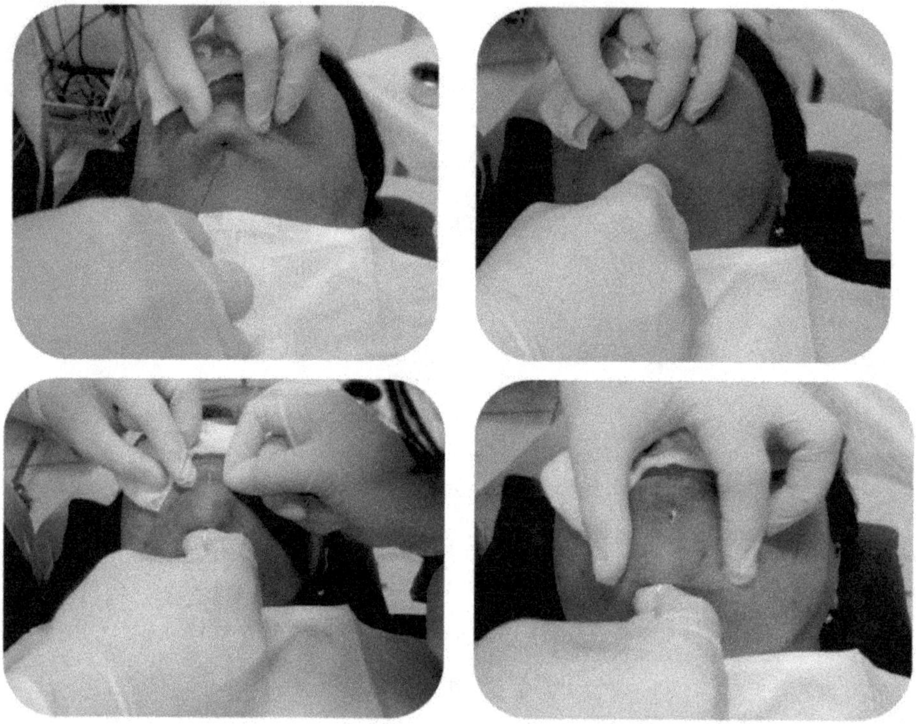

Figure 8. Thread is inserted to the tip of the needle and pulled until thread is seen in the lowermost of the chin.

2.3. Third case

A 30 year old woman came to Aesthetic Central RSAL Dr. Mintohardjo with the desire to perform chin lift because she feels her chin is lacking beauty and sagging.

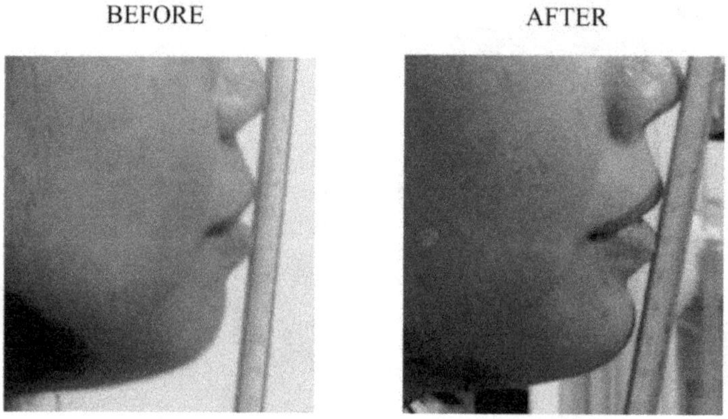

Figure 9.

From anamnesis, no chronic medical history is found like diabetes mellitus, hypertension, heart disease, or bleeding disturbances. In terms of physical examination, no abnormality to the chin is found. Routine laboratory blood test is within normal limits. Thereby, chin lift can be performed using Serdev method after the patient read, understand, and agree to sign a medical consent.

2.4. Fourth case

A 39 year old woman came to Aesthetic Center RSLA Dr. Mintohardjo with the desire to perform chin lift because she feels her chin is lacking beauty and sagging.

From anamnesis, no chronic medical history is found like diabetes mellitus, hypertension, heart disease, or bleeding disturbances. In terms of physical examination, no abnormality to the chin is found. Routine laboratory blood test is within normal limits. Thereby, chin lift can be performed using Serdev method after the patient read, understand, and agree to sign a medical consent.

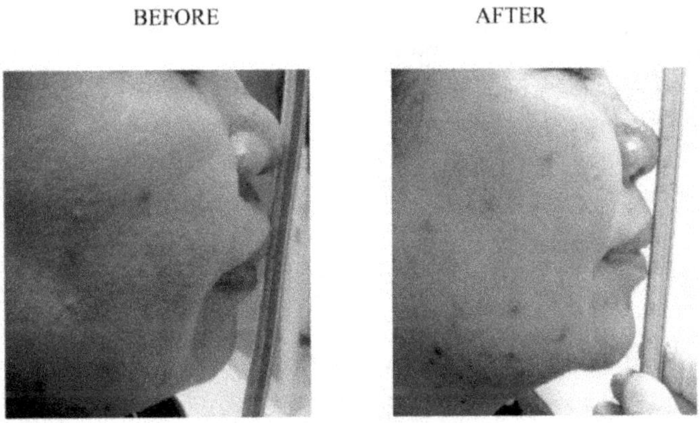

Figure 10.

2.5. Fifth case

A 45 year old woman came to Aesthetic Center RSAL Dr. Mintohardjo with the desire to perform chin lift because she feels her chin is lacking beauty and sagging.

From anamnesis, no chronic medical history is found like diabetes mellitus, hypertension, heart disease, or bleeding disturbances. In terms of physical examination, no abnormality to the chin is found. Routine laboratory blood test is within normal limits. Thereby, chin lift can be performed using Serdev method after the patient read, understand, and agree to sign a medical consent.

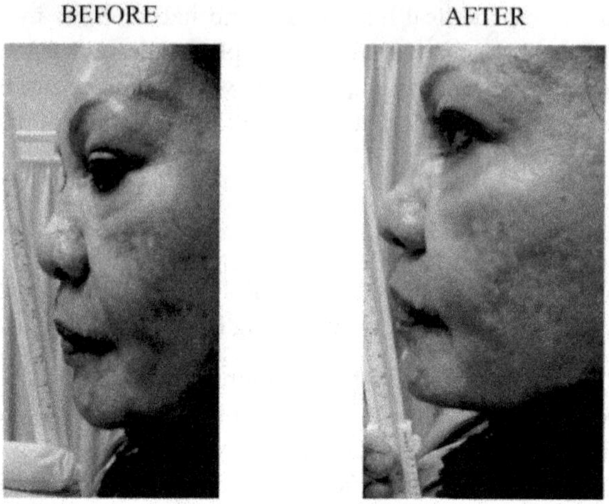

Figure 11.

3. Discussion

Chin enhancement is a surgical procedure to improve the shape or increase the size of the chin. For several decades, various methods and materials are used to enhance the chin. This includes implanted specimen from the body, transplantation of the bone and cartilage, fat, fascia, tendons and skin are the first materials used for this kind of procedure. A variety of alloplastic are then used to lift the chin. The polymer is used as a bone replacement. Sincethe 1950s, materials that can be used to enhance a small chin include silicon, collagen injection, expanded politetrafluoroetilan (e-PTFE), high density plyethylene (HDPE), polidimetiloksan (PDMS), proplast, and hyraxypatile porous block (PBHA) [1,2,7,8,9]

There are many injections available in the market over the last decade. But the materials are foreign for the body thus causing complications. Complications that occur include infection, position that is not fitting, parastesi, absorption, rejection, migration, implant, erosion of soft tissue, asymmetry, and indentation. [1]

There are no materials found that are perfect for the face, therefore a study is conducted to determine a method that is much more effective and less complicated. Surgery without implant is introduced by Dr. Nikolay P. Serdev, an aesthetic expert from Sofia, Bulgaria, which has become popularly known as Serdev method. This method is an operation without implant and only usesthread to pull/stitch soft tissue in the chin. This technique is done by changing the angle of the chin and keeping the chin align to the jaw line thus providing a better result. [1,10]

The advantages of Serdev method compared with other methods is that the result can be seen after the surgery, complications is minimal, more natural results, long-lasting, and can be applied to other areas of the face and body. [10,11]

Serdev thread is a woven polycapromide that is semi-synthetic, antimicrobial and non-absorbable. The result is more natural looking chin because an implant is not inserted and the operation only uses thread that is stitch to the soft tissue. The method can be used to correct flabby chin and does not cause scarring. [1,12]

Serdev method only requires a short amount of time and also requires only local anesthesia. The duration of the operation is dependent upon the area that is to be operated, the level of flabbiness, and the expertise of the doctor. Results can be seen immediately after the operation, but still accompanied with mild ederma. The pain will disappear by itself, and patients are recommended not to overly manipulate the chin. Serdev thread is not visible in the suface of the skin and the result can last 10-20 years. [1,12]

The report discusses cases for five women between the ages of 30 to 40 years old that complain sagging to the chin. From medical history record and check-up, there are no systematic diseases found or other contradiction, thus chin lift with Serdev method is chosen by patients.

Chin lift performed to the five patients are satisfactory with no complications after the operation. The patients are able to perform their usual daily activities after the operation. Although the patients are given antibiotic to prevent secondary infection and analgetic if in pain.

Author details

Meity Hidayani and Dali Amiruddin
Dermatovenereology Department Medical Faculty of Hasanuddin University Wahidin Sudirohusodo General HospitalMakassar, Indonesia

Syarief Hidayat
Dermatovenereology Department Mintohardjo Navy Hospital Jakarta, Indonesia

4. References

[1] Serdev NP. Chin enhancement and form correcting using a suture of the soft tissue. *Intern Jof Cosmetic Surg.* 2002:11(1); 16-25
[2] Serdev NP. Chin enhancement using serdev suture. Available from www.google.com
[3] Serdev NP. Chin form correction and augmentation using simple suture. *Int J AesthCosm Beauty Surg.* 2001;3(1):42-66
[4] Pachigolla R, Calhoun K. Chin and malar augmentation. Available from www.google.com
[5] Serdev NP. Serdev Suture. Available from http://en.wikipedia.org/wiki/Serdev_suture
[6] Anonyme. Chin augmentation, nasal, and facial plastic cosmetic surgery institute and laser centre. Available from www.google.com
[7] Serdev NP. Principles of face beautification in liftings: aesthetic proportions, volume and angles. Available from www.what11.com

[8] Anonyme. Chin augmentation. Available from www.veri.google.com
[9] Berman M. Chin and cheek augmentation. Available from www.google.com
[10] Serdev N. Scarless suture liftings. Available from www.google.com
[11] Anonyme.Scarlessserdev suture miniinvasive suspension lift and volume technique suspension lift and volume techniques. Available from www.drserdev.com
[12] Anonyme. Facelift with minimally invasive threadlift enhancement. Available from www.parkwayaesthetics.com

Chapter 7

Serdev Technique for Cervicoal Flaccidity and Mandibular Definition Utilizing "Serdev Sutures"

Roberto Tulli

Additional information is available at the end of the chapter

http://dx.doi.org/10.5772/56202

1. Introduction

Working with cosmetic surgery, in 25 years I performed several techniques for facial flaccidity beyond the plastic surgery that were presented in congresses and workshops with the goal of minimizing scars leading to a pos-op with less trauma, less edemas, aiming good results in medium average time.

Since I met Doctor Nikolay Serdev in 2001 during the International Congress of Esthetic Medicine in Brazil I became very interested in a new technique for facial flaccidity, developed by him, which lifts and fix mobile fascias to immobile fascias/periosteum, with semi-elastic threads from Bulgaria. That procedure was baptized as "Serdev Sutures".

After analyzing for years the follow up and results of "Serdev Sutures" procedures for cervical flaccidity, I decided to combine two techniques that would give an excellent retraction of lower SMAS – platysma, sunken skin aspect especially in the submandibular zone improving the jaw line.

I started to perform this technique on selected patients, observing their complaints carefully and thinking if I could give them long lasting results and what anatomic structures I should handle to obtain an harmonical retraction of platysma and surrounding tissues, as dermis and epidermis, always respecting the natural look of the patient.

2. Aim

The aim of modern aesthetic surgery is to create aesthetic forms and proportions for the face and body with the purpose of beautification. In the Aesthetic Cosmetic Surgery rejuvenation which means the same of beautification, by giving the right proportions and angles, typical for young people. In the last decade surgery was renovated, based on the experience of many specialties, increased technology and computer devices.

Lower face lifting techniques to repair the laxity and ptosis of tissues were submitted to invasive procedures with visible scars pre and retro auricular. Recently these techniques were replaced by more simple procedures. One of these is the scarless "Serdev Suture" liftings used in this case to restructure and reposition the "subdermal facial mask". The idea of lower SMAS–platysma face-lift using semi-elastic long term absorbable sutures is to tighten and elevate the lower face and neck, together with facial soft tissues without unnecessary incisions. As we know that soft tissues and skin are attached to the SMAS and platysma, lifting and fixing them in better position, aims repositioning of other facial structures as well. In young patients where no real ptosis exist, heavy faces, not well-expressed cheekbones, mandible arch, bad proportions, angles and sad look should be corrected.

One cannot expect the same results from this technique as from other excision surgery. However the suggestion for carrying out this technique under local anesthesia and that patient leave the clinic at the end of the procedure and rapidly recover their normal life is encouraging.

Results and duration vary from person to person according to each case, state of skin and subcutaneous tissue. There is no unique procedure in aesthetic cosmetic surgery for perfection of beauty. Other mini-invasive techniques as peelings, PRP, liposowing and fillers can be an addition to "Serdev Suture" techniques to keep significant results and satisfaction.

3. Anatomy

With age, loosening of SMAS and facial fascias, atrophy of ligaments due to the gravity, causes sagging of the neck and results in an aged face. Jawing is caused by displacement of the SMAS and aging of the skin. (Figs. 1 and 2)

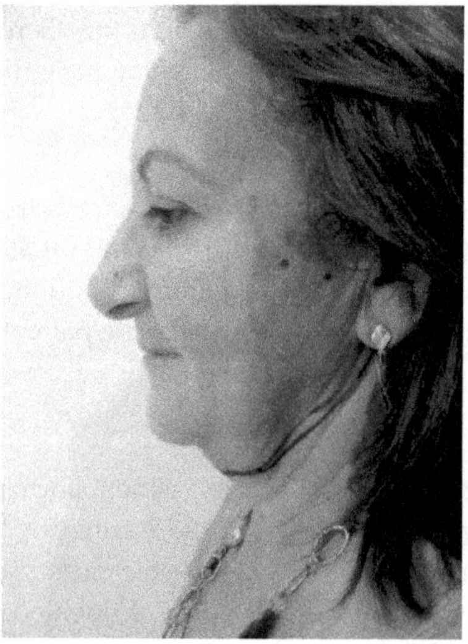

Figure 1. Example of jawing caused by displacement of the SMAS and aging of the skin

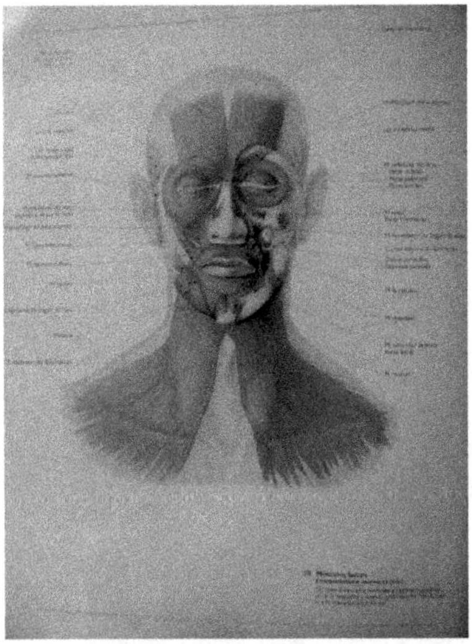

Figure 2. Example of jawing caused by displacement of the SMAS and aging of the skin

The neck is a face related area and an important part of the aging face. The SMAS is a fibro-muscular layer that connects platysma and galea and acts as a suspension for the overlying facial skin. (Fig. 3)

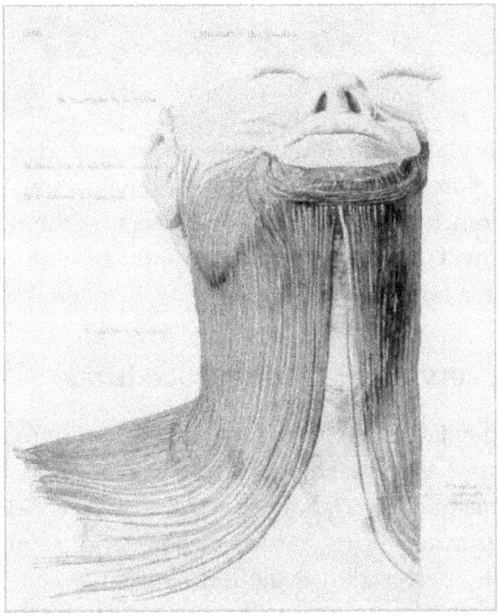

Figure 3. SMAS is a fibro-muscular layer that connects platysma and galea and acts as a suspension for the overlying facial skin

Performing face lift surgery, the continuity between aponeurotic facial fascia and the platysma is an anatomical fact that is very useful for surgeons. The SMAS lies deep to the subdermal plexus of vessels and superficial to the motor nerves of the facial musculature. It provides a suspensory sheet, which distributes forces of facial expression, mimetic and overlying skin. The idea that suspending this layer leads to a better long-term suspension has become common. (Fig. 4)

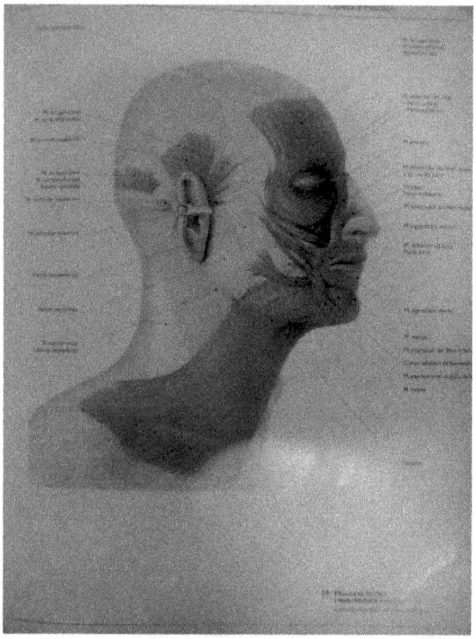

Figure 4. Side view of SMAS

SMAS overlies the parotid gland in mandibular angle and tends to be substantial and easy to handle, because the parotid gland, zeugmatic major and minor muscles protect underlying facial nerve branches. With regard to protecting the facial nerve structures, we can accept that Serdev lower SMAS-platysma face-lift "by sutures only" or "with retro-lobular incision" is done in a fairly secure area.

4. First technique for cervical flacidity procedures

The first proposed by Serdev technique was done with a 1cm retro auricular incision, careful dissection of subcutaneous tissue reaching platysma, clamping it and traction it with a mosquito. It fixation to mastoid periosteum was done with a 3-0 thread. After a time the same technique was performed with Serdev needle and semi elastic thread, without incisions, using only a tinny perforation at the retro auricular zone and some centimeters in front of the sternocleidomastoid muscle. Results depend on the flaccidity status of the skin, fat tissue amount and not too much hanging skin in the submandibular zone.

From this point, desiring to develop a technique that could give patients a good result, despite of high level of flaccidity in the submandibular zone, and aiming also a better definition of jaw line, I increased some alterations on classic techniques.

5. Surgical technique

The skin perforation points as well as fixation to colli fascia, mastoid or occipital periosteum should be planned previously, while the patient is sited or standing up in the surgical room, after photographing the face in standard protocol, the patient is asked to lay down marking the points where the needle will pass with a special surgical pen. The main points are marked over mastoid, 4cm from the sternocleidomastoid muscle, over the platysmal bands if they are visible and at the same places on the other side. Lidocain 2% with adrenaline is used to numb the region. (Fig. 5)

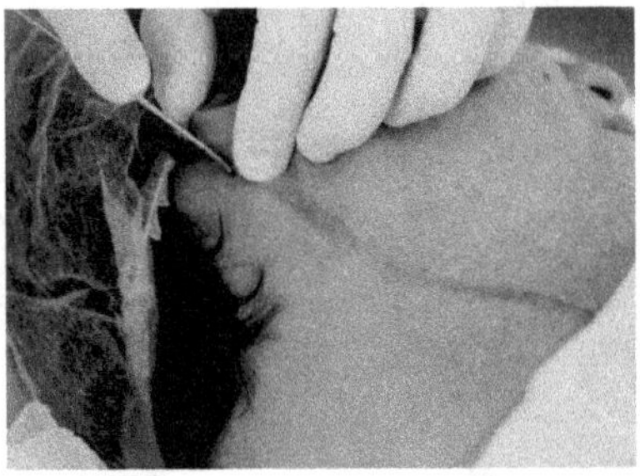

Figure 5. Administering the Lidocain 2% in order to numb the region

I start with a tiny incision using a scalpel blade number 11 from where a Serdev needle number 60 is introduced to reach the mastoid periosteum. Having a good tangential fixation to mastoid I move the needle towards subcutaneous tissue superficial to sternocleidomastoid muscle. Attention should be paid to superficial vessels as well as to the internal jugular vein and artery, passing above the sternocleidomastoid muscle avoiding any nerve and vessel damage (Fig. 6).

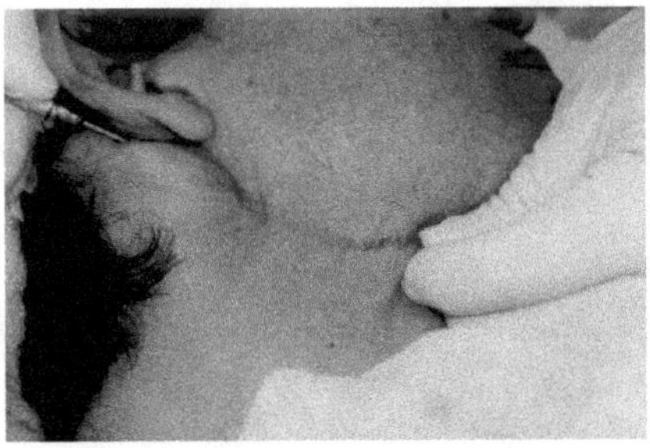

Figure 6. Incision using scalpel blade number 11

With a twisting movement I continue moving, pointing the tip of the needle down to reach platysma that is punctured in a zigzag way and getting out through the skin marks in a 90 degree angle avoiding dermal damage. (Fig. 7)

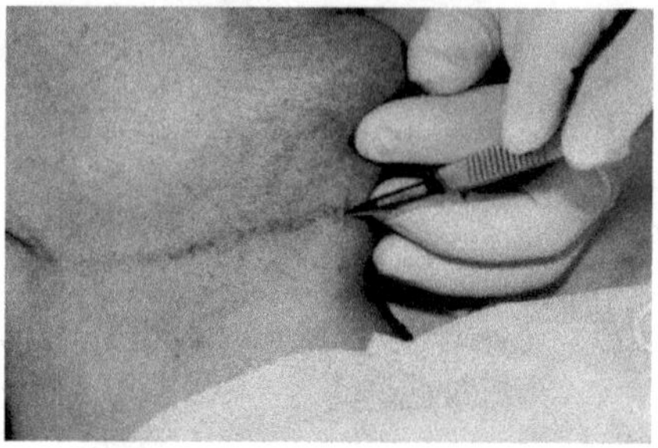

Figure 7. Reaching platysma

The needle is loaded with a number 2 semi-elastic thread and the needle is pulled through the first entry point. This thread has to be long enough to reach both sides twice. (Fig. 8)

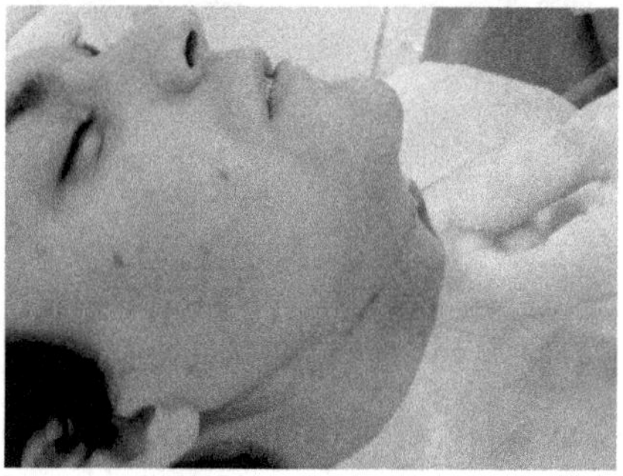

Figure 8. Placing a number 2 semi-elastic thread

The procedure goes along the same way using a Serdev needle 140 zigzag through platysma and additional skin perforations, until it reaches mastoid periosteum of the opposite side where the other thread's end will be exteriorized (Fig. 9).

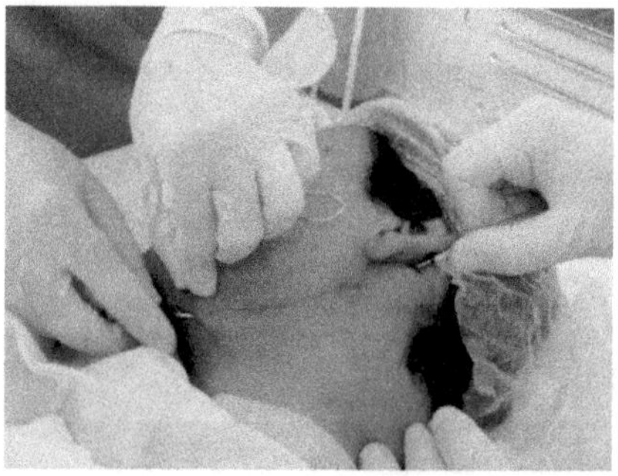

Figure 9. Reaching mastoid periosteum on the opposite side

Enough thread should be present to return until the submenthal mark is reached, where both thread ends will be tied with three knots which are made while the patient is sited, with medium elastic tension. (Figs. 10a and 10b)

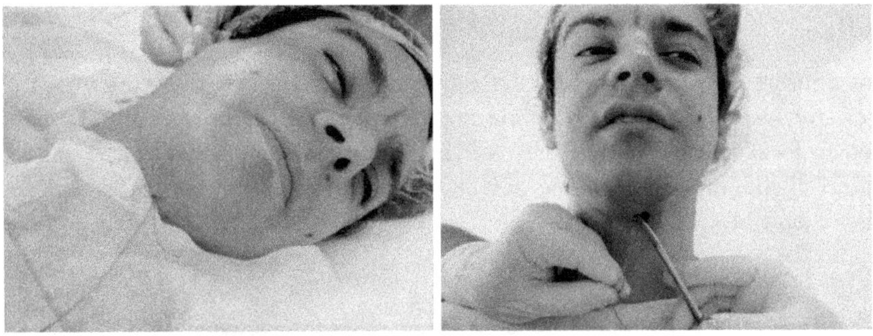

(a) (b)

Figure 10. Tying the knots

This will direct the skin flaccidity upwards improving the anatomical mandibulo-cervical angle, the mandibular line, and the sagging neck as well. (Figs. 11a and 11b)

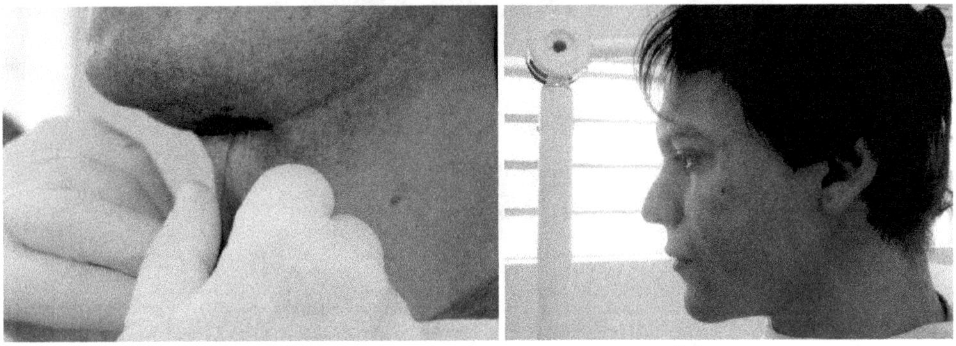

(a) (b)

Figure 11. Placing the patient is a sitting position will direct the skin flaccidity upwards

Possible skin dimples can be managed by pulling the skin laterally and away from the suture using a "mosquito" instruments. (Fig. 12.)

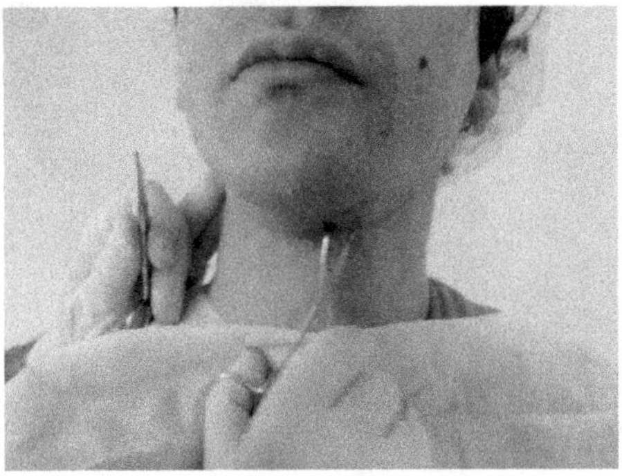

Figure 12. Using "mosquito" instrument

6. Results

The Serdev Suture for platysma generally shows excellent results. There are no visible scars, no sign of any operative intervention and no "operated" appearance at all. The patients are submitted to local anesthesia and the method is minimally invasive, that means, without severe surgical cuts or incisions. The day after the procedure the patient is back to normal life. (Figs. 13. and 14.)

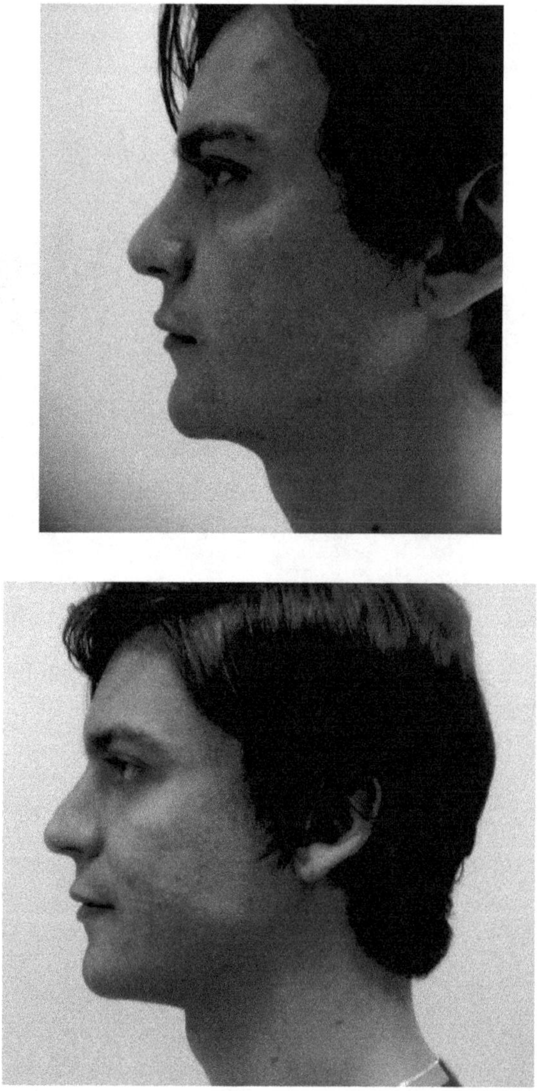

Figure 13. Example of before and after the procedure

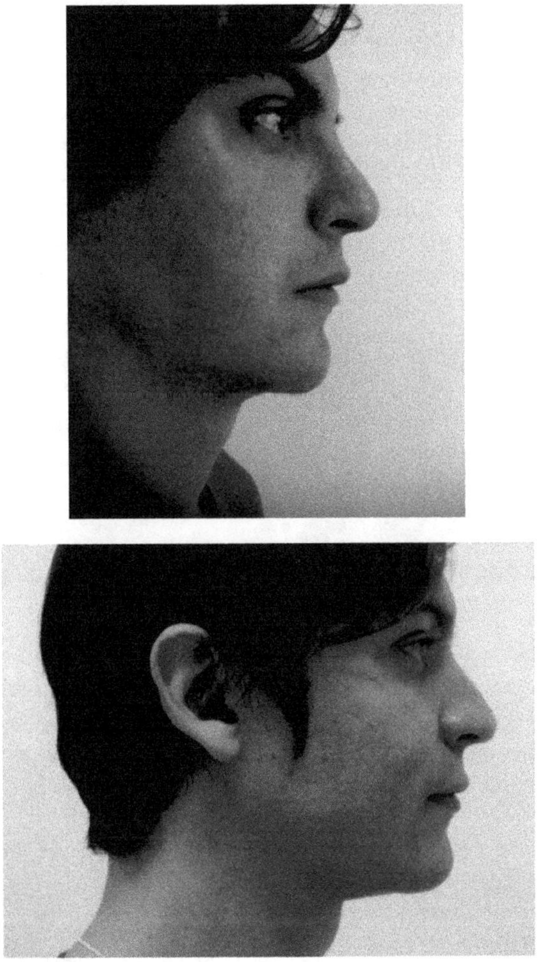

Figure 14. Example of before and after the procedure

Having performed seventeen patients with an indication of the modified technique over the past two years, some complications were observed, such as: two patients had pain in the first two days in front of the sternocleidomastoid, one of which also showed shrinkage the skin in this area. Detachment of the dermis with 18 gripped needle has been successful in improving the pain the day after. The other patient, from outside São Paulo, visited a plastic surgeon on her town who removed the thread.

Other four patients complained of discomfort in the mastoid region. Infiltration of 0,2ml of Dexametazone plus 0,2ml of 1% Lidocaine with epinephrine symptoms improved significantly after two days. One patient reported inflammation and infection at the place of the knot. Antibiotics and drainage of localized collection solved the problem without having to remove the thread. The degree of patient's satisfaction is high due to the simplicity of the technique and immediate results. Weekly follow up helps to solve complications.

7. Discussion

Beautification and immediate social activity are the first and most important patient's requirements. Classic rhytidectomy, in the past years were replaced by minimal invasive procedures with hidden incisions within the hair, extending around the earlobe and retroauricular area. Subperiosteal endoscopic surgeries have also been proposed. In recent years, with increasing demand of patients due to modern lifestyle, requiring less invasive surgical procedures with no visible scars, the Serdev's Sutures were developed, which give patients an optimal solution for face and neck beautification while preserving the natural appearance at the same.

In the case of medium flaccidity in the lower region of the SMAS and platysma, the first Serdev technique is recommended. In cases of excess sagging of the neck and laxity in the submental area, the extended modified technique (Serdev - Tullii), is a valid alternative to stretch the neck, the lower SMAS and platysma, anchoring them to the retroauricularly positioned mastoid. Also, the laxity of the submental area is affected by the suture elevating the hole area.

When the facial skin is also very flaccid, dermal rejuvenation techniques are employed (PRP, Peelings), to improve skin tonus prolonging the results.

If there is excess fat located in the submental region, first we should perform an ultrasonic liposuction with local anesthesia. The skin will retract sticking largely to the deep plane, avoiding extended surgeries. After months it could be necessary to add the first Serdev suture technique as a complement. Also, an submental incision would be performed with plications of the platysmal bands fixating one above the other with two folds.

8. Conclusions

The "Scarless submental platysmal suture band" using skin needle perforations only, or in combination with the Serdev suture lift techniques in lower face and neck "by hidden retro-lobular incisions" provide a safe and effective method for beautification of flaccid neck and submental area, as an independent procedure or combining with other techniques of rejuvenation in order to solve face and neck ptosis and aging appearance.

The platysmal Serdev – Tullii suture band in the submental area achieves a bidirectional lower face and neck lift, correction of submental area laxity. It is a safe and effective procedure that gives a pleasant result, the patient obtains a younger appearance maintaining a natural and harmonic expression without plastic surgical incisions. After the surgery there is minimal swelling and business people can work normally.

This much desirable effect of the method is immediate, without visible scars and fulfills patient's desires.

In cases of localized submental fat, the ultrasonic assisted liposuction in combination with our method is helpful to give the good definition of the cervicomandibular angle.

Author details

Roberto Tullii
Clínica Valian, Sao Paolo, Brazil

9. References

[1] Mitz V, peyronie M. The superficial muscculo-aponeurotic system (SMAS) in the parotid and cheek area. Plast Reconstr Surg 58: 80-88, 1976

[2] Brennan HG. Rhytidectomy: Mandibular and submandibular contouring. Facial Plastic Surgery Clinics of North America 1(2): 181-96, 1993.

[3] Baker DC, Conley J. Avoiding facial nerve injuries in rhytidectomy. Anatomical variations and pitfalls. Plast Reconstr Surg 6: 781-95, 1979

[4] Owsley JQ. SMAS-platysma facelift. A bidirectional cervicofacial rhytidectomy. Clin Plast Surg 3: 429-401, 1983

[5] Serdev, N.P. Forehead Subperiosteal Masklift in Combination with McIndoe Facelift Technique and Profile correction. The 7th IPRAS Congress European Section, Berlin, Germany, June 2-5, 1993

[6] Serdev, N.P. Temporal SMAS lift without skin excision in: Lip Augmentation During Mask and SMAS Lift Procedure, AAARS Annual Meeting, New Orleans, USA, October 5-9, 1994

[7] Serdev, N.P. Temporal SMAS Lifting of the Face. Life Surgery Workshop. Unidad Medica Clinica Del Country, Bogota D. C., Colombia, November 8-10, 1999

[8] Serdev, N.P. SMAS Liftingof the Face by Minimal Incisions – the Serdev Tecnhique. Life Surgery Workshop sponsored by International Academy of Cosmetic surgery and the Balkan Academy of Cosmethic Surgery, held at the Krilig Clinic in Caracas, Venezuela, November 12-18, 1999.

[9] Serdev, N.P. Principles of Face Beautification, Ier Congresso International de Cirurgia Cosmetica, Buenos Aires, Argentina, 31 Octubre – 1 de Noviembre 1999

[10] Serdev, N. P. Temporal SMAS lift, Lecture and Life Demonstration, 1st World Congress of Cosmethic Surgery with Life Demonstrations, Edsa Shangri-La Manilla and Quezon City Medical Center, Febuary 25-27, 2000

[11] Serdev, N. P. Temporal SMAS Lifting of the Face, Combined with Liposuction and Chin Augmentation Using Suture. Life Surgery Workshop, Tel Aviv, Israel, April 20-24, 2000

[12] Serdev, N. P. Principless of face beautification, The 3-rd World Congress of ISAS, Tokyo, April 8-10, 2000, 9W58

[13] Serdev, N. P. Lifting del SMAS con Una Pequenna Incision Temporal, VIIIas Journadas Mediterraneas de Confrontaciones Terapeuticasen Medicina y cirurgia Cosmetica, Sitges, Barcelona, March 16-19, 2000

[14] Serdev, N. P. Facial Rejuvenation by Minimal Skin Incisions, International Congress "Refiinments in Aesthetic Surgery" Oradea, Romania, June 22-24

[15] Gasparotti M. Superficial liposuction: a new application of the technique for aged and flaccid skin. Aesthetic Plast Surg 1992, Spring;16(2):141-53

[16] Gasperoni C, Salgarello M. MALL liposuction: the natural evolution of subdermal superfiction liposuction. Aesthetic Plast Surg 1994, Summer, 18(3): 253-7
[17] Perssonelle, J. G. Cosmiatria A Ciência da Beleza, 2004
[18] Kopf Maier, P, Wolf Heidegger Atlas na Anatomia Humana, Volume 2, Ed: 5, 28-36
[19] Rees and LaTrenta, Aesthetic Plastic Surgery, Cap. 28 "Composite Rhytidectomy" (Sam, T. Hamara, M.D.) 1994
[20] Rees and LaTrenta, Aesthetic Plastic Surgery, Cap. 26 "The Classic Operation" (Thomas D. Rees, M.D) 1994
[21] Serdev, N. P. Year 1994, Sutures suspension for lifting or volume augmentation in face and body (English version), Int.J.Cosm.Surg. 2001, Volume 1, Number 1, 2561-2568.

Chapter 8

Suture Lifting and Liposculpture Integration in the Creation of Facial Esthetic Harmony

Ronald Feiner and Chedly Bouzouaya

Additional information is available at the end of the chapter

http://dx.doi.org/10.5772/51246

1. Introduction

Youthful esthetic facial enhancement can be created with natural and scarless outcomes if innovative and minimally invasive surgical principles are properly employed. Feminine facial beauty can be characterized through mathematical, geometric and architectural constructs. However it is the triad of esthetically revealed eyes, curvaceous undulating cheek-lip landscape and a well defined jawline that hallmarks radiant feminine appeal.

In the contemporary setting numerous minimally invasive and non-invasive treatments are available for facial rejuvenation and beautification. Judicious use of soft tissue fillers, botulinum toxin, skin lasers, photothermics, platelet rich dermal stimulant therapies, chemical peels and bioactive topical applications have variously enabled cosmetic practitioners to exploit an intensifying non-invasive treatment armamentarium. In concert with these treatments, blepharoplasty using radiofrequency technology can be considered as a minimally invasive procedure. In lower lid blepharoplasty, the transconjunctival approach does not result in external scars at all. In the upper lid incision scars are very small and in time barely detectable when hidden in the natural upper eyelid crease.

It can be argued that traditional invasive rhytidectomy is a comparatively overly aggressive and in many circumstances obsolete procedure that should be reserved for relatively elderly case presentations or reconstructive situations. We have found the utilization of percutaneous suture lifting of flaccid or ptotic facial tissues can provide for a natural scarless alternative to invasive rhytidectomy surgery with the added advantage of respecting natural tissue vectors and contours. This is particularly important as the overly common "windswept" appearance associated with outcomes of traditional rhytidectomy can be avoided using percutaneous sutures without excision.

Furthermore, in appropriate cases the disciplines of liposculpture and percutaneous suture lifting can be synergistically integrated to attain a natural and esthetically pleasing facial harmony for the patient.

2. History

Historically there has been a steady evolution of percutaneous lift methods. Some techniques unfortunately did not achieve sufficient outcome durability and were accompanied by side effects and complications that included thread migration and extrusion. Rachel et al conducted a retrospective study reviewing 29 cosmetic patients evaluating the morbidity associated with a polypropylene barbed thread lifting technique and its long-term effects. This study demonstrated adverse events in 69% and early recurrence in 45% of the patients. The adverse events that occurred most commonly were pain, dimpling, visible threads, and foreign body reactions. [1]

Abraham et al in their study claimed that thread lift procedures provided only a limited, short term improvement that may have been largely attributed to post procedural edema and inflammation. Furthermore they asserted that the examined thread lifts relied on a similar basic technique involving subcutaneous placement of cogged threads along a planned trajectory, the threads being pulled to achieve the desired skin lift, secured and trimmed at the entry point. [2]

However such studies do not apply to certain well sustained and successful percutaneous thread lift techniques. Technique integrity necessitates methods that must be ingenious in anatomical design, providing for acceptable long term tissue suspension outcomes without significant side effects and risks.

The authors have found the percutaneous suture technique concepts invented by Serdev, N fulfill such requirements. Serdev has devised percutaneous suture lift techniques that are differentiated by the amalgamation of firmly anchored fixation of suspended lax soft tissues and non-barbed polycaproamide sutures with an extended period of absorption delay. [3]

Furthermore Serdev techniques often incorporate relatively deeper anatomical suture passes that enhance outcomes while avoiding impacts and potential injury to critical neurovascular structures. The authors are not aware of any other percutaneous suture lift design constructs that incorporate such innovative features that serve to reinforce the security, viability and extended duration of the desired tissue suspension. *(Detailed descriptions of the Serdev techniques authored by the inventor can be found elsewhere in this book.)*

3. Correction of anatomical pathology in midface aging

The authors regard enhancement of the eyes and midface as being critical to successful and youthful facial beautification. However the aging midface has always been a challenging region for cosmetic surgeons. Traditional techniques are complex and variably incorporate invasive rhytidectomy, malar implants and midface elevation with intraoral, temporal incisions or transcutaneous lower blepharoplasty incisions. Wulc & Hartstein wrote that "many of the procedures that have been innovated over the past 20 years are complex and are associated with steep learning curves and new complications. Some of these complications are difficult to manage. Some surgeons are sceptical of the longevity of the procedures designed to correct changes in this area. Many have adopted a particular procedure, only to have abandoned midface surgery altogether for any of these reasons."[4]

However all surgical considerations must take into account the pathological basis for midface aging which is characterised by changes in the central third of the face.[5] Structural changes develop with rhytid formation, progressive soft tissue ptosis and tissue atrophy.

The ideal youthful face is a proportional construct featuring a curvaceous convex into concave "S" shaped facial landscape known by the architectural definition of the "Ogee" curve.[6]

The youthful midface is characterized by prominent cheeks with a smooth transition between the lower eyelid-cheek interface which is an important aesthetic continuum and also a significant indicator of facial beauty. It is important to appreciated the lid-cheek interface is situated above or at level of the orbital rim in youth but with aging descends below the orbital rim. With midface aging the malar fat pad can atrophy and descend inferomedially over the SMAS with the development of a sulcus below the inferior eyelid. Correction involves vertical or superolateral elevation of an adequately volumized malar fat pad in order to restore a youthful midface esthetic.[7], [8]

The retaining ligaments of the malar fat pad and midface consist of the orbital retaining ligaments and lateral orbital thickening.[9] It should also be considered in relation to lower eyelid fat pad herniation that additional to the anterior migration that occurs through a weakened orbital septum, orbitomalar ligament fatigue permits an inferior migration of orbital fat. The diminished integrity of these facial retaining ligaments is fundamental in the pathogenesis of the soft tissue ptosis.

Suspension of the malar fat pad, suborbicularis occuli fat (SOOF) along with reconstitution of the orbibomalar ligament re-mounds the midface and supports (from below) the lower orbital soft tissue structures. With aging, sulcus formation occurs in the osseous insertions of these elongated ligaments, creating sunken appearance in this region.

Laferriere et al reported a percutaneous suspension technique of the malar fat pad anchored to deep temporalis fascia, repositioned it in a more youthful position. It was observed that this minimally invasive technique produced a long lasting elevation that would be a welcomed addition to midface rejuvenation. [10]

However the Scarless Serdev suture[R] percutaneous midface technique ("Cheekbone Lift") appears to be a unique construct on the basis that an inherent percutaneous ligamentous repair is established within the actual procedure. Unlike the case in traditional open surgery where invasive dissection and ligament release is often required before securing tissue elevation, Serdev's percutaneous midface technique does not necessitate ligamentous interruption prior to mobile tissue elevation. The lax mobile tissues to be lifted may include the malar fat pad, SOOF and what Serdev describes anatomically as "mobile muscle-cheek SMAS flap or fascial tube of buccal fat pad (also called Bichat's fat pad)". *(Detailed descriptions of this and other Serdev techniques authored by the inventor can be found elsewhere in this book.)*

It is important to appreciate that these facial soft tissue structures are elevated and suspended by suture fixation variously to the zygomatic periosteum "and in selected cases to orbital rim periosteum or temporoparietal tendon insertion and underlying periosteum, or upper temporal line periosteum and temporal fascia". [11] Thereby ligament laxity is not interrupted but instead effectively repaired with a concurrent elevation and fixation of these lax soft tissues. The procedure is conceptually ingenious while elegant in its simplicity.

Complimentary to the cheekbone lift is the concept of the Serdev Scarless Serdev suture[R] midface lift that sutures loose zygomatic SMAS extension to temporoparietal tendon insertion and underlying temporal periosteum. This technique achieves remarkably firm and secure fixation. [12] Naturally mounded or previously enhanced cheekbone tissues are elevated into a natural and youthfully vectored position. In essence the mid and lower face is securely suspended in a diagonal superolaterally directed elevation. This provides for a naturally inclined correction of the tissue fall induced by aging.

4. Synergistic integration of suture lifting and liposculpture

While the suspension of the aging midface is a key region for the restoration of youthful aesthetics, the authors have observed that enhancement of the midface is often more achievable after liposculpture has been performed in appropriate cases of submandibular soft tissue redundancy. This is an important consideration in the quest to optimize esthetic outcomes and was observed recently by Bisaccia et al who described the use of specialized 3-0 polypropylene sutures with absorbable cones to suspend platysma with combined, on occasions, with neck liposuction techniques to elevate sagging tissues of the face and neck, concluding that the technique had proven to be a useful addition to facial rejuvenation. [13]

Liposculpture is a very effective method of rejuvenation in the lower face, particularly in the submandibular region and jowls. It is a viable and minimally invasive alternative to traditional surgical face lifting particularly when combined with well anchored percutaneous suture lifting techniques as in the methods described by Serdev.

From an historical perspective, cosmetic surgeons performing formal face lifting have long recognized the need to consider concurrent neck liposculpture in appropriate cases of submandibular adipose accumulation. Adamson et al. observed that obtaining ideal results with cervico-facial rhytidectomy had frustrated facial plastic surgeons due to the difficulty of removing local excesses of adipose tissue in the submental, submandibular and other facial regions. They noted that open and closed liposuction techniques were being developed in conjunction with face lifting to improve the definition of the facial, mandibular and cervical contours. [14]

Over the several years we have observed that submandibular liposculpture not only improved the target anterior neck and lower face aesthetic but also seemed to improve the midface aesthetic. This is particularly so in younger patients. We have noted that certain other procedural strategies can be synergistic in the attainment of aesthetic facial harmony. Analysis of a patient's potential for an harmonious fascial aesthetic can focus the surgeon's treatment strategy. In suitable cases facial treatment favoring elimination of any prominent anterior neck laxity, ptosis and/or fat accumulation is preferable before attempting other aesthetic procedures for midface and perhaps even upper face enhancement.

This observation is consistent with Fournier's philosophy of esthetic semiology which implies that an interaction or interrelationship may exist between neighbouring tissues. [15] Fournier made particular reference to the contribution of the gravity, weight, hypertrophy or ptosis of the buttocks on the generation of lateral thigh or "saddlebag" deformity. Furthermore in cases where isolated volume reduction of the buttocks alone eliminated the anatomically inferior saddlebag deformity, the term "pseudo-saddlebag" deformity was coined. Fournier indicates that, along with other factors, errors in liposculpture technique can include miscalculation of the exact cause of a targeted fat accumulation. In order to determine the nature or aetiology of age related accumulation or ptosis of fat in many regions of the body, Fournier proposed that an analysis of various passive tissue maneuvers or active muscle contractions should made to assess tissue semiology. As the human body is naturally appreciated in the vertical perspective, the most obvious semiologicical factor to consider is gravity. Fischer, G. described performing liposculpture on a theatre table that is engineered to tilt vertically, enabling the effect of gravity on the tissues to be best appreciated during the actual procedure. Some other practitioners take the opportunity during the procedure to intermittently stand the patient in order to assess this effect. Fischer terms his technique "orthostatic liposculpture". [16]

Accordingly the impact of gravity must always be factored in any treatment plan. Such considerations relate to the expected influence of the gravity and weight of a superior tissue region on inferior location. However we have observed how the reduction of the inferiorly located submandibular adiposity can improve a superiorly located midfacial ptosis or projection insufficiency. We have termed this rather unexpected observation to be an example of "gravity inverted aesthetic semiology". Another example of this "gravity inverted" tissue interrelationship is the creation of the superiorly located "axillary roll" (or perhaps better phrased as "pseudo-axillary roll") in certain cases of the inferiorly located breast hypertrophy.

Zins et al concluded that young patients with minimal sub-platysmal fat can be treated by liposuction alone, reserving surgical skin excision for patients with severe skin excess or laxity. [17] However in most of these circumstances percutaneous suture lifts without recourse to skin excision provide for excellent tissue elevation, minimal trauma and without the imposition of scars for the patient.

5. Methodology

Traditional techniques are utilized for submandibular liposculpture with the aspirated fat (platelet rich plasma (PRP) enhanced) for transfer grafting to the midface if there is an indication of significant tissue atrophy in that region.

Fundamentally we have observed that closed suture lifting outcomes can be enhanced due to less strain imposed on the sutures. In other words we are "asking less" of the sutures by lightening the tissue load burden on them, diminishing the risk of suture fatigue and tissue suspension failure. Accordingly in appropriate cases, correction of a coexisting submandibular laxity by liposculpture lays the foundation for improved outcomes in minimally invasive closed suture face lifting and ultimately in other facial enhancement procedures.

Outcomes are readily observed clinically. We postulate that this midface enhancement is perhaps greater than one may expect from subtraction of sub-mandibular weight or the gravity "pull" effect alone. Indeed the subtracted tissue weight loss is generally minimal (20-60 grams fat). As Fournier suggests the totality of the aesthetic improvement is semiologic, possibly influenced by the interplay of factors such as physical mass, muscle tone, vascular, biochemical and hormonal changes in the altered regional tissue balance.

The following outlines our treatment method of a submandibular laxity/adipose accumulation in the aesthetic enhancement of both lowerface and midface disharmony.

All procedures are undertaken in the clinic operating theatre under local anesthetic tumescence (Klein type) alone. [18] Some patients elected to have a pre-med of oral Lorazepam 1mg 1hour before the procedure. We use one and two hole 1.5mm, 2mm & 3mm diameter liposculpture canulae and use a criss-cross (fanning) liposculpture technique. The liposculpture is performed anterior to the platysma. The marginal mandibular nerve and indeed all major vessels, nerves and endocrine gland structure lie deep to the platysma. We have found that the progressive development of a fibrous mesh support that occurs over several months is as important as the actual volume of fat removed. We have encountered no significant infections, bleeding or neural damage with this technique.

Following the liposculpture (either contemporaneously or a later date), suture lifting in the cheek and/or midface is undertaken in manner of the Serdev methods described earlier.

There seems to be a logical advantage when possible in delaying suture lifting until after the maturation of the liposculpture occurs over several months as swelling is diminished and tissue contraction maximized. The ptosed and redundant submandibular neck tissues can be seen to have been elevated and the mentocervical angle generally improved to 90-120 degrees. This is inherently associated with elongation of the neck which in itself is a very pleasing esthetic phenomenon. The soft tissue neck redundancy and ptosis having been corrected allows for powerful and secure percutaneous suture lifting, theoretically possible in all methods. However our own experience favors the combined cheekbone lift and midface lift in the manner of the aforementioned Scarless Serdev Suture^{R} methods. *[Figures 1. & 2.]*

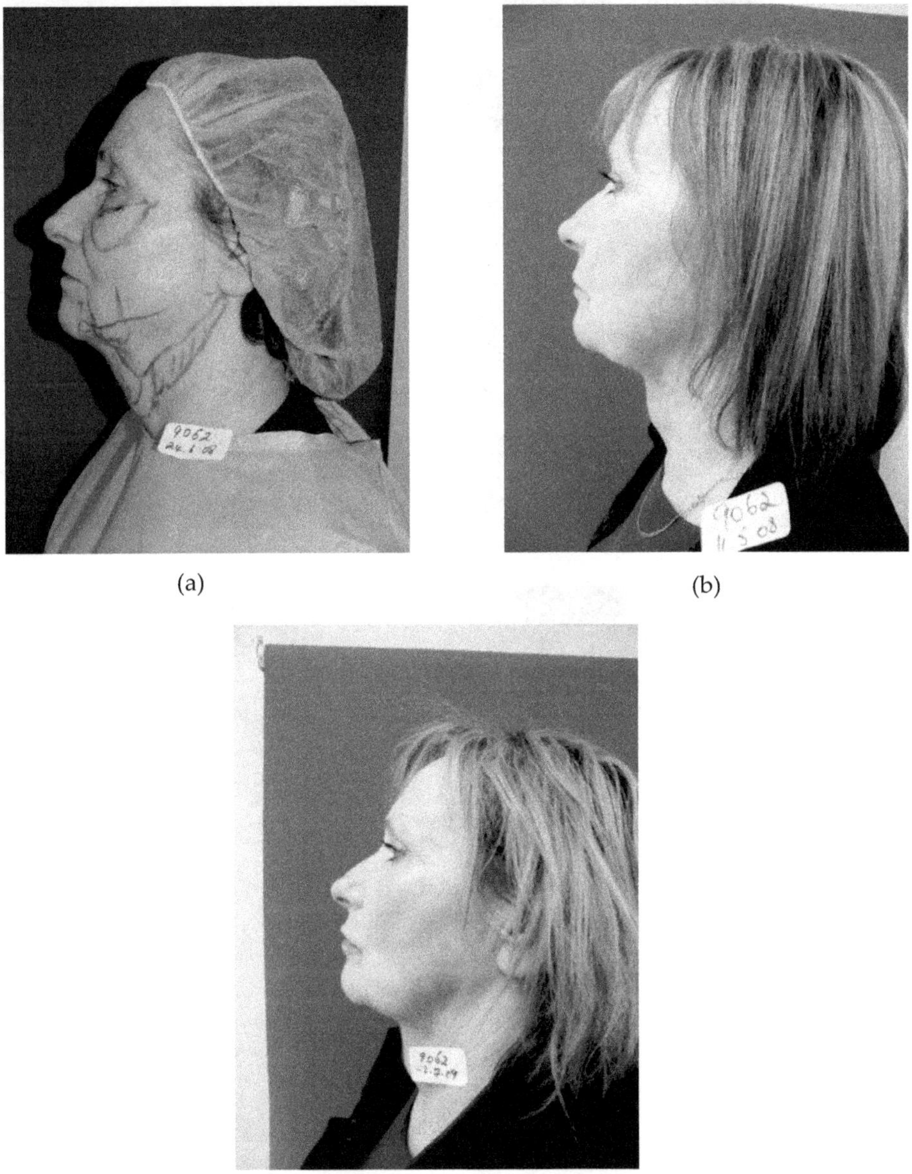

(a) (b)

(c)

Figure 1. 60 year old patient with midface atrophy and ptosis with associated with submandibular adipose accumulation and laxity. Note natural scarless outcome with esthetic angles and contours.

(a) Prior to treatment

(b) Post submandibular liposculpture

(c) Post subsequent Serdev type percutaneous cheek and midface suture lifts

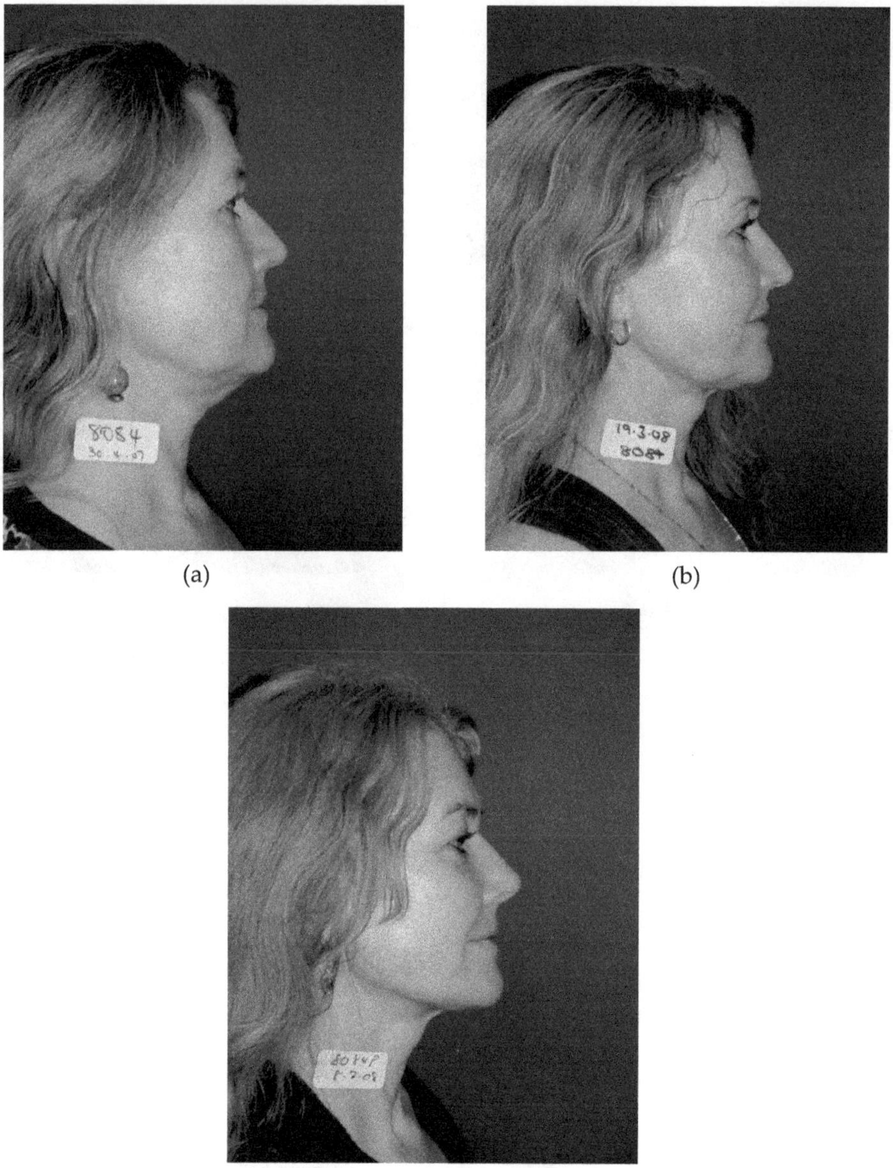

(a) (b)

(c)

Figure 2. 50 year old patient with midface atrophy and ptosis with associated with submandibular laxity. Note natural scarless outcome with esthetic angles and contours.

(a) Prior to treatment

(b) Post submandibular liposculpture with fat transfer graft to midface (plus Serdev type percutaneous suture brow lift)

(c) Post subsequent percutaneous cheek and midface suture lifts (plus Serdev type percutaneous nasal tip lift and lip augmentation by hyaluronic fillers)

Risks and major side effects are few when these techniques are properly mastered.

The combined risks and side effect profile of both treatment methods include infection, vascular trauma, neurological trauma, endocrine gland trauma and suboptimal outcomes.

In practice we have only experienced very occasional and trivial side effects that have resolved either spontaneously or with minor interventions. Specifically with percutaneous suture lifting, capture of dermal tissue in the sutures can result in skin tethering. However with experience and careful technique this risk can be minimized and if necessary corrected by tissue manipulation or even careful subcision.

Importantly for patient acceptance, both minimally invasive facial suture lifts and liposculpture techniques are easily achievable under local anesthetic alone. If required local anesthesia can be augmented by mild sedation.

6. Conclusion

The universal popularity for non-invasive aesthetic facial enhancement using commercial soft tissue fillers, botulinum toxin and skin photothermics/ lasers is well justified with excellent outcomes possible in the hands of creative surgeons. However none of these therapies can significantly elevate or suspend ptotic soft tissues.

Accordingly many surgeons continue to advocate formal invasive face lifting in such circumstances, resulting in permanent scars, significant risks and all too often unnatural looking outcomes. We find such invasive methods unnecessary as well performed and technically advanced percutaneous suture lifting can produce very pleasing and natural outcomes without scars.

While some percutaneous suture lift treatment failures have been reported in the literature, the authors have attained very pleasing outcomes using some of the innovative percutaneous suture lifting techniques in the manner outlined in this chapter. In cases of moderate to heavy submandibular fat accumulation, significantly improved suture lifting outcomes are likely if prior or contemporaneous submandibular liposculpture is undertaken.

Finally it worthy to observe that utilizing minimally invasive techniques places a high demand on the innovative instincts and skills of the treating surgeon. Patient expectations are for a significant esthetic facial enhancement to be achieved without the imposition of scars. Limited surgical field access makes this objective particularly challenging. Non-invasive procedures such as percutaneous suture lifting generate the quest for creative design that inevitably requires review and adaption. Ultimately elegant procedures yielding excellent surgical results predominate and are in turn a tribute to those surgeons who both invent and successfully modify them.

Author details

Ronald Feiner

Minimally Invasive Cosmetic Surgeon "Cosmetica Medical Aesthetic Clinic" Shire Central Building, Sydney, Australia

Chedly Bouzouaya
Occuloplastic Surgeon Belvedere Centre, Tunis

7. References

[1] Rachel JD, Lack EB, Larson B "Incidence of complications and early recurrence in 29 patients after facial rejuvenation with barbed suture lifting" Dermatologic Surg. 2010 Mar; 36(3):348-54
[2] Rima F. Abraham, Robert J. DeFatta, Edwin F. Williams III "Thread-lift for Facial Rejuvenation: Assessment of Long-term Results" *Arch Facial Plastic Surgery*. 2009; 11(3):178-183.doi:10.1001/archfacial.2009.10
[3] Serdev, Nikolay "Serdev suture techniques in Cosmetic Surgery ". International Journal of Cosmetic Surgery 6 (1): 408–503. (2006).
[4] Morris E. Hartstein (Editor), Allan E. Wulc (Editor), David EE Holck (Editor) Preface "Midfacial Rejuvenation" Pub: Springer Edition: 2012
[5] Yousif NJ. "Changes of the midface with age". *Clin Plastic Surg*.Apr 1995 22(2):213-26.
[6] http://www.merriam-webster.com/dictionary/ogee
[7] Graf R, Groth AK, Pace D, Neto LG.Facial rejuvenation with SMASectomy and FAME using vertical vectors. *Aesthetic Plast Surg*. Jul 2008; 32(4):585-92.
[8] De Cordier BC, de la Torre JI, Al-Hakeem MS, Rosenberg LZ, Costa-FerreiraA,Gardner PM, et al. Rejuvenation of the midface by elevating the malar fat pad: review of technique, cases, and complications. *Plast Reconstr Surg*. Nov 2002; 110(6):1526-36; discussion 1537-40
[9] Gamboa GM, de la Torre JI, Vasconez LO Surgical anatomy of the midface as applied to facial rejuvenation. *Ann Plast Surg*. Mar 2004;52(3):240-5.
[10] Laferriere KA, Castellano RD. Experience with percutaneous suspension of the malar fat pad for midface rejuvenation.Facial Plast Surg Clin North Am. 2005 Aug;13(3):393-9.
[11] Serdev, Nikolay "Serdev Suture Methods on the Face" Int. Journal Cosmetic Surgery Volume 8 No.3 Pages 1504-1553
[12] Serdev, Nikolay "Midface lift-The Protocol" Int. Journal Cosmetic Surgery Vol 11 No. 3 Pages 9-10
[13] Emil Bisaccia et al Dermatologic Surgery Volume 35, Issue 4, pages 645–650, April 2009
[14] Adamson PA; Cormier R; Tropper GJ; McGraw BL Cervicofacial liposuction: results and controversies.) J Otolaryngol. 1990; 19(4):267-73
[15] Pierre F. Fournier MD, Liposculpture the syringe technique, Arnette, Paris, 1991, Pages 185-187
[16] Giorgio Fischer; Via della Camiluccia, Rome, Italy; "Liposuction Principle and Practice" –"Orthostatic Liposculpture" 10.1007/3-540-28043-X 31_Melvin A. Shiffman and Alberto Di Giuseppe Pub. Springer Berlin Heidelberg
[17] Zins JE; Fardo D "The "anterior-only" approach to neck rejuvenation: an alternative to face lift surgery." Plast Reconstr Surg. 2005; 115(6):1761-8
[18] Klein J.A, Anaesthesia for liposuction in dermatological surgery. J Dermatol Surg Oncol 1988 Oct: 14 (10): 1124-32

Chapter 9

The Holistic Scarless Rejuvenation of the Face

M. B. Des Fernandes

Additional information is available at the end of the chapter

http://dx.doi.org/10.5772/56203

1. Introduction

This chapter will concentrate on the holistic approach to harmonious facial rejuvenation by concentrating on the procedures that should accompany every face-lift procedure. In particular I will concentrate on facial rejuvenation in younger adults or those who do not need a full facelift with excision of skin. However, the principles of holistic rejuvenation of the face remain the same.

Rejuvenation of the face is commonly asked for yet, sadly, often not delivered. A Face-lift is not automatically facial rejuvenation. Surgeons who concentrate on surgery only fail to recognize that the very best surgery done without any attention to the skin will deliver only a semblance of rejuvenation and very often a disharmony between structure and surface appearance. For real rejuvenation, one needs to pay attention to the skin in particular and restore *naturally young,* and not just *smoother* skin. As aesthetic surgeons we have to be sure that our patients get the best advice for rejuvenation. This is my experience and when a patient comes for facial surgery I explain that there are three important steps that we should always attend to:

1. First of all we need to make sure that our patients use skin care that can actually rejuvenate skin. The only molecule so far described in the history of skin care that actually rejuvenates skin physiologically as well as in appearance is vitamin A. We do not need to use retinoic acid to get these effects because we can use the pre-cursors of retinoic acid e.g. like retinyl palmitate to get exactly the same end-result without the irritation normally encountered when using retinoic acid. However, there are very few products available that contain effective quantities of vitamin A. One way to ensure that you are recommending a product with sufficient vitamin A is to choose a product that presents vitamin A in gradually increasing doses till the maximum dose is reached. We have at the same time to remember that skin care alone cannot make photodamaged skin return to younger skin. This is where we need to add regeneration of youthful skin through skin needling.

2. The second step for the most convincing, scarless rejuvenation of the facial skin is Collagen Induction Therapy (CIT) by skin needling to generate platelet-derived growth factors and regenerate skin (P-CIT). [1] This is the only process yet described in the medical literature that causes regeneration of skin and the normal latticework matrix.
3. Finally, a simple face-lift without attention to the mid-face will not produce a convincingly younger face. The mid-face is the key to a youthful appearance because it not only addresses the naso-labial folds, but also rejuvenates the lower eyelids and lifts up the corner of the mouth. In fact the mid-face-lift addresses most of the concerns of many people seeking a face-lift. The ideal situation is where the intervention occurs at an earlier rather than a later time and the facial tissues can be lifted by sutures or threads and repositioned in their youthful position. [2]

2. Restoring the skin surface through scientific skin care

Vitamin A is a normal component found in our skin and is absolutely essential for healthy skin. [3] However, vitamin A is rapidly destroyed by exposure to light because it is in fact a natural sunscreen and absorbs UVA and UVB rays [4]. As a result our skin develops a chronic, progressive and unrelenting deficiency of vitamin A that manifests as pigmented blotches, wrinkles, thin skin, and pre-cancerous lesions that eventually develop into skin cancer. This is exactly the sort of person who may present to you for a face-lift. Fortunately, by restoring normal levels of vitamin A we can reverse these effects and create healthier skin. The earlier the patient starts to use Vitamin A topically, the better. Do not waste time thinking about Alpha hydroxyacids except to enhance the effects of vitamin A products. Only vitamin A has this power to rejuvenate the skin cells and restore more normal function.

While sunscreens can give protection, the safety of the skin depends to a large extent on the quantity of vitamin A and other antioxidants in the skin. Keep the skin rich in Retinyl palmitate (RP) because it is the major form of cellular vitamin A. RP is relatively non-irritating and is converted into every possible metabolite of vitamin A. As a result, when used topically at adequate dosage, it affords us the most acceptable method of vitamin A replacement. Research shows us that Retinyl palmitate plays a role in preventing skin cancer [5] and squamous skin cancer cells have an impaired ability to esterify retinol [6]

Doctors generally think retinoic acid is the only effective vitamin A but retinyl palmitate, as described above, is the major form of vitamin A in the human body and skin [3]. Retinyl esters are de-esterified to retinol, which is then oxidised by alcohol dehydrogenases to retinal and finally retinoic acid [7]. There seems to be a feedback mechanism whereby retinoic acid production is controlled by increasing or decreasing the esterification of retinol to retinyl palmitate. [8] The ratio is tightly controlled with the retinyl esters being 91% and retinol, retinal and retinoic acid each at 3%. By increasing the RP one automatically increases the quantity of retinoic acid that is the molecule that interacts with the DNA.

Guide your patients to healthier, lovelier skin by using products containing vitamin A, especially RP. [9] [10] [11]. Make sure that the creams are adequately supported by antioxidant vitamins at the same time. Pay particular attention that they contain vitamin C (preferable in its ester form and particularly ascorbyl tetra-isopalmitate. Vitamin C and E are the dominant antioxidant vitamins of the skin [12].

Figure 1 shows the degree of photo-damage often seen in "sun-worshipping" people who may come to you for surgery and Figure 2 shows the changes that can be expected from using topical vitamin A as retinyl palmitate in doses that I recommend. The skin is clearly healthier.

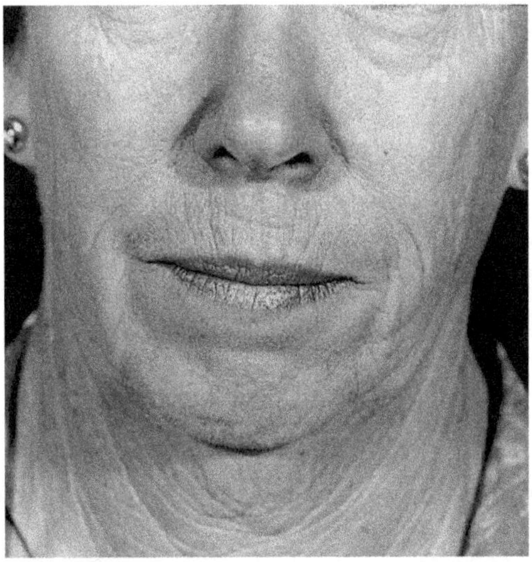

Figure 1. Before using vitamin A, C and antioxidant skin care.

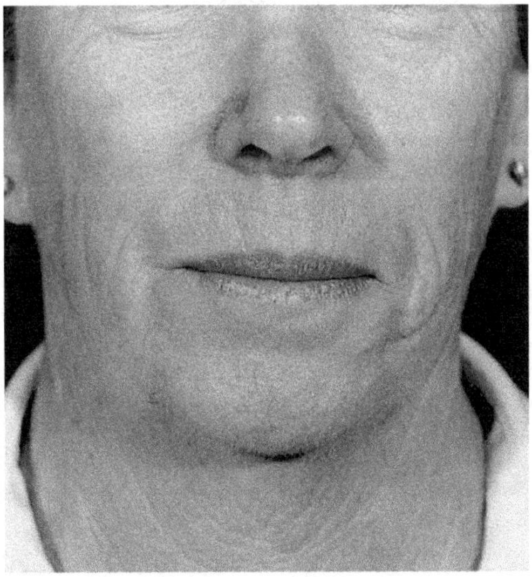

Figure 2. Six months after using vitamin A, C and antioxidant skin care.

Clinical effects of topical retinyl palmitate

- It affects the genes of the stem cells so that the keratinocytes grow and look more normal. It increases the growth of the basal layer (growth layer) of skin cells that causes thickening of the epidermis. Not only does the skin get thicker; it also heals faster because the cells are growing faster.
- Vitamin A improves the horny layer, so it makes the skin more resistant to environmental pollution. [13]
- Melanin in keratinocytes becomes more evenly distributed. [14]
- The production of melanin by melanocytes is generally reduced to the normal constitutional colour of the skin.
- The production of sebum is decreased in oily skin. [15]
- Vitamin A supports and potentiates the Langerhans cells of the skin. [16]
- It affects the fibroblast cells, the most important cell in the dermis, particularly the genes for the production of collagen. Healthier collagen is formed and unhealthy collagen is removed by enzyme activity. [17]
- It increases the secretion of natural moisturising factors by the fibroblast cells of the dermis into the space between the cells, allowing the skin to retain more water with some puffing out of the wrinkles. These natural moisturising factors filter up into the epidermis between the cells. Glycosaminoglycans are some of the chemicals created by the fibroblast to help retain moisture. [18]
- The blood supply to the deeper layers of the skin is improved, which means that nutrition of the skin is improved. The skin also assumes a healthier colour.

Vitamin A should be used twice daily and if used during daylight hours it should be accompanied with anti oxidant vitamins like vitamin C, E and beta carotene, so that it is better protected from ultra violet light. Vitamin A metabolism is strongly tied to vitamin C, and vitamin C is essential for the proper function of vitamin E. The concept of the balanced use of these vitamins as the main way of maintaining skin health is becoming more and more certain with current research work. Our skin is constantly exposed to light and light destroys certain essential chemicals in our skin. We can never escape this fact. A reliable UVA and UVB sunscreen with sun protection factor SPF 15 – 20 should be used at the same time in preference to high SPF products over 30. Vitamin A should also be replaced every evening as a topical application to the skin to try and address the loss of vitamin A from being in light. Because we cannot prevent the damage to the vitamin A in the skin, it is essential to replace the vitamin A each day so that we minimise the signs of photoaging that are really also the signs of accumulative vitamin A and antioxidant deficiency of the skin.

Recommended skin care regime:

Select a skin care regime that offers vitamin A as retinyl palmitate especially, or retinyl acetate, retinol or even retinaldehyde. I prefer a heavy bias towards retinyl palmitate and the vitamin A should be offered in a series of creams that increase from low levels right up to 50,000 i.u. per g., which is the maximum permitted dose for vitamin A in cosmetics in the European Union. You cannot start at high doses because that would induce a retinoid reaction that would dissuade the patient from using the product. Start on the lowest and even that levels will still give excellent changes [19]. Then for maximum results gradually build up to the strongest permitted concentration. The simultaneous use of stable versions of vitamin C and other antioxidants is essential. Peptides such as Matrixyl are particularly valuable in giving tighter smoother skin. The patient ideally should start this skin care regime before surgery and continue forever afterwards to maintain the best, healthiest skin.

The effects of topical vitamin A and C and antioxidants and even peptides can be enhanced by using a device that punctures only the stratum corneum[1] Even greater tightening of the skin may be obtained as witnessed by Figures 3 and 4 which show skin before being treated with vitamin A and antioxidants[2] and the Skin-Roller and then the appearance after one year. This demonstrates tightening that is normally only achieved after heavy peels or intensive treatments with fractional laser or radio-heating devices. However, this was done by the patient herself with a simple device that caused absolutely no pain or discomfort.

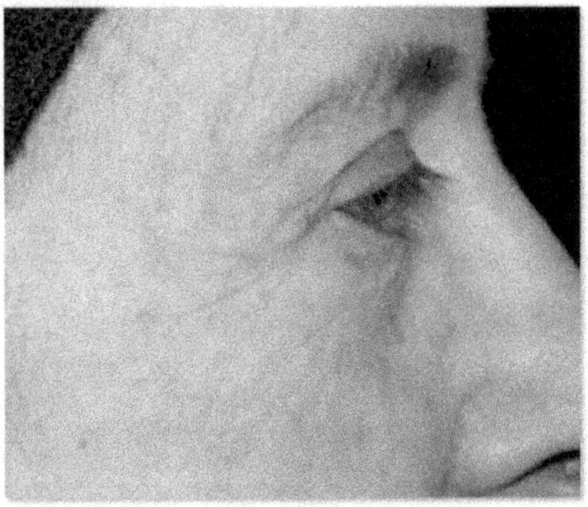

Figure 3. photo-damaged skin before starting vitamins A, C and antioxidants.

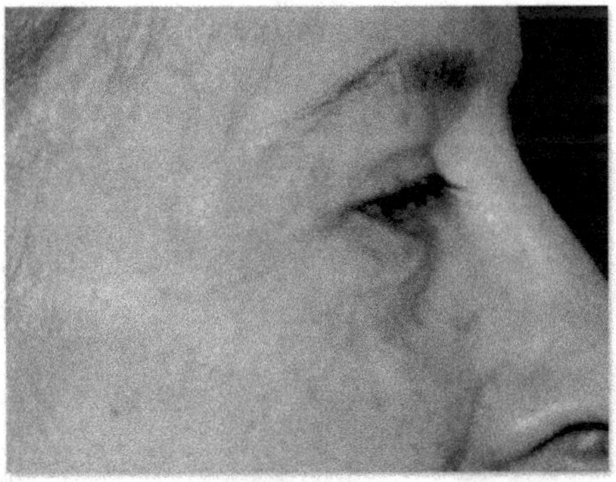

Figure 4. One year later with no surgery peeling or anything else except daily skin care enhanced by using the Cosmetic Skin Roller

[1] The Environ Cosmetic Skin-Roller

[2] Environ Skin Care

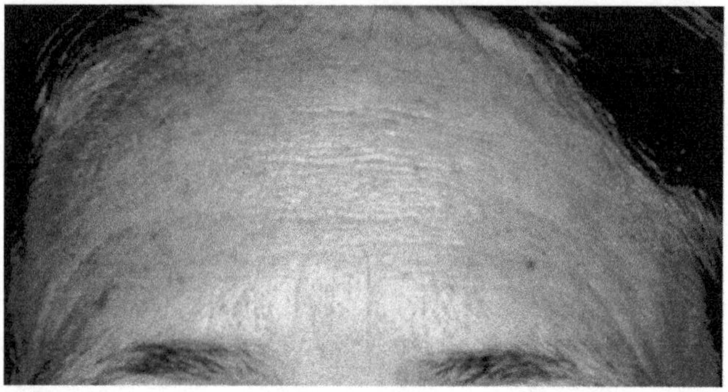

Figure 5. Lower face before needling with 3 mm Roll-CIT

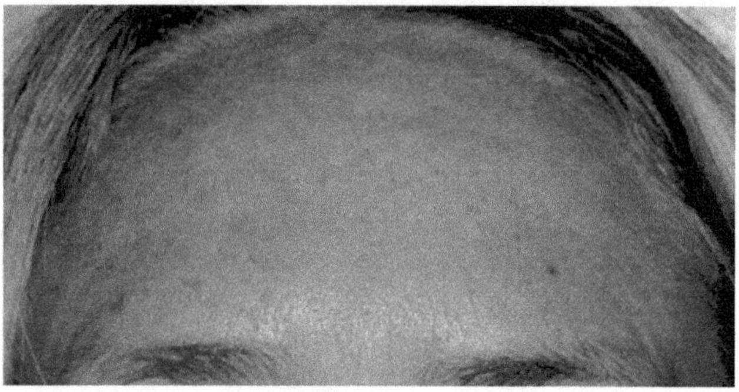

Figure 6. After Roll-CIT and skin care.

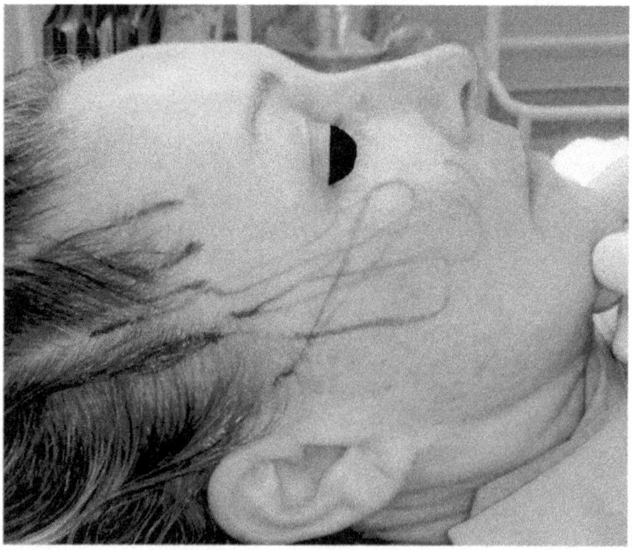

Figure 7. Markings for suture loops of the cheeks. In this case a number of loops have been marked in case they will be needed to get full tightening of the facial tissues. Generally by adding the Silhouette sutures, one can avoid adding extra loops.

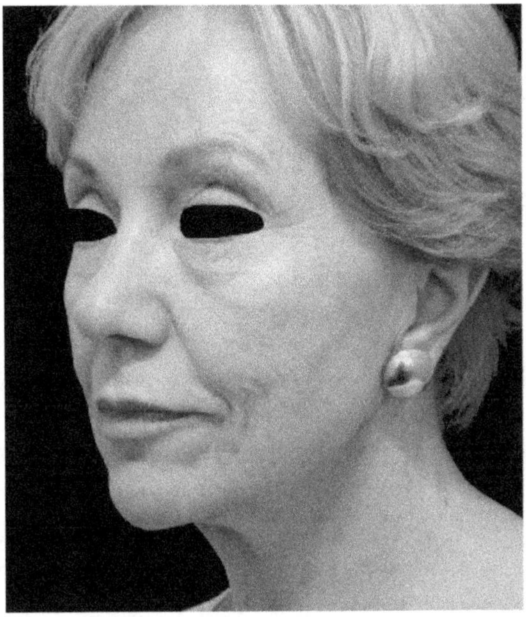

Figure 8. This patient has had a face-lift but was not given a mid-face-lift and is unhappy with the result. One can understand this because the corners of her mouth turn down and she still has a heavy naso-labial fold.

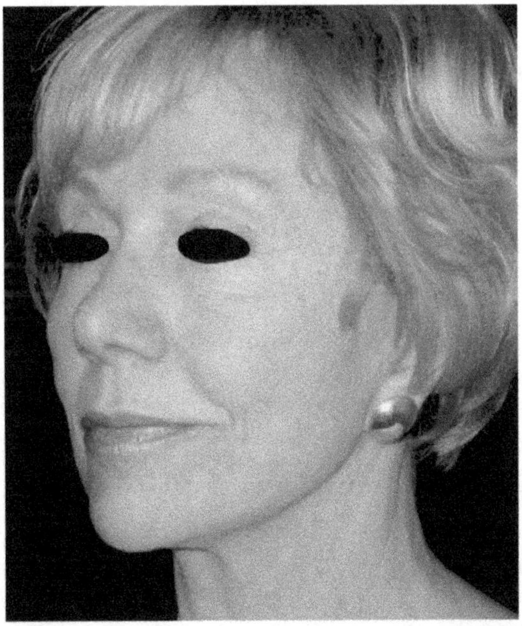

Figure 9. One year after a scarless suture suspension mid-facelift only and skin care with vitamins A, C and antioxidants enhanced by the use of the Cosmetic Skin Roller.

Summary of Skin Care

Vitamin A, particularly as retinyl palmitate, is probably the safest way to protect skin from solar irradiation and may also be used for protracted periods to rejuvenate skin. The ideal treatment would be to apply topical vitamin A to the skin starting at an early age, soon after our first exposure to light, and continuing the daily replenishment of vitamin A into old age. Not only would this maintain healthy young looking skin, but most likely would also protect against cancer.

While skin care can make a big difference and when used under ideal conditions, may hold back the clock of photoaging, most patients present to us with well established damage and skin care needs to be supplemented with a more radical and new technique that actually regenerates younger skin.

3. Regenerating skin through percutaneous Collagen Induction Therapy (p-CIT)

Needling skin is rapidly becoming an established method to rejuvenate skin and refine scars that is competing with ablative and minimally ablative procedures. [1] While the technique may seem new, we actually have centuries of experience of needling skin because tattooing has been practiced in both "civilized" and "primitive" cultures all around the world. Needling stands above all other currently used treatments because it has been shown to be the first method described, as far as we can determine, that conclusively regenerates tissue and restores the natural lattice-distribution of collagen of the dermis. Neither fractionated laser or any other treatments induce regeneration of tissue. To date it is the only described skin treatment that regenerates elastin [20]. It has a wide list of indications and can be used on all ages and all different coloured skins with safety.

To achieve results one has to cause bleeding of the skin because it is the release of platelets that stimulates the regeneration of tissue, and the degree of improvement is directly related to the amount of bleeding. Since I first started needling in 1994 I have been searching how to get the best out of needling.

Here are my guidelines:

I always insist that the patient should use topical vitamin A and C and antioxidants for at least three weeks before the procedure. I persuade my patients to use a device with needles protruding only 0.2 mm as a "rolling massage" system so that only the stratum corneum is punctured and this allows better action of the applied vitamin A etc. See figure 3 and 4

I first started experimenting with needling of the skin in the early 1990"s and by 1996 started the micro-needling of skin in the way that we now do it.

I called the process Collagen Induction Therapy and that term is used around the world and usually abbreviated to CIT. [21] [22]

Then I recommend **The Medical Roll-CIT** that has needles that protrude 1.0 – 1.5 mm so that the needles will penetrate right down into the dermis and rupture the tiny arcade capillaries in the dermal papillae (rete pegs). Bleeding releases platelets and the platelets in turn release growth factors and particularly TGF-Beta-1, 2 and 3. TGF-beta-1 and 2 soon disappear after needling in direct contrast to the levels seen after a surgical incision. TGF-beta-3 disappears within 24 hours after a surgical incision whereas with needling it is raised for more than two weeks and that seems to be responsible for regeneration [23] of tissue and natural lattice arranged collagen fibres and elastin.

Generally I recommend that the patient should have six sessions of needling done once a week under topical anaesthesia, or if they prefer, then they could have one intensive session done with nerve block and local anaesthetic infiltration. The difference is that with the lighter sessions under topical anaesthesia, they can return to work the very next day whereas after an intensive needling, they will be swollen and bruised for about four days.

I use a unique cream-form of low concentration TCA cream[3] that I apply for 20 minutes before and then for only four minutes after the needling session. I believe this gives me better results. I do this to clean the skin and reduce the chance of an infection in people with acne spots. The second reason for doing this is that I deduce that lower pH levels induce the release of growth factors from the keratinocytes.

The technique for needling is simple and has been well described. [21] Basically one keeps rolling until one has made as many holes as one can either physically or when topical anaesthesia is used, until the patient finds it uncomfortable.

By doing skin care and then skin needling I can offer my patients a safe way to get smooth clear healthy younger-looking skin without any risks. The results, according to many observers, outrank the results achieved with fractionated lasers and radio-frequency devices etc.

I have used iontophoresis and sonophoresis of vitamin A and C immediately after the needling treatment to maximize the induction of healthy collagen. Iontophoresis also tends to reduce the swelling of the skin and I also recommend it after all facial surgery. Low Frequency Sonophoresis can be used to enhance penetration of peptides to induce more collagen and elastin production.

In summary, Skin needling

1. Tightens skin laxity and restores normal skin tension in the early stages of ageing. Some patients who are worried about face-lift surgery may be satisfied with simple Percutaneous CIT. The arms, hands, abdomen, thighs, and buttocks can also be treated to give total rejuvenation. In fact this has become the only "anti-ageing full body treatment that we have.
2. Treats fine wrinkles. The interesting feature about skin needling is that it sets up a metabolic mechanism that replaces photo-damaged fibres and re-invigorates cells to regenerate skin. As one would expect, this cannot happen overnight, so it is not

---

[3] Environ Acid Cream Mask

surprising that the regeneration phase is prolonged and there is continual improvement over many months. I believe the best time to judge the final result is about one year after the needling sessions. Our photographs show that the three-month picture is not as good as the six-month picture and the photograph at the end of the year is the best. This is quite different from the commonly used soft lasers etc. where the best time to take the post-intervention picture is within three months after the treatment otherwise the results become more difficult to see.

3. Reduces Acne scarring and it is gratifying to see that previously scarred skin is slowly replaced by normal looking skin. Interestingly enough, histology shows reduction of scarring and restoration of the normal architecture of the skin.
4. Stretch marks respond well to skin needling even when they have become "silvery" after a long time. This however, is not a problem with facial work except in rare cases where there are stretch marks on the neck.
5. Scars are always improved - even if they are white, old scars they can become more skin coloured.
6. Burn scars – both flat and hypertrophic scars can be treated with success and de-pigmented areas are restored to even normal coloured skin.

Advantages of PCI

1. PCI does not damage the skin. The epidermis remains intact. Histology done at 24 hours, a week, and several months after needling fail to show any signs of damage.
2. Any part of the body may be treated. It is excellent for rejuvenating hands so that younger looking hands can accompany facial rejuvenation.
3. Skin becomes thicker as has been repeatedly demonstrated in histological studies. The epidermis is thickened by vitamin A and antioxidant creams but the restoration of a healthy lattice of collagen and elastin results from skin needling. We have never seen excessive deposition of collagen or any sign of scar collagen after skin needling.
4. The healing phase is short. With milder needling under topical anaesthesia, the patients can normally return to work the next day. Most patients select this form of needling but some people choose intensive needling because of time constraints and even do needling at the same time as the scarless minimally invasive face-lift. That way their healing period from needling over-laps with the healing of the facial lifting.
5. Not as expensive as laser resurfacing.
6. The skin does not become sun sensitive so this can be done any time of the year.
7. Can be done on people who have previously had laser resurfacing, or those with very thin skin. The skin always thickens up so the ugly complication of translucent skin following CO2 laser re-surfacing can be treated. I like these patients to use topical vitamin A for a minimum of three months prior to needling.
8. I have never seen hyper-pigmentation in patients with darker skins e.g. African, Indian, Malaysian, Chinese and Mediterranean skins.
9. Telangiectasia may disappear totally. I think the explanation for this may lie in the fact that the tiny vessels are repeatedly fractured and cannot be easily re-constituted.

10. Does not really have to be done by a doctor but should be done under their supervision. In my office the skin-care therapists and nurses, do the needling and that makes it more affordable for the patient.
11. The technique of Medical Roll-CIT is easy to master and is easily taught by a demo DVD. Medical Focus-CIT is also useful for smaller areas and makes the treatment more affordable.
12. Can even be done with topical anaesthesia.

Disadvantages of PCI:

1. Exposure to blood. If the procedure is done properly there will be exposure to blood so the proper precautions have to followed
2. While we cannot achieve as intense a deposition of collagen as in laser resurfacing, we can repeat the treatment and get even better results that will last even longer. The scar collagen following laser resurfacing is dense and often reflects white through the skin. These scar collagen fibres, as with any other scar, are resorbed over time. It seems that the normal collagen latticework is not affected in the same way and is only damaged by light.
3. Local anaesthetics limit the area that may be treated and in some cases a general anaesthetic is required e.g. when extensive areas or virtually the whole body is needled.

This is a simple technique and with the right tool it is easy and fast to puncture any skin thoroughly. While one treatment may not give the smoothening seen with ablative laser re-surfacing, the epidermis is normalised and if the result is not sufficiently improved it can safely be repeated as often as necessary. The technique can be used on areas that are not suitable for peeling or laser re-surfacing.

Some Pitfalls to avoid.

1. Never use retinoic acid after needling. It irritates the skin and the patient is also less likely to use it properly.
2. Never use Ascorbic acid preparations immediately after needling. Experience has shown me that the ascorbic acid can cause a deep, destructive peel.
3. Never use any strong peeling agents immediately after a peel. The peel will be very much deeper than expected and may cause scars.
4. Needling is painful for about 20 minutes after the operation so, if the procedure has been done with general anaesthesia and without local anaesthetic infiltration, do make sure that the patient is given adequate analgesia before waking up.

Skin Needling induces collagen and elastin induction by employing the body's natural mechanisms that for the first time, as far as we know, produces regeneration of the skin and it's matrix. There is no scar formation and the procedure can safely be repeated until the desired effect is achieved. This can be repeated as often as necessary after face-lift surgery.

4. Lifting the most important component of the face with the scarless Mid-face-lift

Younger patients in their thirties and early forties are presenting to the plastic surgeon because they want to

- Reduce the early tear-trough shadows that run obliquely across their cheeks, and
- Early naso-labial grooves that make them looked tired and jaded. This results from the medio-inferior descent of malar fat and Sub Orbicularis Oculi Fat. There is a loss of the "ogee" curve of the face and in order to restore a youthful appearance to the face the surgeon has to reposition these two essential "padding" structures. However, this is not achieved even with the standard full face-lift, which tends to address the lower face and hardly deals with the mid-face. Improvement of the sagging mid-face can only be achieved by re-positioning of the malar and SOOF pads. We cannot approach this area without causing noticeable scars and because we are aesthetic surgeons we have to try and do this with virtually no scars.

I believe the solution is to anchor the tissues of the cheek with loops of non-absorbable sutures, to the temporal fascia on the side of the head and avoid making visible scars. I call this "Suture Suspension Loops" which I started doing in 1994. Alternatively, or in combination one can use specially designed anchoring threads to lift the midface tissues. After using various types of these threads I prefer Silhouette threads [24] either alone or in combination with suture suspension loops.

Suture suspension Loops

By using a number of 4/0 non-absorbable suspensory suture-loops, positioned in the malar fat pads with a spinal needle, one can easily lift the malar and sub-orbicularis oculi fat to create a youthful lower eyelid and ogee curve to the face. The principle is surprisingly simple and will be described in more detail [2]. However, there are many small tips and I found a rather steep "learning curve" in developing this procedure.

These threads are anchored by using 4-6 stab-incisions in a special pattern behind the temporal and side-burn hairline. Then I define the tissues of the malar fat pads and one easily can see that traction on these tissues will eliminate the jowls and improve the corner of the mouth. This creates the classical "ogee" cheek contour [25]. One of the major advantages of this procedure is that the anchoring area can be marked with silicon or even metallic rings and then at a later date, when the tissues start to sag again, they can be tightened up with a small operation in the temporal area without any signs of surgical intervention in the face. This is a unique feature of the technique and stands out as an important difference from virtually all other facelift operations. This novel idea is derived from the anchoring system for the Silhouette suture-lift.

In some cases it is useful to use the described suture loop to lift heavier tissues of the cheek, but in other cases with very little malar fat, I prefer to use "Silhouette" threads with absorbable cones to lift the cheek. These threads are also anchored onto the same anchoring system as the suture loops. I often use both sutures and threads.

Markings

You must mark the patient in the upright position and draw the guidelines that will give you the most appropriate lift. Some people only need moderate lifting of the actual mid-face whereas many require lifting of the tissues pushing down the corners of the mouth. In these people an extra loop is required.

The first loop should be designed (see figure 7) about 1.5 cms from the naso-labial groove at about the level of the nostril curving on its upper line over the malar arch, infero-laterally to the orbital margin, towards the temple about 2 cms behind the hairline. This point on the temple will be the anchor point. Mark the area where this line reaches the hairline. We will need to make a small stab incision at this point. The inferior part of the loop curves sufficiently to catch a good volume of malar fat and then goes straight up to the temple anchor point. Plan to anchor the Silhouette threads, if they will be used, in the same place.

If there is heaviness of the lower midface, then a similar loop is designed catching tissue more inferiorly but anchored to the same temporal area. If necessary other loops can be added. I prefer often to add another loop in a different horizontal vector just below the lateral canthus as shown in figure 7.

5. Methods and instruments

The following instruments and materials are required:

1. 11 or 15 blade scalpel
2. A 22 (yellow) gauge spinal needle.
3. Sharp pointed fine scissors
4. Fine dissector
5. Toothed "Adson's" forceps.
6. Fine needle-holder to tie the knot.
7. Skin hook to free the skin from the buried thread
8. 4/0 non-absorbable suture. I use a "Provein" polypropylene suture but this could be an elasticised suture as described by Serdev.
9. A Mayo style thick curved suture needle

Surgical technique.

The reason why this technique is called a scarless mid-face-lift is because no incisions or scars are made on the face at all. Only a needle prick is necessary on the facial skin. A stab incision is made on the hairline where the guidelines transect on their way to the temporal anchoring point as shown in figure 7. A slightly larger incision is made at the anchor point so that an anchoring silicon ring marker can be inserted into the depths. These incisions are carefully dissected away from the surrounding tissue so that the skin is totally free.

Push the needle into the skin in the cheek on the most medial part of the upper loop. The needle should be directed perpendicularly into the substance of the cheek fat, then upward towards the orbital margin to catch the greatest volume of cheek fat and finally directed to the upper incision at the hairline. The needle tip is "fished" out with the `Adson's forceps and then the non-absorbable suture is passed through the barrel of the needle till it emerges from the hub. Then the needle and the contained suture are withdrawn until the needle reaches the starting point in the depths of the cheek tissue. The needle is then re-directed in the opposite direction and then towards the lower incision at the temporal hairline. The needle is once again "fished" out and the thread inside the needle is pulled out. The needle can be totally withdrawn and the loop of the suture remains and can be checked to make sure that it pulls the tissues upwards without any retraction of skin. If necessary the suture should be replaced if it is not perfect.

WE now have a suture loop that can be anchored on the temporal fascia by taking each end respectively and then threading it through the mayo needle which is passed from the stab incision through the temporal fascia to the anchoring incision. The loop is tightened carefully with only mild over-correction and knotted. Once it has been knotted a silicon ring is used to mark the knot and the loop is tied onto the ring. I use six throws at least. At a later date if the face tissues become a little loose, one can open the incision again, find the silicon ring and tug it further backwards to restore the tightness.

Any other loops are similarly made and connected to the silicon ring.

I believe that it is necessary to change the vector of pull and introduce horizontal traction at the level of the lower orbital margin. For that reason I place a horizontal loop as shown in figure 7 after the malar lift. This restores a natural curve to the malar area.

Then if necessary, thc uppcr silhouette threads are positioned and tied and also attached to the silicon ring. One needs to bury the silicon ring carefully and without any tension. If necessary I use a deep suture to close the skin as well as a skin suture. The stab wounds do not need to be sutured.

Once you have finished the one side you can easily see the difference between the tightened and the untreated side. I have learned to be sure not to have any traction areas or bumps because I have found that small irregularities do not always disappear. Often these irregularities can be pulled out with the skin hook.

I use this easy and safe procedure for younger patients as well as when I do a full face-lift with skin excision. The recovery can be rapid but some people swell rather more than one expects.

This can be a rather painful operation for about 50% cases in the initial 24 hours. The pain does not seem to be related to the tension of the loops. I tend to prescribe a special program of two unrelated analgesics to be taken alternately at 4-hour intervals. I usually use oral diclofenac as the one and a standard analgesic for moderate to severe pain as the other. That keeps the total daily dose down to minimal levels of each of these agents and also gives great pain relief.

PRE-OPERATIVE CARE – notes I give to the patient

1. To reduce bruising, avoid products that contain ASPIRIN, high doses of Vitamin E, high level Omega Oils and Evening Primrose oil for a period of 4 weeks before surgery. Avoid strong alcoholic drinks prior to surgery. I recommend that you use Vitamin C

1000 mg daily prior to surgery to reduce bruising and facilitate healing. You may use antioxidants, as usual. The use of bovine colostrum is also recommended.

2. It is also my impression that iontophoresis treatment with vitamin A and C by your beauty therapist may promote rapid healing if it is done a day or two before your operation. This may promote lymphatic drainage.
3. Do not smoke before or for a few days after surgery. Smoking interferes with the circulation of your skin. For people who cannot stop smoking, I will still operate because there is no threat of skin necrosis.
4. Wash your hair the night or the morning before surgery. We supply a medicated shampoo.
5. If you develop any signs of infection, pustules or boils on the face or body before surgery, please notify my office. We will be able to stop the infection rapidly.
6. Do not wear any make-up to surgery: this includes mascara and nail polish. If you tint, dye or bleach your hair then this should be done about one week prior to surgery.
7. Wear comfortable loose clothes that you don't have to pull over your head.
8. I always recommend a skin care with vitamin A and C and antioxidants for as long as possible before the operation and then continue post-operatively indefinitely to keep your skin as healthy and young-looking as possible.
9. I recommend Medical Roll-CIT skin needling to maximise the rejuvenation of your skin. Generally a course of six treatments should be done prior to surgery but can be done after surgery and repeated as often as necessary to achieve eradication of fine wrinkles.
10. I have designed a special pillow to remove the distorting pressure on your face that is partially responsible for the aged appearance and the development of the naso-labial grooves and upper lip lines. This pillow will also be essential to help you sleep comfortably after the operation.

POST-OPERATIVELY

1. It is important to remember that even though this delicate, extensive operation has been done under local anaesthetic, you must treat yourself as if it had been done under a general anaesthetic. Do not laugh, talk much, or run about. You have had a very large operation and you must rest properly. The fine suturing of the deep muscle layer and the re-positioning of the facial fat must be protected from rupturing in the first 2 weeks. Failure to take care may compromise the long-term result.
2. If you have had an intensive medical Roll-CIT at the same time then apply your topical skin products as normal.
3. Blood may stain the bandages. You may remove the bandages the morning after surgery. Do not remove any facial support that I have placed on the skin. You can have a shampoo one day after surgery.
4. You will be given a special mask to use post-operatively that will prevent distortion of your facial tissues no matter what pillow you chose to use. This also allows you to sleep on your side immediately after the operation. As soon as I have removed the support tapes, then you should use the "facial support mask" to protect the repair.

5. Do not turn your head from side to side but turn your body as a unit. Keep your chin in an elevated position and your head above shoulder level at all times. I prefer that you do not sleep flat. The head of the bed should be elevated with bricks if necessary so that you may sleep comfortably and still have your head elevated.
6. Use the special Pillow to support the face without placing stress on the repair while sleeping.
7. If eyelid surgery has been done at the same time as your face-lift, apply cold eye pads as frequently as possible for the first 48 hours.
8. Swelling and discoloration, and uneven swelling (more on one side than the other) are expected. Bruising and discoloration may rarely persist for 2-3 weeks after surgery. There might also be some lumpiness of the neck or cheeks and this may persist for 6-8 weeks, but it will disappear. In unusual cases it may be necessary to anaesthetise areas and tug on the skin.
9. Swelling may be improved by having Lymphatic drainage by a qualified skin-care therapist. A Facial treatment involving pulsed iontophoresis and low-frequency-sonophoresis is recommended a few days after surgery to reduce swelling and promote a tighter skin.
10. Avoid strenuous activity, getting overheated and sunbathing for 2-3 weeks.
11. Excessive swelling or pain should be reported as soon as it is noted.
12. If you have pets then please be particularly careful not to allow them close to you during the early stages of healing. Their hairs etc. can contaminate your scars and cause an infection.
13. Generally you may use topical vitamin A and C products again within a day or two of the operation.
14. You will have had a major operation so please remember to be gentle with yourself. Many people laugh in the initial phases after the operation and are euphoric but then become depressed as they realize the gravity of the operation, and the local anaesthetic. You should not be surprised to feel a little depressed about a week after the operation. Slowly, as the swelling in your eyes disappears, you will regain your confidence, and feel much happier.
15. You may drive as soon as you feel comfortable and safe to do so.
16. Usually, after a scarless facelift with or without intensive Roll-CIT needling, the patients feel comfortable to be out socially by about 5-7 days.
17. If the forehead has been lifted, you may have bruised eyes for 10-14 days.

6. Conclusion

It is easier to achieve impressive results when one ensures that the patient who wants a face-lift for rejuvenation, first treats their skin with vitamin A and C to get the youngest skin possible and reverse as much of their photoaging as possible. By adding six sessions of Roll-CIT done with topical anaesthesia one can make the skin actively more vital and convincingly younger. Finally, one can do a scarless mid-face-lift or total scarless face-lift with or without upper blepharoplasty or forehead lift and achieve a holistic and truly scarless rejuvenation of the face.

Author details

M. B. Des Fernandes
Renaissance Surgical Clinic, Cape Town, The Renaissance Body Science Institute, South Africa
Department of Plastic Surgery, Groote Schuur Hospital, University of Cape Town, Cape Town, South Africa

7. References

[1] Fernandes, D., Percutaneous collagen induction: an alternative to laser resurfacing. Aesthet Surg J, 2002. 22(3): p. 307-9.
[2] Hudson, D.A. and D.B. Fernandes, Caveats for the use of suspension sutures. Aesthetic plastic surgery, 2004. 28(3): p. 170-3.
[3] Randolph, R.K. and M. Simon, All-trans-retinoic acid regulates retinol and 3,4-didehydroretinol metabolism in cultured human epidermal keratinocytes. J Invest Dermatol, 1996. 106(1): p. 168-75.
[4] Antille, C., et al., Vitamin A exerts a photoprotective action in skin by absorbing ultraviolet B radiation. J Invest Dermatol, 2003. 121(5): p. 1163-7.
[5] Moon, T.E., et al., Effect of retinol in preventing squamous cell skin cancer in moderate-risk subjects: a randomized, double-blind, controlled trial. Southwest Skin Cancer Prevention Study Group. Cancer Epidemiology, Biomarkers and Prevention, 1997. 6(11): p. 949-56.
[6] Guo, X. and L.J. Gudas, Metabolism of all-trans-retinol in normal human cell strains and squamous cell carcinoma (SCC) lines from the oral cavity and skin: reduced esterification of retinol in SCC lines. Cancer Res, 1998. 58(1): p. 166-76.
[7] Bailly, J., et al., In vitro metabolism by human skin and fibroblasts of retinol, retinal and retinoic acid. Exp Dermatol, 1998. 7(1): p. 27-34.
[8] Kurlandsky, S.B., et al., Auto-regulation of retinoic acid biosynthesis through regulation of retinol esterification in human keratinocytes. J Biol Chem, 1996. 271(26): p. 15346-52.
[9] Idson, B., Vitamins in cosmetics, an update: 1. Overview and vitamin A. Drug Cos Ind, 1990. May, 1990.
[10] Counts, D.F., F. Skreko, and J. McBee, The effect of retinyl palmitate on skin composition and morphometry J Soc Cosmet Chem, 1988. 39(44): p. 235-240.
[11] Hill, D.L. and C.J. Grubbs, Retinoids and cancer prevention. Annu Rev Nutr, 1992. 12: p. 161-81.
[12] Lin, J.Y., et al., UV photoprotection by combination topical antioxidants vitamin C and vitamin E. J Am Acad Dermatol, 2003. 48(6): p. 866-74.
[13] Goffin, V., et al., Topical retinol and the stratum corneum response to an environmental threat. Skin Pharmacol, 1997. 10(2): p. 85-9.
[14] Ortonne, J.P., Retinoid therapy of pigmentary disorders. Dermatol Ther, 2006. 19(5): p. 280-8.
[15] Shalita, A., The integral role of topical and oral retinoids in the early treatment of acne. J Eur Acad Dermatol Venereol, 2001. 15 Suppl 3: p. 43-9.

[16] Murphy, G.F., S. Katz, and A.M. Kligman, Topical tretinoin replenishes CD1a-positive epidermal Langerhans cells in chronically photodamaged human skin. J Cutan Pathol, 1998. 25(1): p. 30-4.

[17] Varani, J., et al., Vitamin A antagonizes decreased cell growth and elevated collagen-degrading matrix metalloproteinases and stimulates collagen accumulation in naturally aged human skin. J Invest Dermatol, 2000. 114(3): p. 480-6.

[18] Edward, M., Effects of retinoids on glycosaminoglycan synthesis by human skin fibroblasts grown as monolayers and within contracted collagen lattices. Br J Dermatol, 1995. 133(2): p. 223-30.

[19] Watson, R.E., et al., Repair of photoaged dermal matrix by topical application of a cosmetic 'antiageing' product. Br J Dermatol, 2008. 158(3): p. 472-7.

[20] Aust, M.C., et al., Percutaneous collagen induction-Regeneration in place of cicatrisation? J Plast Reconstr Aesthet Surg.

[21] Fernandes, D., Minimally invasive percutaneous collagen induction. Oral Maxillofac Surg Clin North Am, 2005. 17(1): p. 51-63.

[22] Fernandes, D. and M. Signorini, Combating photoaging with percutaneous collagen induction. Clin Dermatol, 2008. 26(2): p. 192-9.

[23] Aust, M.C., et al., Percutaneous collagen induction-regeneration in place of cicatrisation? J Plast Reconstr Aesthet Surg, 2010.

[24] de Benito, J., et al., Facial rejuvenation and improvement of malar projection using sutures with absorbable cones: surgical technique and case series. Aesthetic plastic surgery, 2011. 35(2): p. 248-53.

[25] Little, J.W., Volumetric perceptions in midfacial aging with altered priorities for rejuvenation. Plastic and reconstructive surgery, 2000. 105(1): p. 252-66; discussion 286-9.

Chapter 10

Midface Thread Lifting: Method of Internal Suturing

M.A. Sulamanidze, G.M. Sulamanidze and C.M. Sulamanidze

Additional information is available at the end of the chapter

http://dx.doi.org/10.5772/56583

1. Introduction

The past two decades have seen rapid development of aesthetic surgery of the aging face, especially its middle zone [1, 2, 3, 4, 5, 6, 7, 8], which has always been preceded by considerable prerequisites: the patients reported, and the surgeons agreed that the visual signs of the facial aging are most sharply pronounced exactly in this region. At relatively stable high contour of the zygomatic areas, early (in the relatively young age) sliding down and ptosis of soft tissues of suborbital and buccozygomatic areas, appearance of the lachrymal groove and suborbital fold, worsening of the nasolabial fold have always been considered as sign of a dull, flabby, ageing face. The growing demand for interventions aimed at eliminating such deformities has always been pushing the surgeons toward improving the classic and developing newer surgical techniques of contour plasty and lifting of the middle facial area. Amongst them are: open and endoscopic SMAS, supra- and sub-periosteal face lifting, contour plasty with various implants, lifting of the suborbicilaris oculi fat (SOOF), skin peelings, the Curl Lift, APTOS THREAD, and others.

Possessing some or other certain advantages, each of them has its own disadvantaged, which do not allow of carrying out the manipulation or operation in all the cases, irrespective of the scope and nature of the deformity.

For instance, face lifting, especially SMAS, supra- and sub-periosteal, is technically difficult to perform, it should be carried out by a highly qualified specialist, and is fraught with severe complications, it is characterized by a long rehabilitation period, leaving visible scars. Besides, from these approaches, using the known suturing materials it is difficult to perform qualitative stitching of the suborbital and buccal areas, especially their medial portions (the nasolabial fold, upper portion of the lachrymal groove) since this zone is rather remote from the edge of the wound [1, 4, 8]. For this purpose it is necessary to mobilize and stitch soft tisues of these sites through intraoral additional access [6].

SOOF lifting requires the suborbicular ocular fat pad to be identified and mobilized through an inconvenient and insufficient transconjunctival access, sutured, which is not that easy to perform by the currently available suturing material, and what is important that this method allows of removing deformity of the subocular region only [6].

Application of solid or shell implants envisages carrying out rather an invasive operation, requiring the presence of the implants themselves, which must often have individual sizes and shapes [5].

The injection administration of various permanent and long-term filling agents is connected with leaving under the facial skin foreign, allogenic artificial substances, which rather often leads to suppurative and other complications [5, 7].

Autolipolifting is most preferable but to achieve permanent long-lasting results, this manipulation should be carried out repeatedly. Besides, the use of this method seems inappropriate for plump faces and is impossible in the absence of donor fat in lean patients [5, 7].

By using any peeling, one may attain contraction of the skin, improvement of its structure, to result in some tightening of flabby tissues, but neither lifting, nor a new contour will be attained [5].

Publication of the data concerning the Curl Lift gave hope that a new simple, easy method was found to lift soft tissues in general, and those of the middle facial zone, in particular. However, practical application showed that the outcomes of this-type operation did not persist over time. The causes seem to consist in incompetence of the suture applied in the temporal area, rather large length of the thread used, and what is more important – underestimation of the anatomical peculiarities of the middle facial zone, consisting in the presence of the reference points in zygomatic regions [8].

The APTOS THREAD method, with technically correct operation performed, is the most minimally invasive and at the same time rather effective. But thoughtlessly pursued marketing policy, underestimation of the issues related to specialists training, flooding of the market with poor-quality copies of the threads, the appearance of diversified and impossible to understand on what grounded modifications have lead to the appearance of a great number of inefficient outcomes in patients and even complications and respectively to a certain decrease in the interest on behalf of certain part of surgeons in this promising method. A particular negative role in this was played by seeming simplicity of carrying out the manipulation, and the necessity of rather brittle, specific post-operative management of the patients [5].

The present study was aimed at improving the cosmetic effect of surgical treatment of patients suffering from ptosis of soft tissues of middle face area, at increasing the reliability and duration of the obtained results, at decreasing severity and duration of the rehabilitation period.

2. Materials and methods

In our practice, we have used the method of carcass stitching and lifting of flabby soft tissues (subcutaneous fat) of the middle area of the ageing face with special suturing material to be followed by stable fixation in a new, aesthetically more advantageous position.

This method, we called it APTOS NEEDLE (application for invention PCT/RU 2004/000525), unites the possibilities of several methods, i.e.: Curl Lift, and APTOS THREAD.

From the Curl Lift method we borrowed the idea of the double-edged needle and the appropriate technique of subcutaneous passage of the needle, while the scope, level and scale of stitching soft tissues of the subocular and buccozygomatic areas without mobilization thereof were taken from the APTOS THREAD method.

The technique of the method was devised on the basis of studying the topographic anatomy and with due regard for pathogenesis of age-specific deformities of the middle facial area [2].

To implement the idea of APTOS NEEDLE in the midface area we proposed a special, disposable double-pointed curved needle with the thread for suturing (polypropylene 4/0), atraumatically factory-connected with the needle in the middle (Fig. 1).

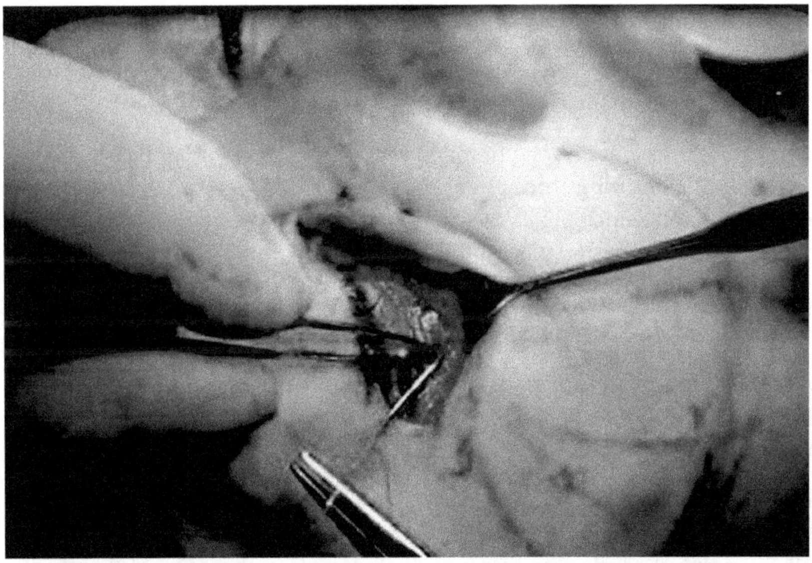

Figure 1. A photo of APTOS NEEDLE for suturing of subocular and buccozygomatic soft tissues.

APTOS NEEDLE possesses a possibility of bilateral passability thus providing its passage under the skin along the polygonal or long contour without its complete emergence to the skin surface. It allows of passing the needle underneath the skin and subcutaneous stitching of soft tissues, without skin retractions, to finally yield an even pulled up contour.

The minimally invasive technology of midface soft tissues lifting we have developed, may be used both independently through a puncture or a small cut of the skin near to the lateral angle of the lid slit, and in a combination with the classical and transconjunctival blepharoplasty.

3. Operational technique

Depending on the ptosis degree and gravity of tissues for lifting of the subocular and buccozygomatic areas, we perform stitching with 2 or 3 sutures. The methods of marking differ respectively (Figures 2, 3).

Along the lower wrinkle "crow's foot", which corresponds to the position of the lateral edge of the orbital bone, we mark the place of inserting the APTOS NEEDLE, i.e. the place where knots are applied after stitching (Fig. 2, 3 – point 1). Usually it is enough to make a puncture here with a thick needle in order to create the channel for passing the APTOS NEEDLE. But, since in this point after application of the knot cutaneous retractions appear, during the period of mastering the operative technique by the surgeon and gaining experience, it is allowed to make a 2-3-cm-long cut with the blade of scalpel № 11 in order to have some view for correct application of the suture. In future, the scar of this cut is completely invisible, since it coincides with the natural fold of the skin. In case of applying this technique on the eyelids, previously subjected to the operation of the classical blepharoplasty this place coincides with the scar being present from the previous operation.

Then, we mark the points of drawing out the needle for the first, second and third sutures, to be connected between themselves with lines, as shown in Figures 2 and 3.

As we see from Figures 2 and 3, the first and second sutures overlap between each other. It is done so that while suturing through on the place of the overlap the tissues be pulled up and fixed more reliably, since ptosis of soft tissues is more pronounced in this area. Besides vectors of lift have different direction and the result of operation is more long-term.

The third seam is imposed only proceeding from aesthetic expediency. Figure 3 shows that the third suture is stitched only through one point (point 6).

In the overwhelming majority of cases, we used infiltration anaesthesia through the marked points along the marking – a 1-percent lidocain solution with epinephrine solution, 4-6 ml for one side.

The operation begins from a puncture of the skin with an ordinary injection needle 1.2 mm in diameter (18 G), or from a 2-3-mm-long cut to be made near the lateral angle of the lid slid (Fig. 2, 3 – point 1). Under the finger-mediated control, the point of the needle (scalpel) is moved to the bony edge of the orbit and using scraping movements creates an area with detached periosteum. After taking out the needle (scalpel), it is advisable to widen the channel by means of a pair of thin mosquito-type forceps. Into this channel, APTOS NEEDLE (from any side) is inserted so that it should slide along the edge of the bone and get a hold of the detached periosteum. Using the fingers of the free hand to impart the

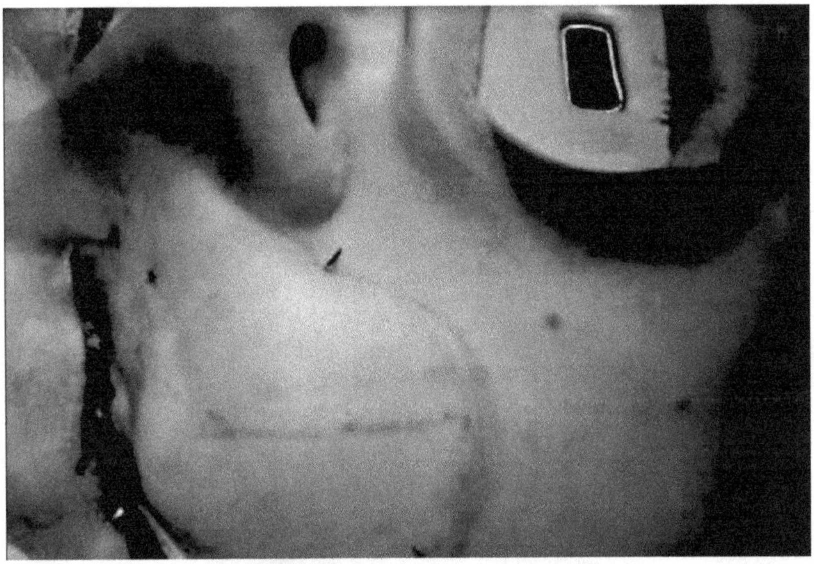

Figure 2. Schematic marking for suturing of midface soft tissues – option I.

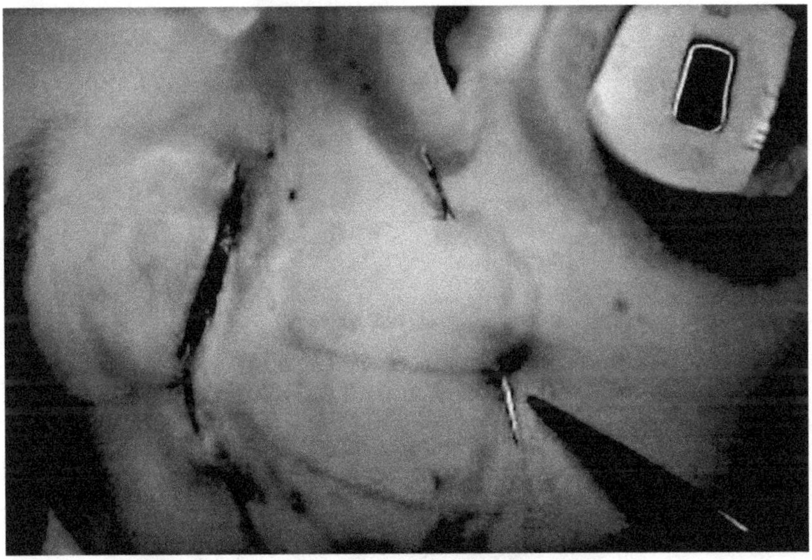

Figure 3. Schematic marking for suturing of midface soft tissues – option II.

tissues of the suborbital and buccozygomatic areas the pulled-up position, high contour, the needle is passed to point 2 near the base of the wing of nostril and brought to the surface over there. The needle is carefully taken out from under the skin but not fully, so that the second pointed end remained inside the tissues at a depth of 0.5 – 1.0 cm. Then, the APTOS NEEDLE is turned by 90 degrees and with the second pointed end is carried towards point 3. Here, also the needle is thrust out and pulled out incompletely. Then, the needle is turned again by 90 degrees and returned to the side of the first puncture (Fig. 2, 3 – point 1). In this case also, the fingers of the free hand are used to impart the pulled up position to the soft tissues. The point of the needle is placed into contact with the periosteum at the level of the bony edge of the orbit to be pulled out through the previously created channel (Fig. 2, 3 – point 1). In this place, the both ends of the thread are pulled up and tied with several knots. It is important to prevent the tissue from entering the knot in the depth of the channel, otherwise in this place there would be skin retraction and even lowering of the lateral angle of the lid slit. The second important moment is straining the suture so that to obtain optimal lifting of this portion of tissues with slight hypercorrection.

The second suture, and if need arises the third suture are applied in a similar manner, according to the marking. Taken together, they should create a newer, higher, aesthetical more favourable contour of the soft tissues with smooth transition to the adjacent areas.

In the same manner, the operation is performed on the collateral side and, naturally, of great importance is achieving symmetry of the left and right sides.

Depending on the individual peculiarities, other variants of suturing are also possible. For example, in rare cases when the lachrymal groove is rather protracted and deep, the usual suturing is not enough with the necessity to apply an additional suture precisely along this contour (Fig. 4).

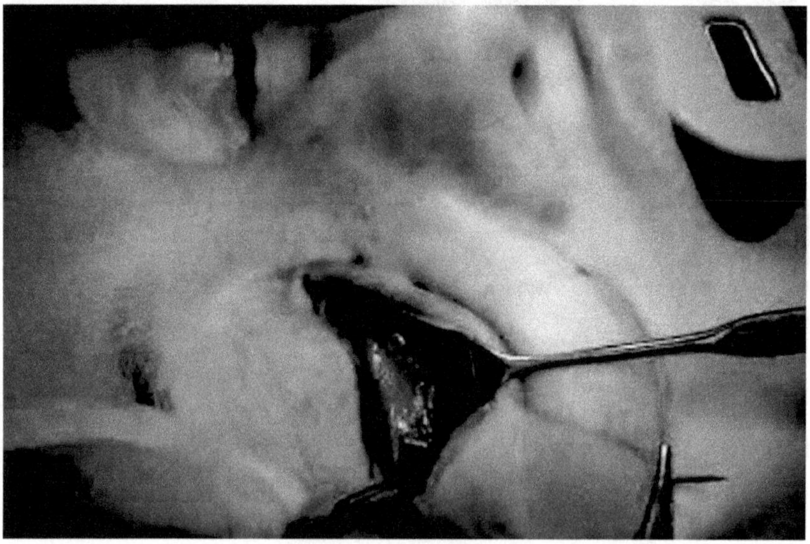

Figure 4. Schematic marking for additional suturing of the lachrymal groove only.

Usually, the operation is easy and rapid to perform, with minimal injury inflicted to the tissues, and the outcome of the intervention is visually seen as early as on the operating table (Fig. 5).

A strip of a sterile adhesive patch is applied onto the wound (or puncture) after the operation for 1 – 3 days, or one seam is imposed - prolen 6/0.

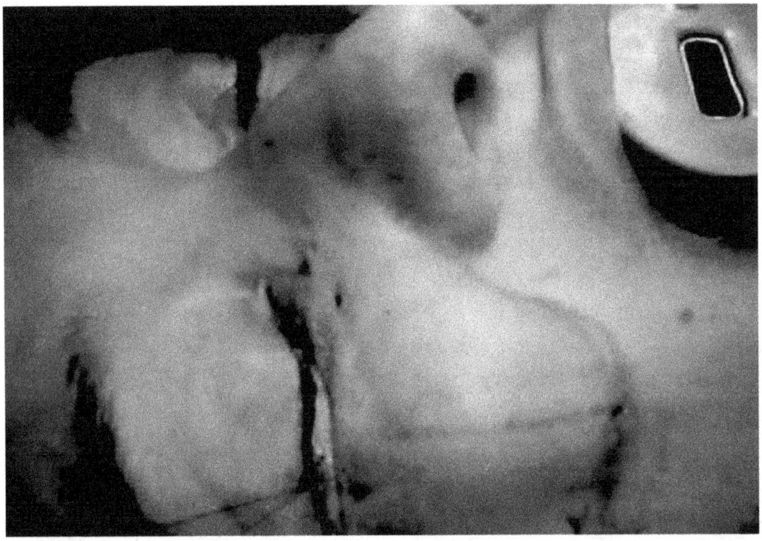

Figure 5. Photo of patient N… immediately after suturing of subocular and buccozygomatic areas.

If the operation is performed through the transconjunctival access, after isolating and dissecting fatty hernias within the required scope the soft tissues of the subocular and buccozygomatic area are sutured, hence, the sutures should be distributed along the whole perimeter of the lower bony edge of the orbit (arcus marginalis).

The sutures are applied in the similar manner in case of carrying out the operation through the classical approach of lower blepharoplasty (Fig. 6).

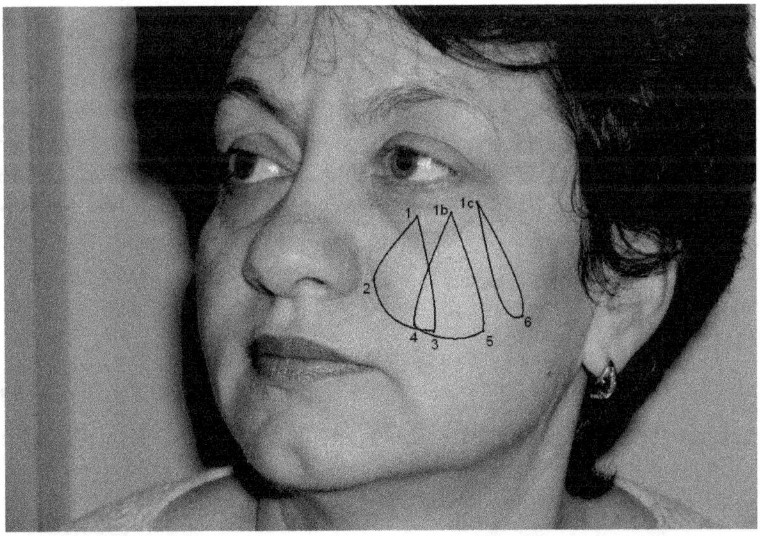

Figure 6. Schematic marking for suturing of midface soft tissues, variant of simultaneous operation with blepharoplasty.

We have been using the method of subocular and buccozygomatic areas lifting - APTOS NEEDLE since May 2003, and have performed by now (November 2004) a total of 144 operations, but in this article we present only the analysis of the cases we managed to follow up one year and more – 77 cases. The patients' age varied from 31 to 56 years, with only six of them being males. A repeated operation aimed at additional correction was required in 4 cases.

4. Discussion

By now, the plastic and aesthetic surgeons have developed a variety of methods for lifting of midface soft tissues, having gained tremendous experience in carrying out similar operations and manipulations.

Surgeons preferring radical interventions believe that ageing of the midface is related to stretching, weakening of fascial nodes (bands) and ptosis of the whole conglomerate of soft tissues, therefore achievement of qualitative and long-lasting rejuvenation of the ageing face requires operations with more or less complete set of such surgical techniques as a wide or endoscope access and mobilization of the skin, mobilization of SMAS or deeper layers of tissues, displacement and fixation thereof in a higher position [1, 4].

At the same time, some of them draw attention to the fact that it is not uncommon that such serious interventions fail to achieve the desired outcome – a high contour of the subocular and buccozygomatic area.

It has been determined that the farther from the cut is the deformity (nasolabial fold, lachrymal groove, ptosis of the medial tissues of the cheek) the more difficult to remove it and to preserve the result, that the only correct decision for qualitative lifting of these areas is local intervention [1, 2, 4, 5].

This fact has led the surgeons to the thought that in many cases, a qualitative and long-term effect may be achieved without mobilization of the skin and subcutaneous tissues, with inconsiderable invasion. To implement this goal, the following methods have been proposed APTOS THREAD, Curl Lift allowing of influencing the deformity in the place of its location [3, 5, 8]. The authors believe that the fascial nodes (bands) do not virtually extend and remain stable during the whole life (zygomatic area), while the tissues that are suspended from under them (buccal, suborbital areas) gradually go down. Following this logic, they try to suture and suspend the ptosed soft tissues to stable portions and achieve good long-term clinical results.

Unfortunately, these methods are not always applicable due to a variety of reasons.

Good outcomes are achieved when using Freeman's method of SOOF lifting. However, this technique removes only the deformity of the subocular region, pulling up inconsiderably the ptosed soft tissues of the whole midface [6].

The APTOS NEEDLE method which we offer for lifting of midface soft tissues accumulates positive qualities of the above mentioned methods. It allows of achieving new aesthetic harmony rapidly, easily, qualitatively and reliably with an inconsiderable operational wound, with even, smooth contours of the skin surface (without skin indrawings) and which requires no excessively delicate postoperative management of the patients (Figures 7 to 29).

Only midface suturing

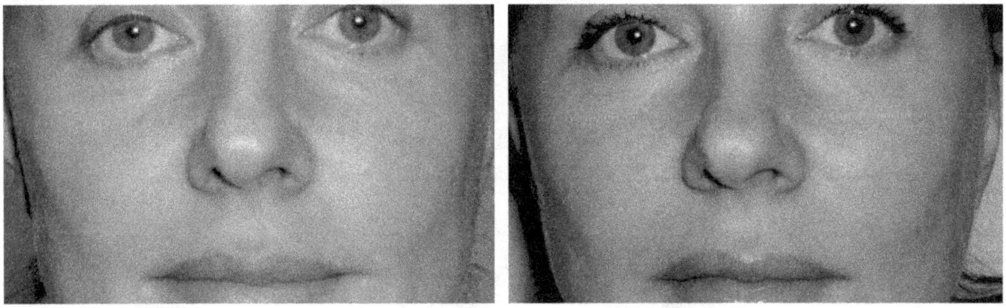

Figure 7. Before and after (4 months)

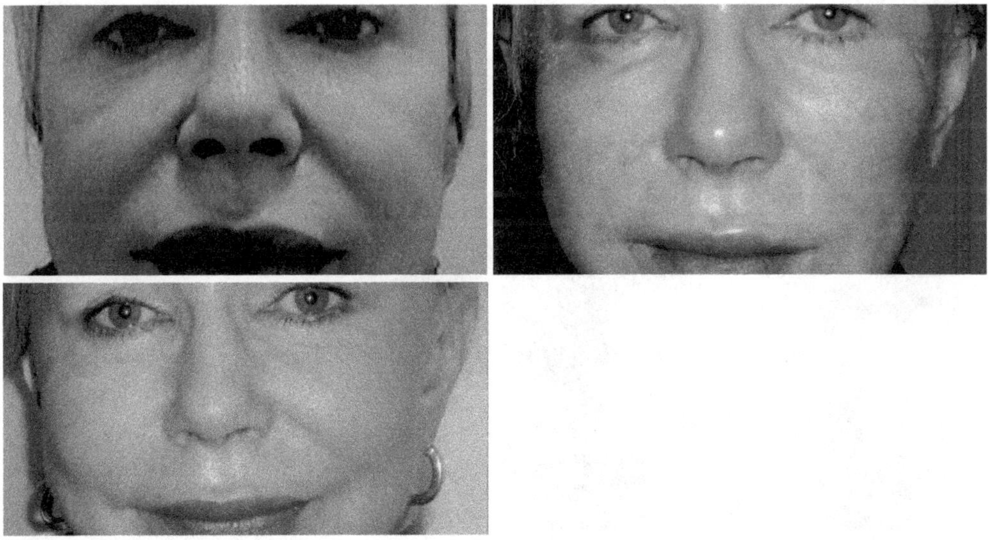

Figure 8. Before, after 4 days and after 1 year.

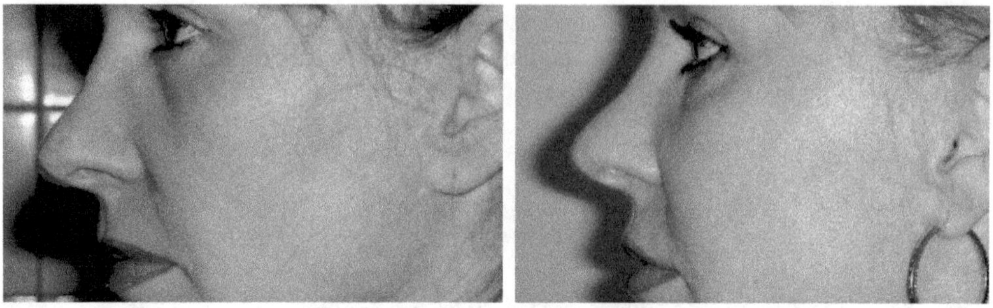

Figure 9. Before and after (1 year).

Simultaneous operation with blepharoplasty

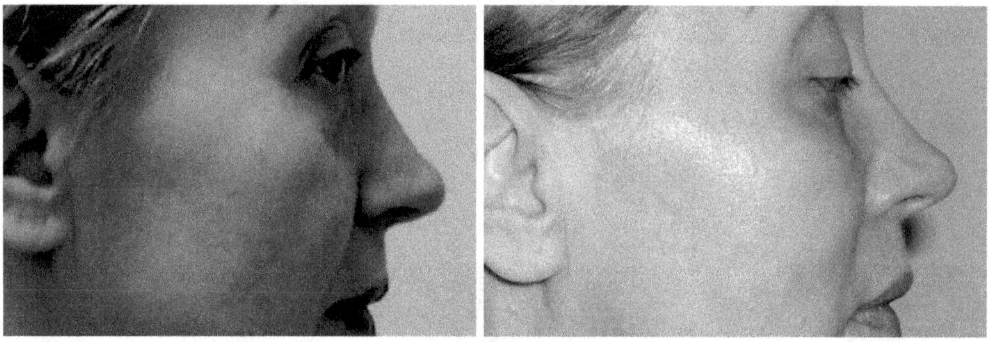

Figure 10. Before and after (4 months).

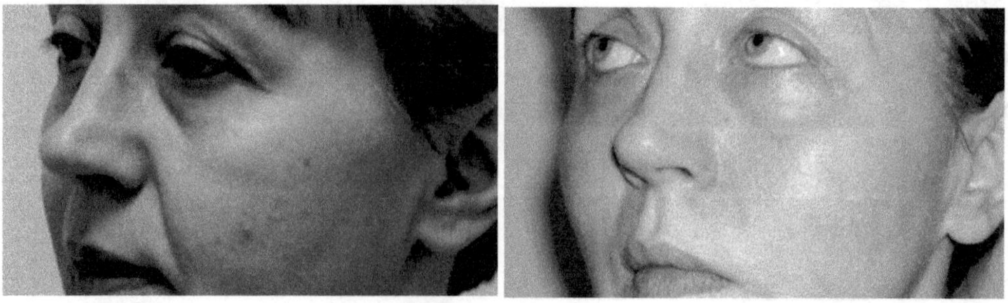

Figure 11. Before and after (4 months).

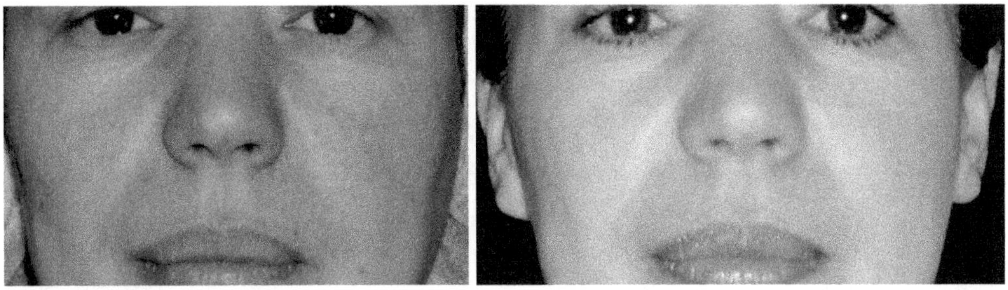

Figure 12. Before and after (1 year).

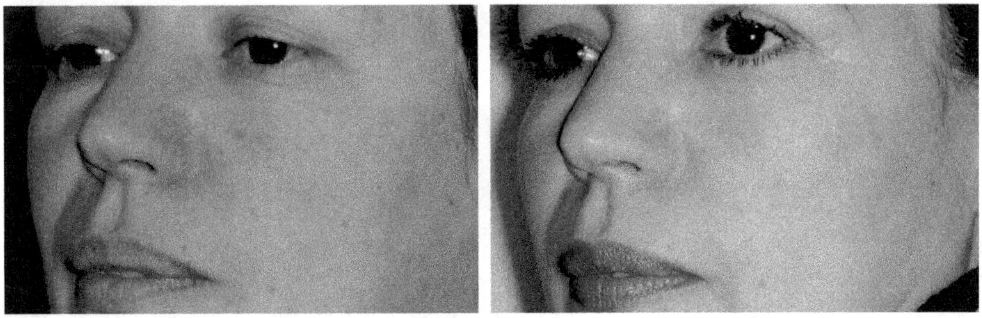

Figure 13. Before and after (1 year).

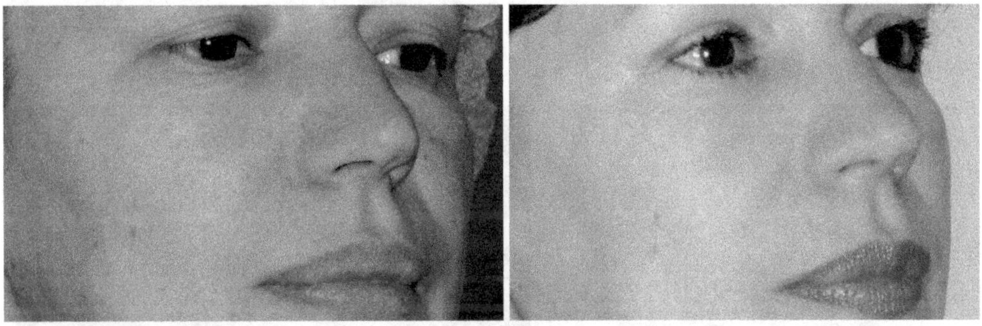

Figure 14. Before and after (1 year).

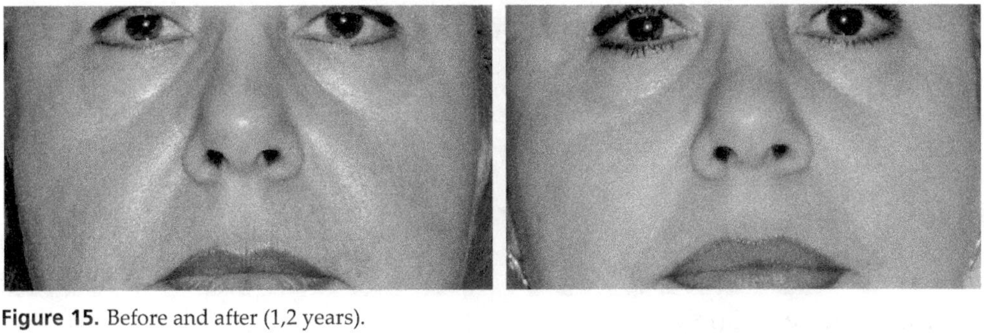

Figure 15. Before and after (1,2 years).

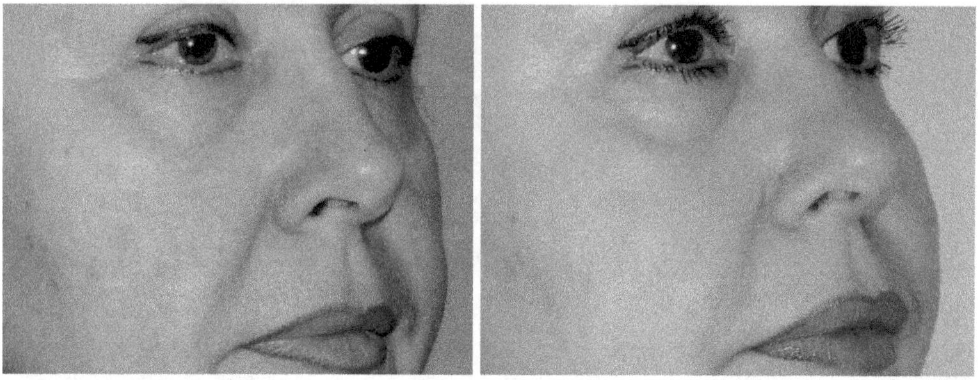

Figure 16. Before and after (1,2 years).

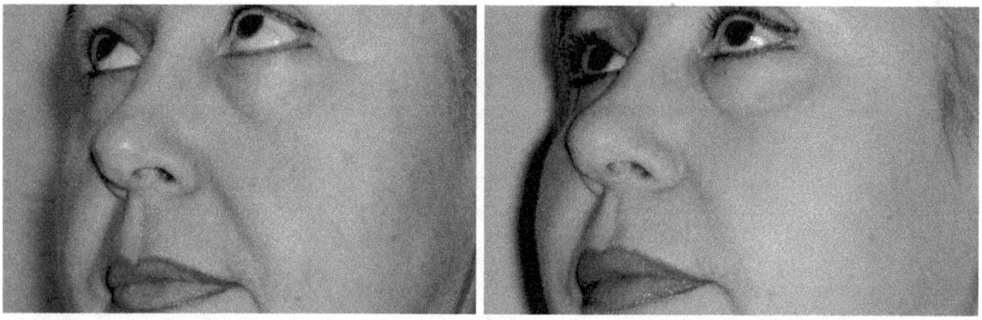

Figure 17. Before and after (1,2 years).

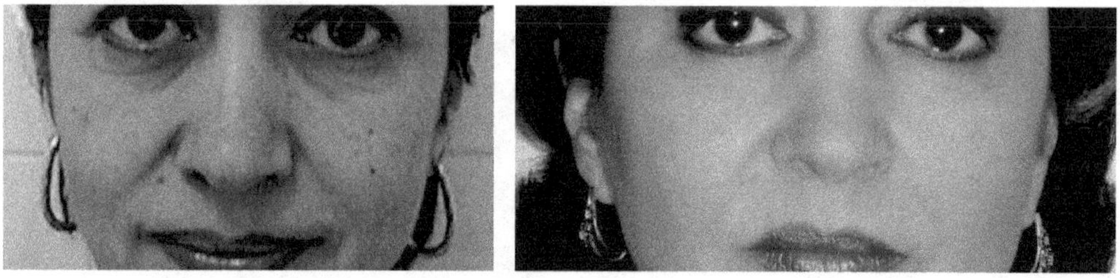

Figure 18. Before and after (1,5 years).

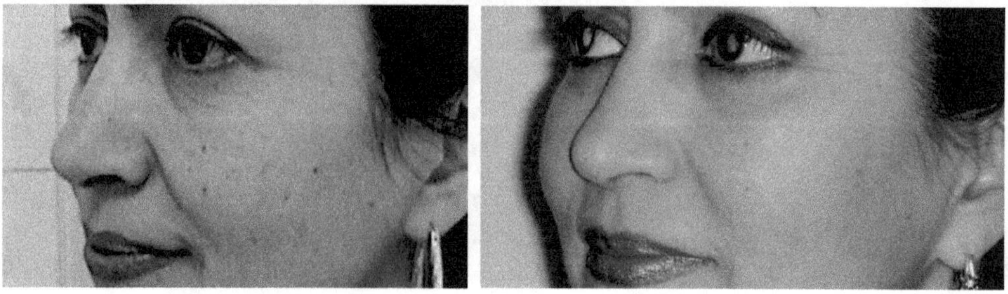

Figure 19. Before and after (1,5 years).

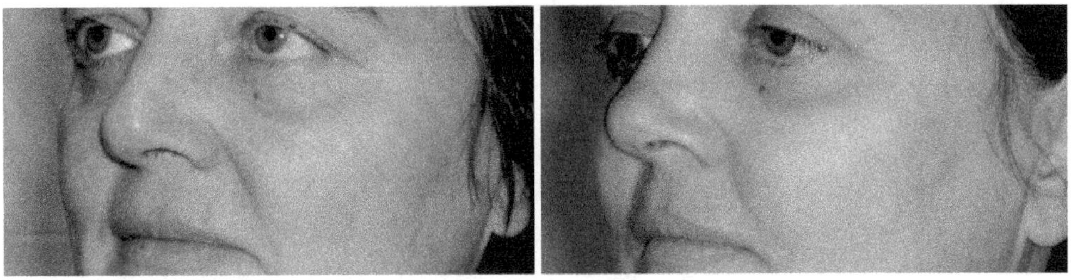

Figure 20. Before and after (1,5 years).

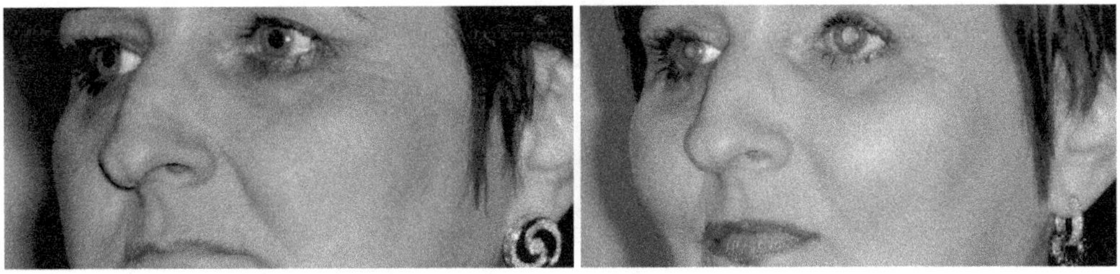

Figure 21. Before and after (1,6 years).

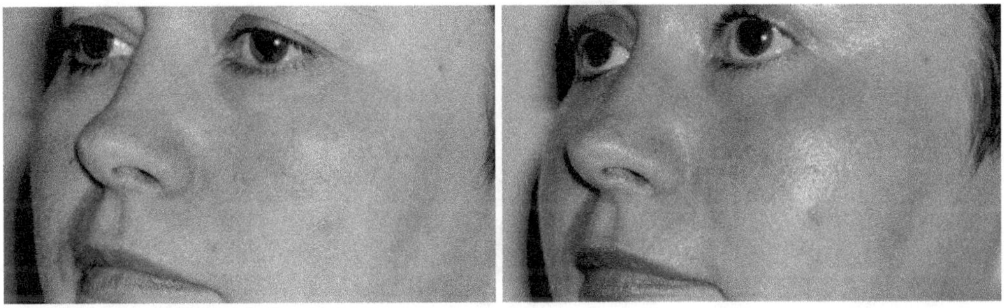

Figure 22. Before and after (1,7 years).

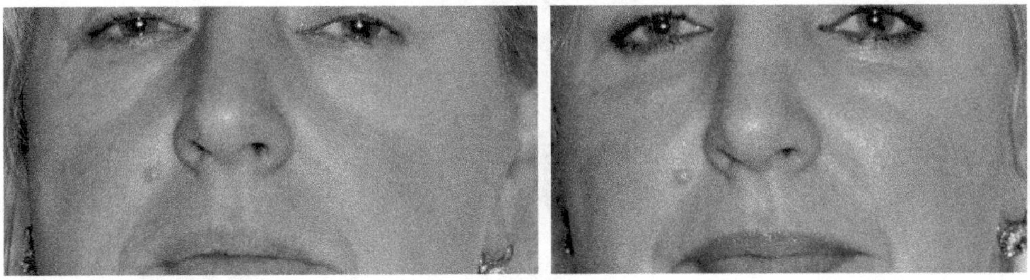

Figure 23. Before and after (1,7 years).

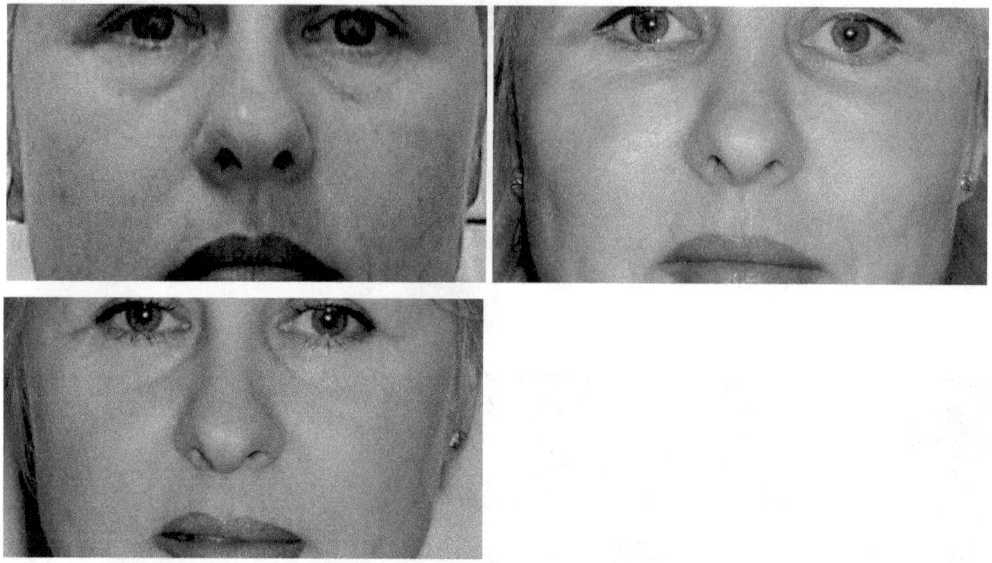

Figure 24. Before, after 5 months and after 1,9 years.

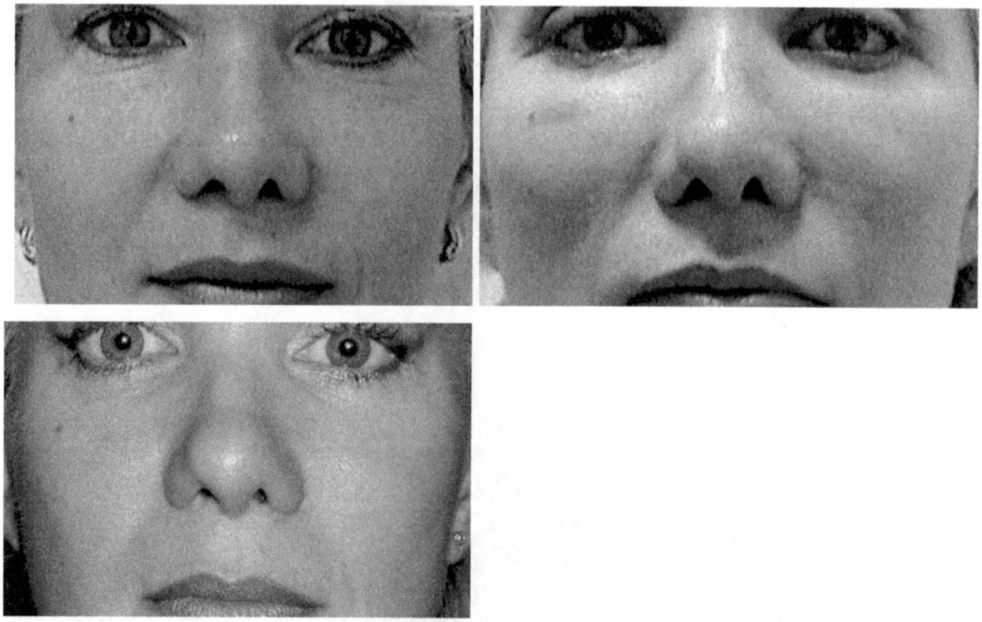

Figure 25. Before, after 5 days and after (14 months).

Simultaneous operation with transconjunctival blepharoplasty

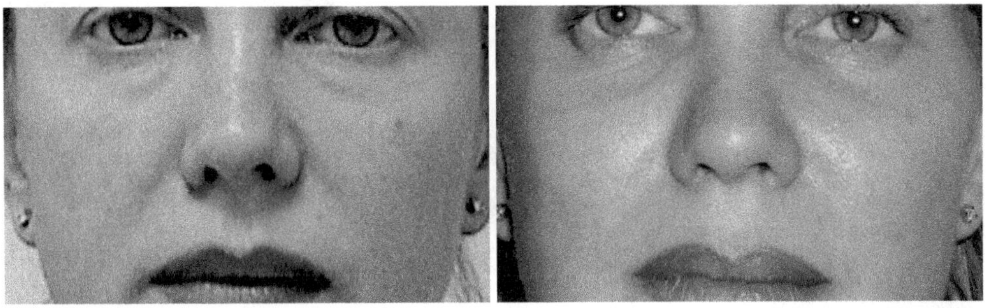

Figure 26. Before and after (1 months).

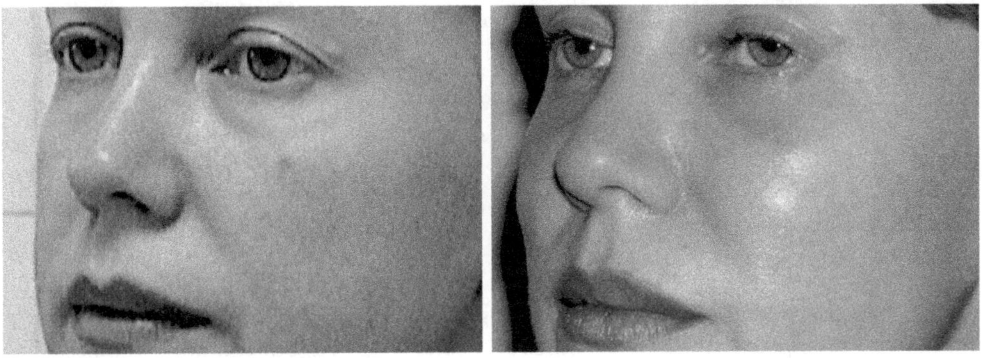

Figure 27. Before and after (1 months).

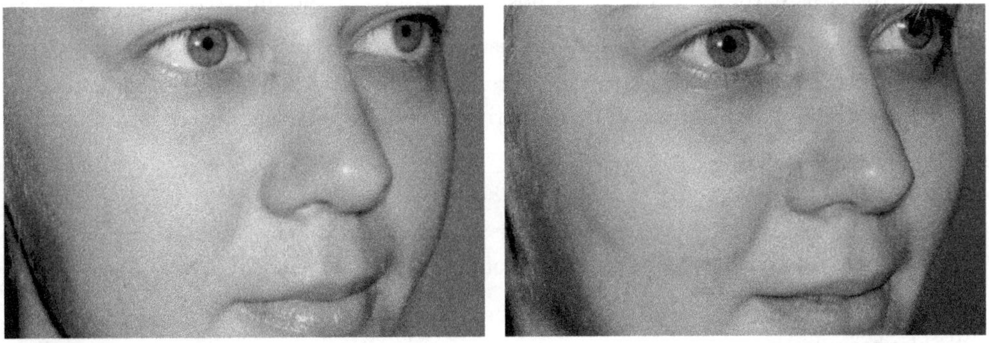

Figure 28. Before and after (6 months).

Simultaneous operation with blepharoplasty (man)

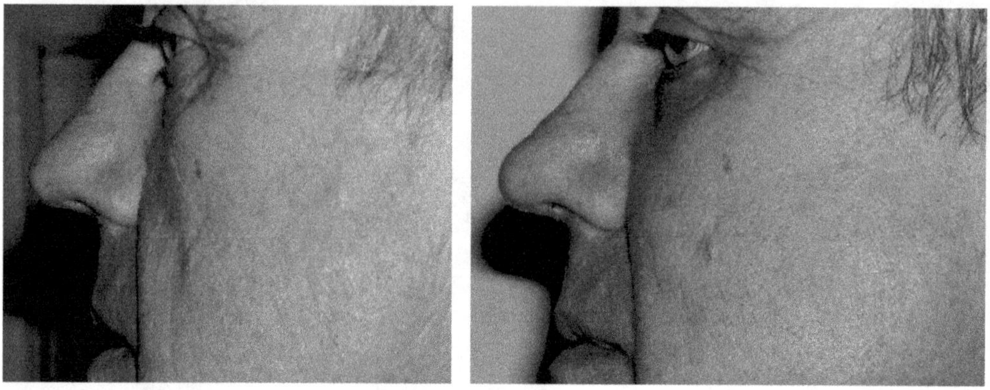

Figure 29. Before and after (2 months)

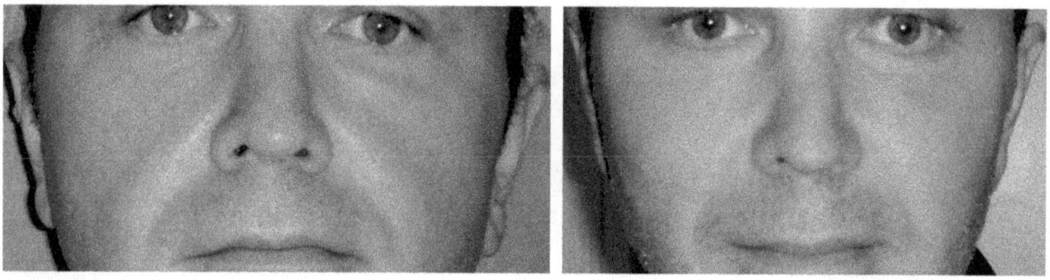

Figure 30. Before and after (1 year).

The immediate postoperative period up to 14 days was uneventful in the majority of the patients. Linear haemorrhages along suturings were noted in once case, with no skin indrawings in the places of needle's entries and exits observed, but contour roughness was noted in 14 patients. These unpleasant manifestations were corrected spontaneously or by means of prescribing appropriate resolving therapy. Only one woman had her social rehabilitation during one month (Fig.), with the rest patients being satisfied with the obtained result as early as within 10-18 postoperative days. No other complications were noted.

Both the short-, and long-term outcomes were good and persistent. In only four cases, we had to repeat intervention, however it was during the period of mastering the technique:

- due to excessive hypercorrection;
- due to asymmetry;
- due to patient's displeasure who did not expect such radical facial alterations;
- in order to remove the right-sided ptosis of the angle of lid slit.

While gaining experience, we noted that when combining the APTOS NEEDLE method with blepharoplasty (both traditional, and transconjunctival) in the majority cases it is necessary to refuse dissecting fatty hernias, or to remove them but in a considerably lesser amount than when using blepharoplasty alone. This is explained by the fact that elevated upper soft tissues of the midface create high contour immediately in the suborbital region, which in turn requires greater completeness of lower eyelids volume. Naturally, in such cases, one has often to redistribute the fatty hernias downwards toward the lachrymal groove and the hollowed-out contour of the orbital edge (suborbital groove).

While carrying out this manipulation simultaneously with the traditional blepharoplasty, there appears a temptation to excise more excesses of the skin, not being afraid of obtaining complications in the form of "round eye" and ectropion. Such an impression is delusive, since pathogenesis of the altered relief of the lower eyelid with age in the majority of cases is related not only to appearance of skin excesses but rather with skin distension due to ptosis of the whole buccozygomatic and subocular regions. Therefore, practically more often there is no redundant skin: on the operating table and within the immediate postoperative period, probably due to oedema, and, consequently at the expense of contraction and distribution of the thin skin of the lower eyelid, which has shed the heavy burden of the whole buccal and subocular regions. Therefore, we warn our colleagues against hasteful steps while solving this problem.

5. Conclusions

The APTOS NEEDLE - method of subcutaneous suturing of midface soft tissues is a simple, minimally invasive, painless, inexpensive, but at the same time reliable method of removing visible manifestations of the ageing face and, according to our experience, provides long-lasting and aesthetically qualitative lifting. Among the major positive qualities of this technique are: lack of coarse cutaneous indrawings in the places of skin punctures, a possibility to suture soft tissues to any depth and in any amount, infiltration anaesthesia, conjugation with other rejuvenating interventions. The rehabilitation period is as short as in using the APTOS THREAD technique, however differing therefrom in that it requires no special guarding measures during 2 – 3 weeks following the operation in order to fix the obtained outcome (such as the advice to exclude active mimic and masticatory movements, facial massage).

The operation is a surgical procedure and despite the seeming simplicity requires high qualification of the specialist involved, good knowledge of the midface anatomy, correct understanding of not only facial aesthetics but the patient's wishes as well.

We are sure that complying with these requirements the operational outcomes would satisfy both the surgeons, and the patients.

Author details

M.A. Sulamanidze, G.M. Sulamanidze and C.M. Sulamanidze
Clinic of Plastic and Aesthetic Surgery, Total charm, Moscow, Tbilisi

6. References

[1] Little J. W., Three-dimensional rejuvenation of the midface: volumetric resculpture by malar imbrication. Plastic Reconstructive Surgery, Jan. 2000 105(1)267-285.

[2] Mendelson B. C., Muzaffar A. R., Adams W. P. Surgical Anatomy of the Midcheek and Malar Mounds, Plastic and Reconstructive Surgery, Volume 110-N3-September 1, 2002, 885-896.

[3] Serdev N., Cirugia ambulatoria de levantamento de gluteos mediante una sutura sin cicatrices de incision. International Journal of Cosmetic Medicine and Surgery, N 1 Marzo 2003-08-05.

[4] Shvyrev S. P., Prevention of tactical and technical errors during the supraperiosteal lift of the upper two thirds of the face, Annals of Plastic, Reconstructive and Aesthetic Surgery (Russia), N 3,4, 1999, 13-27.

[5] Sulamanidze M.A., Fournier P. F., Paikidze T. G., Sulamanidze G. M., Removal of facial soft tissue ptosis with special threads, Dermatology Surgery 2002;28:367-371.

[6] Ramirez O. M., Cervicoplasty: Nonexcisional anterior approach. Plast. Reconstr. Surg. 99:1576, 1997.

[7] Freeman S. M., Transconjunctival Sub-Orbicularis Oculi Fat (SOOF) Pad Lift Blepharoplasty, Arch. Facial Plast. Surg. /vol. 2, Jan.-Mar. 2000, 16-21.

[8] Fournier P. F., Fat Grafting: My Technique, Dermatologic Surgery, volume 26, number 12, December 2000, p.p. 1117 - 1128.

[9] P. Fournier, Les variants dans la technique du Curl Lift, La revue de chirurgie esthetique de langue Francaise, t. XXVIII, n. 117, decembre 2004, 35-38.

Chapter 11

Mastopexy – How to Reach Consistent Results – New Methods

M. Sulamanidze, G. Sulamanidze and K. Sulamanidze

Additional information is available at the end of the chapter

http://dx.doi.org/10.5772/56317

1. Introduction

Ptosis of glandula mammaria is a well-known aesthetic deflection, which gives a woman unpleasant sensations, causing the need for cosmetic surgery in this field to consistently increase over the last several years. The central problem raised by surgeons is the achievement of a longstanding strength of form and a high glandula mammaria position after performing the operation.

There are hundreds of different surgical methods and devices for handling this problem, which are based on more or less significant solution of skin continuity, surgical release of glandula mammaria, cutting out of its parenchymatous tissue in the form of grafts, underrunning for the purposes of getting flexible stroma, cephalic redistribution of glandular tissue and anchoring to structures, such as banding of glandula mammaria musculus or periosteal coverage of feathers. In addition, it is necessary to tolerate the nipple-areola complex to a new higher location, as well as cutting out of glandula mammaria implant proportional to the modified "excipient" for getting stable dermic uplift.

Unfortunately, these approaches are quite often found to be unsuitable and do not clear away the problem of gravity post-operation ptosis over a long-term period. Suspensory skin sags, overcast seams decrease and on the back of the remained nipple-areola complex in the high position, the whole stroma of the glandula mammaria sinks down gradually, making the previously achieved rather good results ineffective (figure 1a, b, c) [1, 2, 3, 4, 5, 6].

In this case there occurs a relative desolation of the glandula mammaria top hemisphere, an overflow of the lower hemisphere, a flattering of glandula mammarias and its spreading on the chest wall. Visible seams aggravate the aesthetic failure of the performed operation.

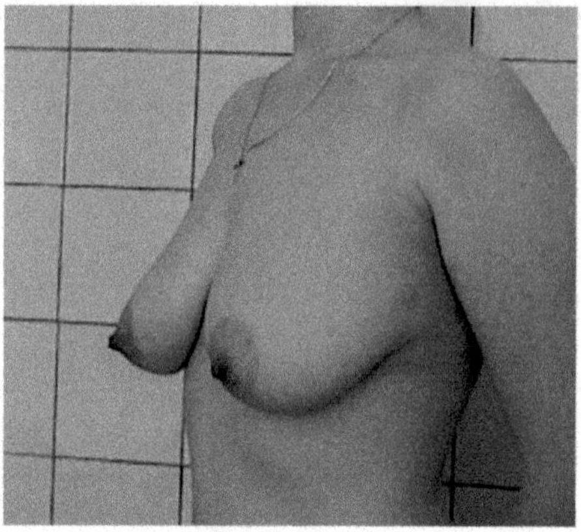

a

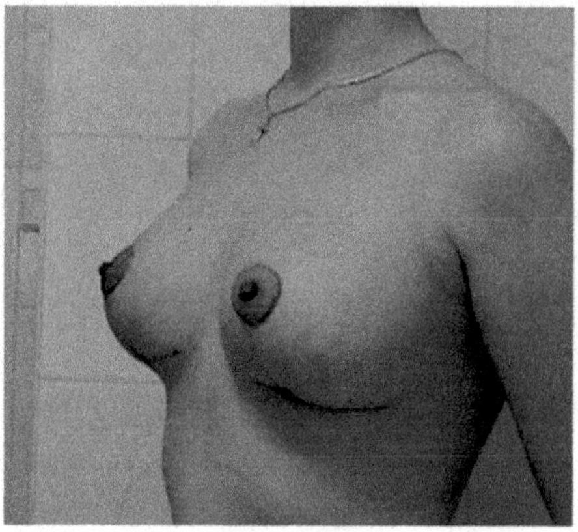

b

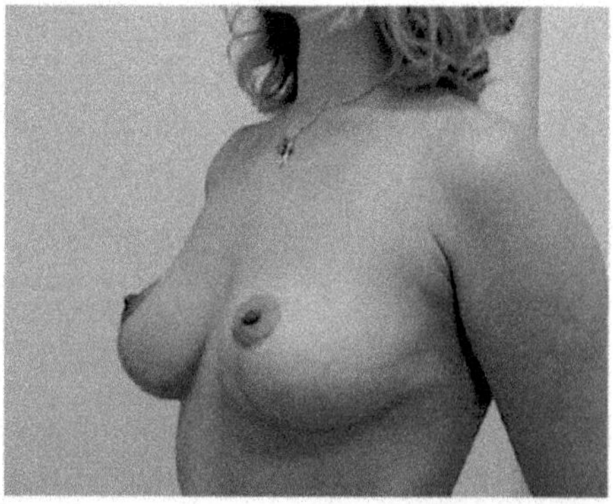

c

Figure 1. The result of classic mastopexy. The sight of the patient before (a); after 2 weeks (b) and a year after the operation (c)

Such results can satisfy neither the surgeon nor the patient and make us doubt the worthiness of the classic mastopexy surgery in most cases of mastoptosis.

Long experience, watching the patients in the post-operation period, analysis of the performed surgeries made it possible to reveal the following reasons of the poor results:

- weakness of architectonics to which the pulled glandula mammaria is attached (banding of glandula mammaria masculus, a periosteal coverage of the feathers);
- incompetence of the overcast surgeon's seams;
- weak effectiveness of the devices which are aimed at supporting the pulled glandula mammaria from the bottom and the sides.

A logical decision was prompted – it is necessary to fix the pulled glandula mammaria to more indurated stable architectonics and provide a strong, steady cradle of the formed glandula mammaria in the lower and lateral portions. Such ideas were put into practice - the original technology was worked out: for the stable anchorage of the glandula mammeria, the technique of hanging the glandula mammeria on the collar bone with the use of special suture material was used, as for the improvement of a glandula mammaria form, strengthening and supporting of the pulled glandula mammaria in the remote post-operation period, cellular endoprosthesis or sutured under-running of the grandula mammaria were used. [7, 8].

The method, which we called "hypodermic bodice", has been successfully used since May 2002 for treating mild glandula mammaria ptosis. The suggested techniques of aesthetic mammoplasty gives an opportunity to get a satisfactory form of a glandula mammaria without post-operation cicatrices or with scarcely noticeable cicatrices in natural places and also to reach the longstanding strength of its form and high catastasis.

2. Materials and methods

A. Materials

During the performance of mastopexy in accordance with the offered method, the following surgical instruments and surgical materials are used.

Aptos Needle DRN 60 is a blunt-ended reflexive needle with an adherent polypropylene needle USP 0, 100 centimeters long. This tool is employed for instilling of the needle around the collar bone and stable anchorage of the glandula mammaria.

Aptos Needle 2/0 is a double-edged needle with a smooth retention suture of prolene 2/0, 100 centimeters long, fixed to the needle in the middle part of it. This unit has a knack for a double-sided patency, it allows to instill the needles under the skin and to perform subdermal under-running of soft tissues according to the broken or the lengthen boundary without skin dimpling with the result of the even pulled boundary (figure 3).

Mersilen specimen-grid holder Ethicon (Johnson & Johnson, USA) is a holder in the thickness of 0.25 millimeters, the diameter of the stroma is 120x85 micron (figure 4).

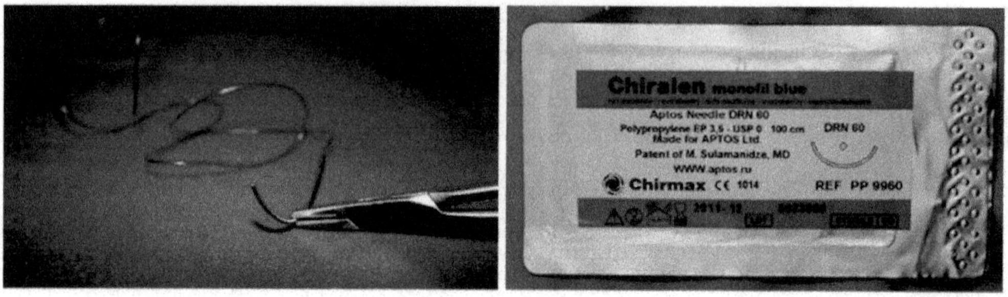

a b

Figure 2. The needle with the suture Aptos Needle DRN 60 for instilling of the needle around the collar bone.

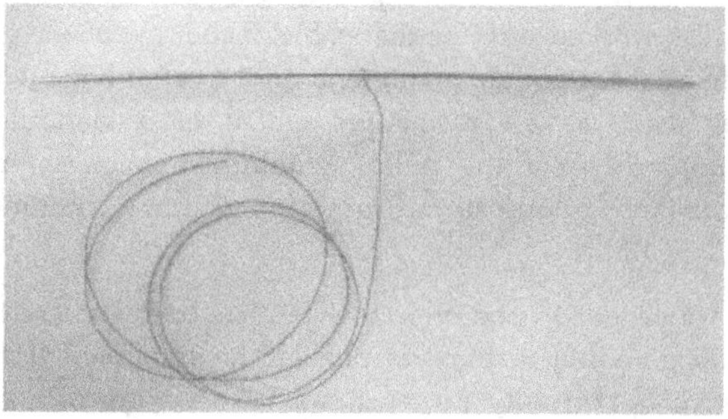

Figure 3. Aptos Needle 2/0 is a needle with the suture for instilling of the glandula mammaria.

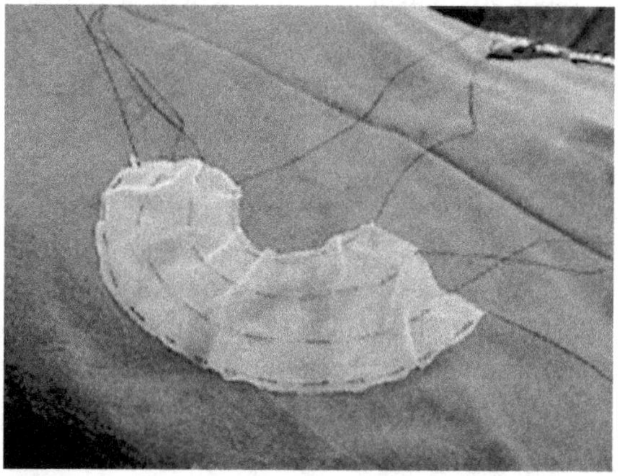

Figure 4. Mersilen speciment-grid holder Ethicon for instilling in the subdermal spatium of glandula mammaria.

Specimen-grid holder Breform (Breform™ Limited, RSA) which is made from a multifilament polyether in the form of a glandula mammaria (figure 5). It allows to make the result of the operation stable.

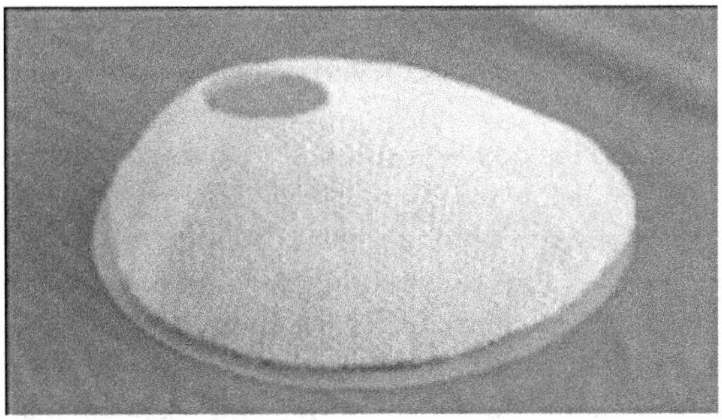

Figure 5. Polyether specimen-grid holder Breform made for anchoraging the results of mastopexy.

B. Methods

Our methods of minimally invasive breast mastopexy consist of anchoring the breasts (with the use of a cellular implant or under-running the breasts with sutures) and the follow-up mastopexy and hanging the breast on the clavicle.

Operational technique of suturing around the clavicle

The operation was performed under general anesthesia. The patient was laid down in a semi-sitting position. Two discissions, of 2-3 millimeters long each, were made along the midclavicular line: one was above the clavicle to its periosteal coverage, the second was lower, at the level of the second intercostal space to the banding of the greater pectorial muscle. The soft tissues were separated by a thin fastener like "mosquito" and hydropreporation of the soft tissues around the clavicle was performed as well (normal saline with epinephrine in amount of 20 ml).

A clavicular acus (Aptos Needle DRN 60) was taken with a heavy acutenaculum. It was inserted in the lower discission by its blunt end, instilled upward subdermal towards the clavicle and agested through the upper discission together with the suture. The suture was pulled with the acus, but the "tail", 10 centimeters long, was left in the lower maim. The acus was turned in the upper maim and the end of the acus was instilled around the collar bone, not separating from the bone. The acus with the suture was egested in the lower maim, where the nodosity with the left "tail" was tied.

Therefore, the path of the clavicular acus went from the lower maim subdermally in the adipose layer to the clavicle, then the path went behind it (postclavicular spatium) and next - under the banding of the internal surface of the greater pectorial muscle to the view of the lower maim, where the acus was egested to the maim through the fibers.

Two interrupted stiches of prolene 6/0 closed the maim over the clavicle at the end of the operation.

The most important stage of the whole operation is instilling of the acus behind the clavicle. In order to do it without any complications, it is necessary to perform the following actions:

- make hydropreporation of the tissues behind and under the clavicle. This will allow moving the attached prescalenic musculus from the bone and enlarge the postclavicular spatium;
- turn the patients' head to the opposite side from where the operation is performed. For the pecroral arch, turn it below maximal. It will allow putting the clavicle forward and providing comfortable position for performing the operation;
- use only the recommended acus for instilling the suture, the bending and the length of which are aimed at the safe performance of the operation;
- move the end of the acus exactly along the bone without stopping the process; the surgeon can achieve it if he/she performs the semicircular movement of the acutenaculum carefully.

Technique of the surgery on insertion of a reticular implant in the hypodermic spatium of the breasts (the method of the "hypodermic bodice")

The surgery was performed under general anesthesia with the infiltration of the hypoderm by means of isotonic solution with adrenalin added.

The respective marking was made beforehand.

The patient was put in the semi-sitting position. Reticular implant was installed through the inframammar and the periareolary access. The length of the discission depended on the method of the surgical release of the cellulocutaneous flap. If this part of the operation was performed with the copper bent blunt-pointed scissors without endoscopic maintenance, the discission was made with the length of no less than 5 centimeters, while with the use of endoscopic equipment or a wire scalpel the length of the discission was no more than 2-3 cm.

Detachment of the flap was done within the lower lateral and medial quadrants of the milk gland. A net was implanted and spread in the underflap area after hemostasis, which was later sewed with the interrupted stitch in the projection of the inframammar fold and the lower edge of the areola. 3-4 pairs of threads which had been sewed to the lateral and medial edges of the net were taken to the wound in the intercostal spatium under skin, where the thread had already been taken around the clavicle. Here they were taken out, pulled, and tied to the ends of the clavicularis thread, lifting the breasts as the result.

At the end of the operation two interrupted sutures were put on the wound in the area of the second intercostal space, while the main wound (under the areola and in the inframammar fold) was sewed in three stages by continuous method.

The important features of this operation are the following:

- the selection of the patients by indication;
- surgical release of the cellulocutaneous flap of such area which allows the net to seize a sufficient volume of the breasts subsequently, especially from the lateral side;
- the installation and straightening of the inserted net in the way that no "recesses" and roughness emerge, and only after that its fixation by the side seams;
- even alternating tightening of the threads with the control of the form of the lifted breasts and their stable tightening to the clavicular thread;

Technique of ligature sawing of the breasts (method of thread lifting of the breasts)

The operation was performed under the general anesthesia with the patient in the semi sitting position.

The respective marking was made beforehand.

The middle clavicular line was drawn from top to bottom through the nipple to the inframammar fold, marking pints on that line: on the level of the second intercostal space (point A), the upper and lower edges of the areola. The distance from the lower edge of the areola to point A was divided into halves, this is where point B was marked, the segments A-B and B- the upper edge of the areola were also divided into halves, where points C and D were marked.

By analogy points A1, B1, C1, D1 were marked below the areola. Oval lines were drawn through these points which outlined the breasts in different levels.

The operation was started with bayonet incisions, 1-1.5 centimeters in depths in points A, B, C, D, which were widened by blunt method with the use of the "mosquito".

Under-running of the breasts was performed with Aptos Needle 2/0. To perform that the point of the needle was inserted in the wound in point A and the thread was taken through under the skin according to the marking. The needle was partially taken out and turned if it was needed, moving it further according to the line of the marking until reaching the point of insertion, and it was taken out in point A. Then the thread was pulled out with its 5-7 centimeters ends left out and taken to the holder.

Under-running of the breasts according to the rest of the lines which had been drawn through points B-B1, C-C1, D-D1 of marking was done by analogy. Therefore, the breasts were fringed with threads in four levels. After that the threads were lifted and the ends were bound together alternately in the form of knots starting from point A to point E.

Afterwards, with the use of the same blunt-pointed needle, the thread for under-running the clavicle (Aptos Needle DRN 60) was tied to the thread from point A to the thread from point C, the thread from C to point B, the thread B to the thread A, and the thread from this point to the thread which was fixed to the clavicle. In this way the breasts were lifted to the aesthetically acceptable form and position.

The important features of this operation are the following:

- the selection of the patients by indication;
- the insertion of the needle hypodermically at the necessary depths without visualization of the thread through the skin;
- under-running of the breasts in the way that in the areas of the entrance and the exit of the turn of the needle there are no retractions of the breasts left;
- even lifting of the threads and their tying together at the same level with the control of the required form.

82 operations of aesthetic mammoplasty of breasts applying the method of sewing the breasts with threads, their lifting, and their suspension to the clavicle, 11 operations with the use of reticular implants have been performed in Total Charm clinics since 2002, in total 93 operations.

3. Results

The indications for undergoing such operations were considered to be:

- a small or a moderate ptosis of milk glands (I-II degree);
- a small size of the milk glands (relative size 1-2.5);
- a small or a moderate excess of skin;
- a small extent of involuntary changes of breasts tissues;

Operative intervention with these methods took place in cases of primary ptosis of breasts or of the recurrence of ptosis in the post-operation period. We have resorted to these methods for preventing the post-operation ptosis of breasts and in the presence of post-operation scars.

In practice, we have applied the first and the second or the first and the third operation.

In any plastic surgery when it is necessary to reduce the area of the skin one of the two well-known methods are used. The first one – resection of the necessary amount of skin in the process of operational intervention, the second one – expecting its retraction, as long as the skin is known to shrink as the result of its release from the function of the long-lasting support of the substructural adipose, parenchymal, and other tissues, the value and the weight of which usually increases with the lapse of time. The second method in particular lies in the basis of some of endoscopic aesthetic operations and methods of thread face lifting. The same characteristic of the skin is taken into account and applied in the operation of "hypodermic bodice".

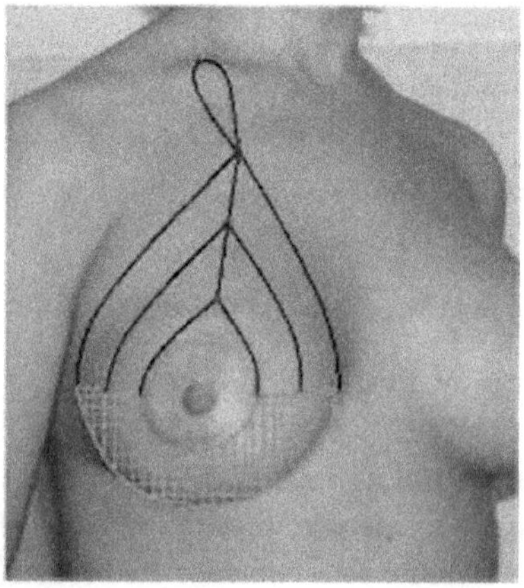

Figure 6. Scheme of marking the breasts for insertion of a reticular implant (the method of "hypodermic bodice").

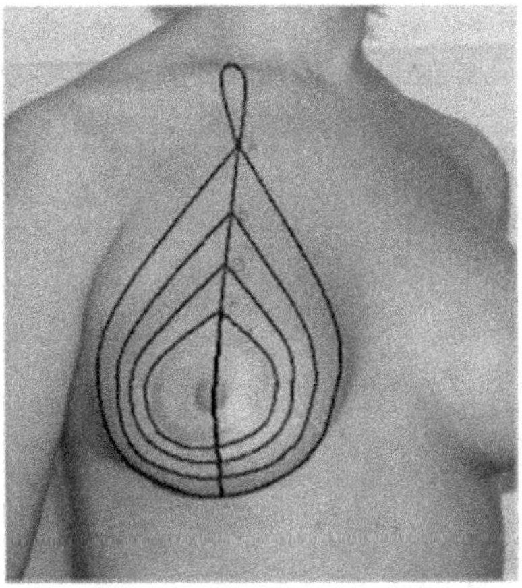

Figure 7. Scheme of marking of the breasts for under-running with the needles and the further lifting of the breasts (the method of the needle breast lifting).

The operational interventions were performed easily without extra trauma, the post-operation period in most cases did not show any after effects, while the aesthetic results were good and stable. In all cases the above mentioned method provided consistent, long-lasting mastopexy.

The presented clinical results confirm the effectiveness of the operations performed (figures 8-13).

4. Complications

During the whole period of performing the operations we witnessed the following complications and unpleasant evidences:

- the case of failure of the hypodermic knot in point B from the left side on the 3rd day after the operation. As a result, ptosis recurrenc of the left breast and obvious skewness of the milk glands occurred (figure 14a);
  Under the infiltrational anesthesia the wound in this place was opened, the ends of the threads were found and a new stable knot was put in place. The post-operation period did not show any complications and the final result was satisfying (figure 14b);
- the case of acquiring an atrophic indrawn scar, which was resolved with the method of lipofilling (figure 15a);
- some cases of skin indrawing in the places of the needle turns or of the skin-deep needle conduction. The defects were eliminated with the help of massage and the method of lipofilling;

We try to examine regularly the patients who were operated with these methods, as long as the methods are new and require special attention. We are usually interested in the following issues in the post-operation period: the condition of the milk gland near the reticule; the invasion of the reticule by the fibrous tissues; the condition of the clavicle; its stability, and the condition of the milk glands during menses, pregnancy, labour, lactation, and during the following period (figure 16).

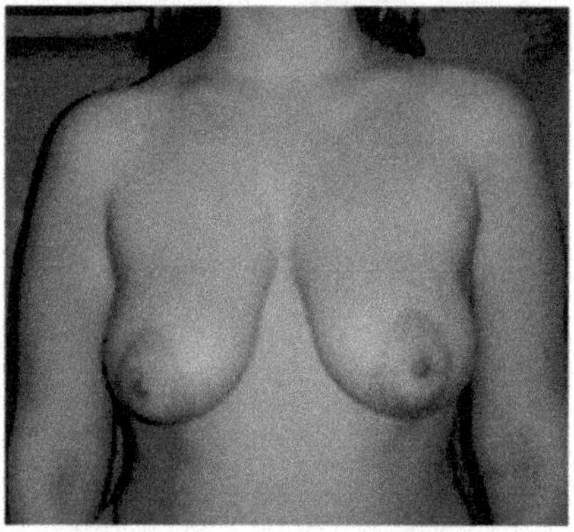

a

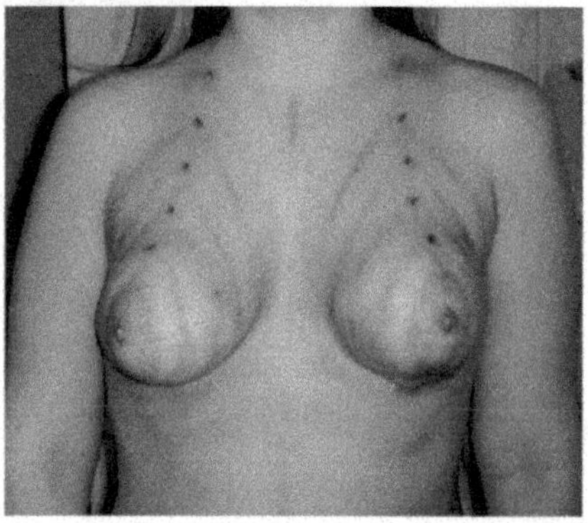

b

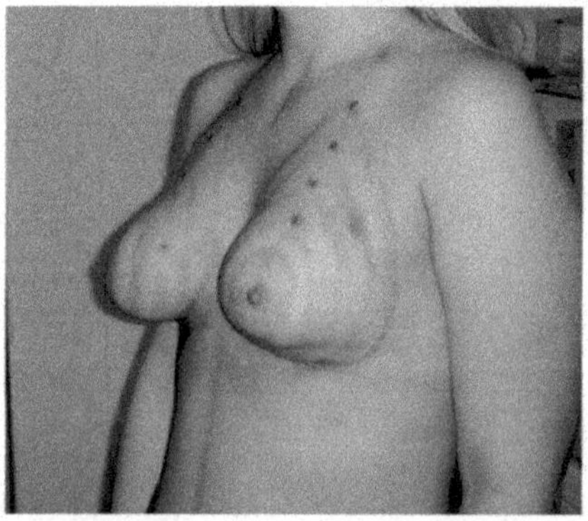

c

Figure 8. Patient A., 32 years old, before (a,b) and in 2 days after (c,d) the thread breasts lifting.

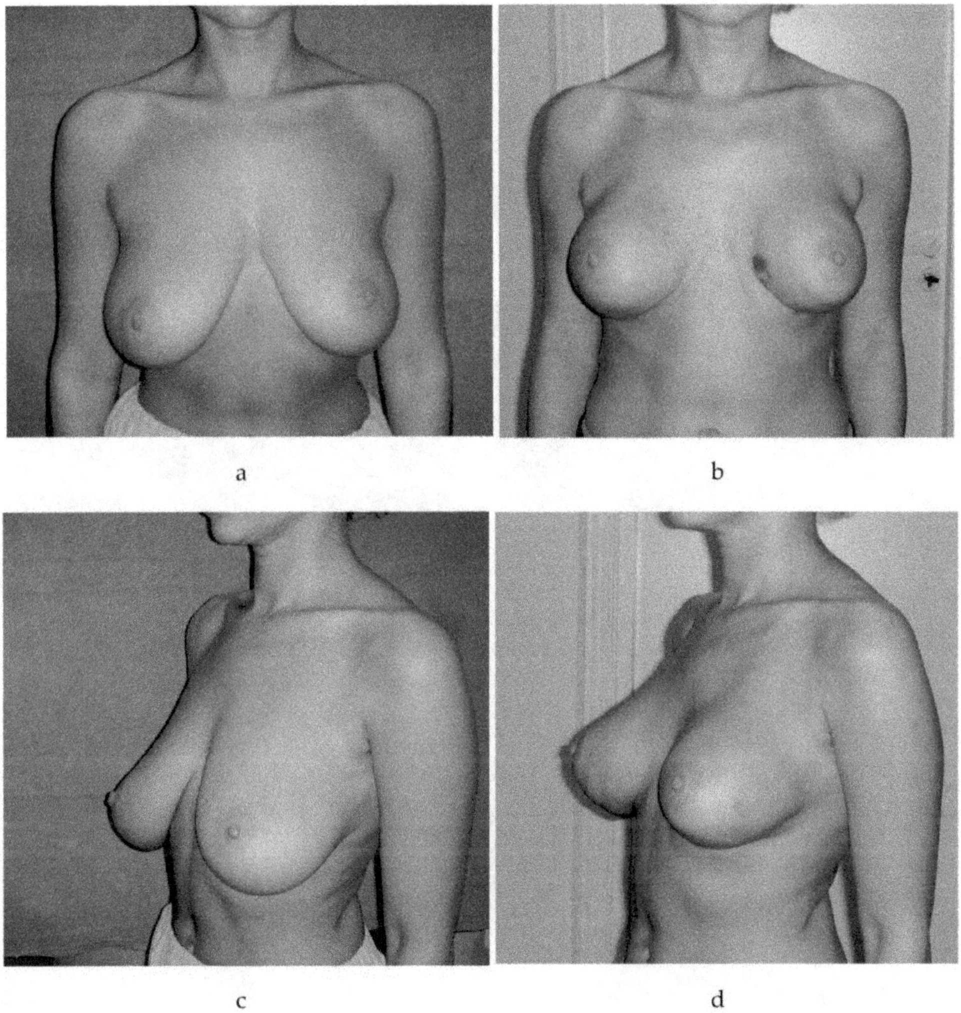

Figure 9. Patient B., 44 years old, before (a,b) and in 10 days after (c,d) the thread breasts lifting;

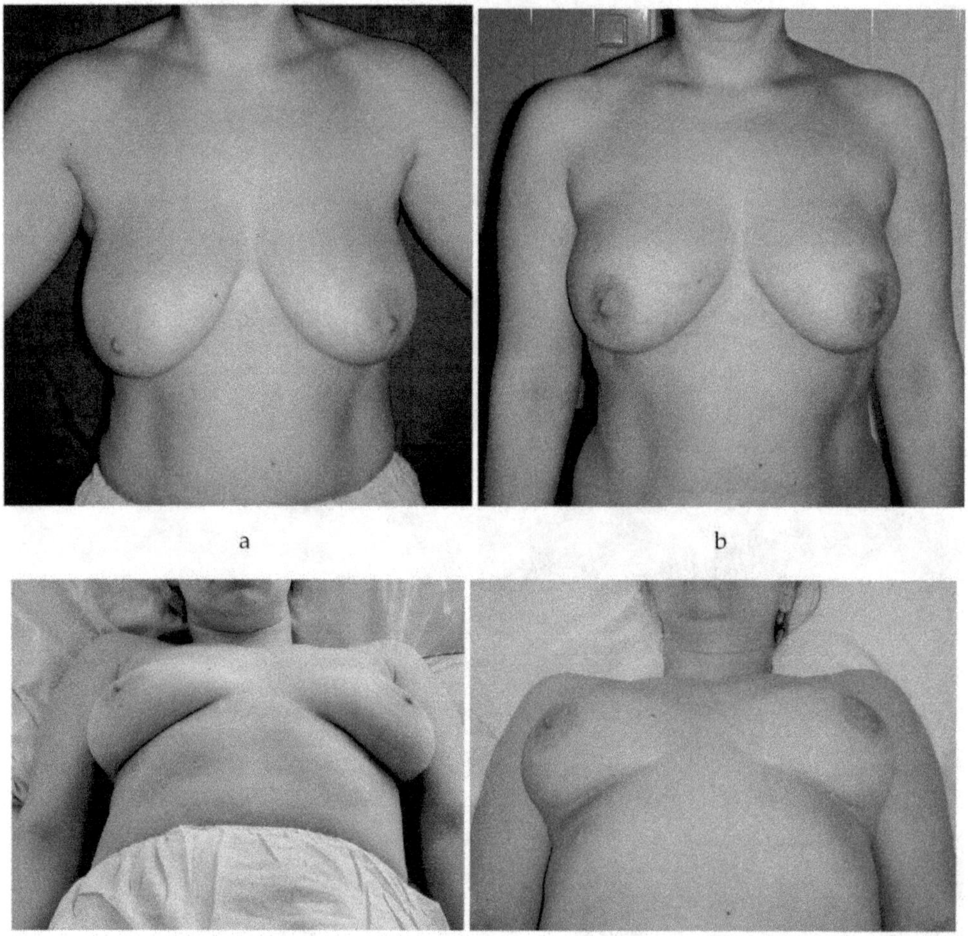

Figure 10. Patient C., 34 years old, before (a,b) and in 2 years after (c,d) the thread breasts lifting;

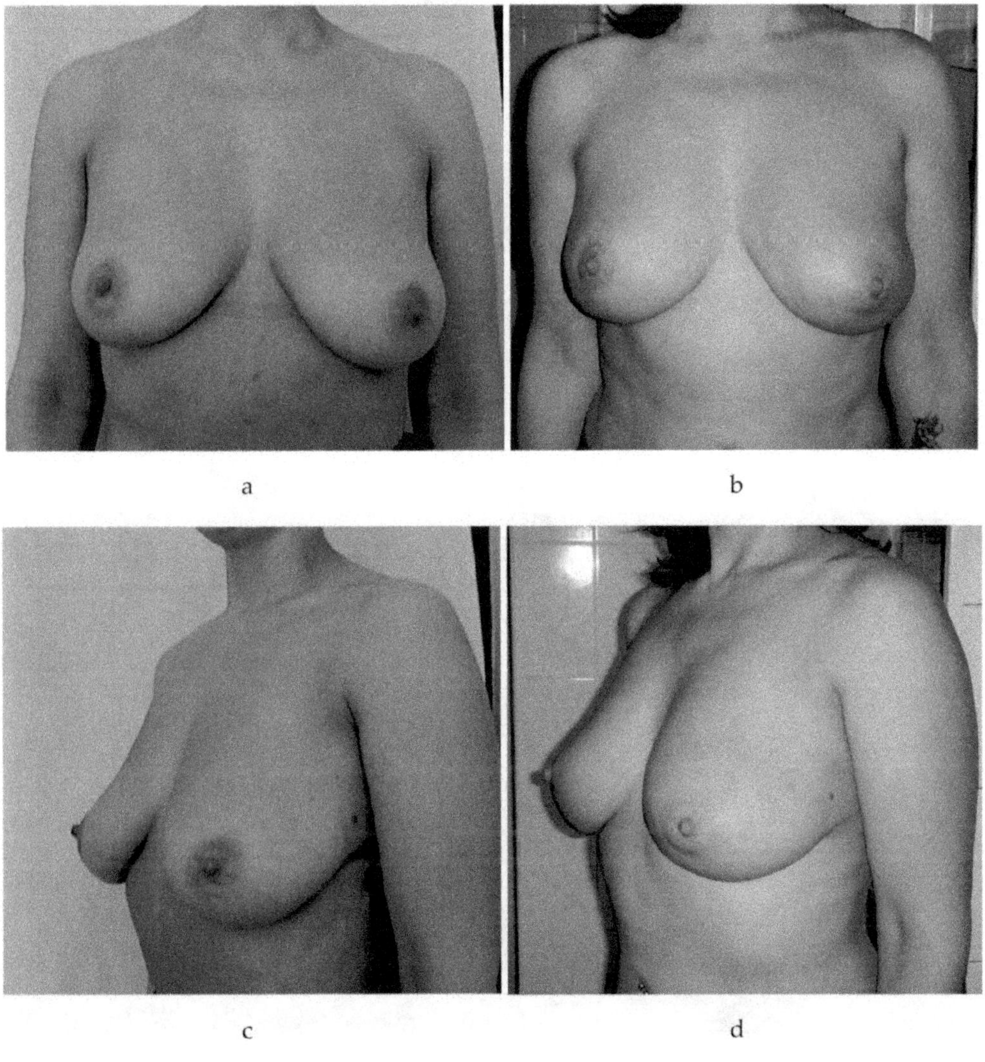

Figure 11. Patient D., 34 years old, before (a,b) and in 5 years after (c,d) the operation with the use of a reticular implant.

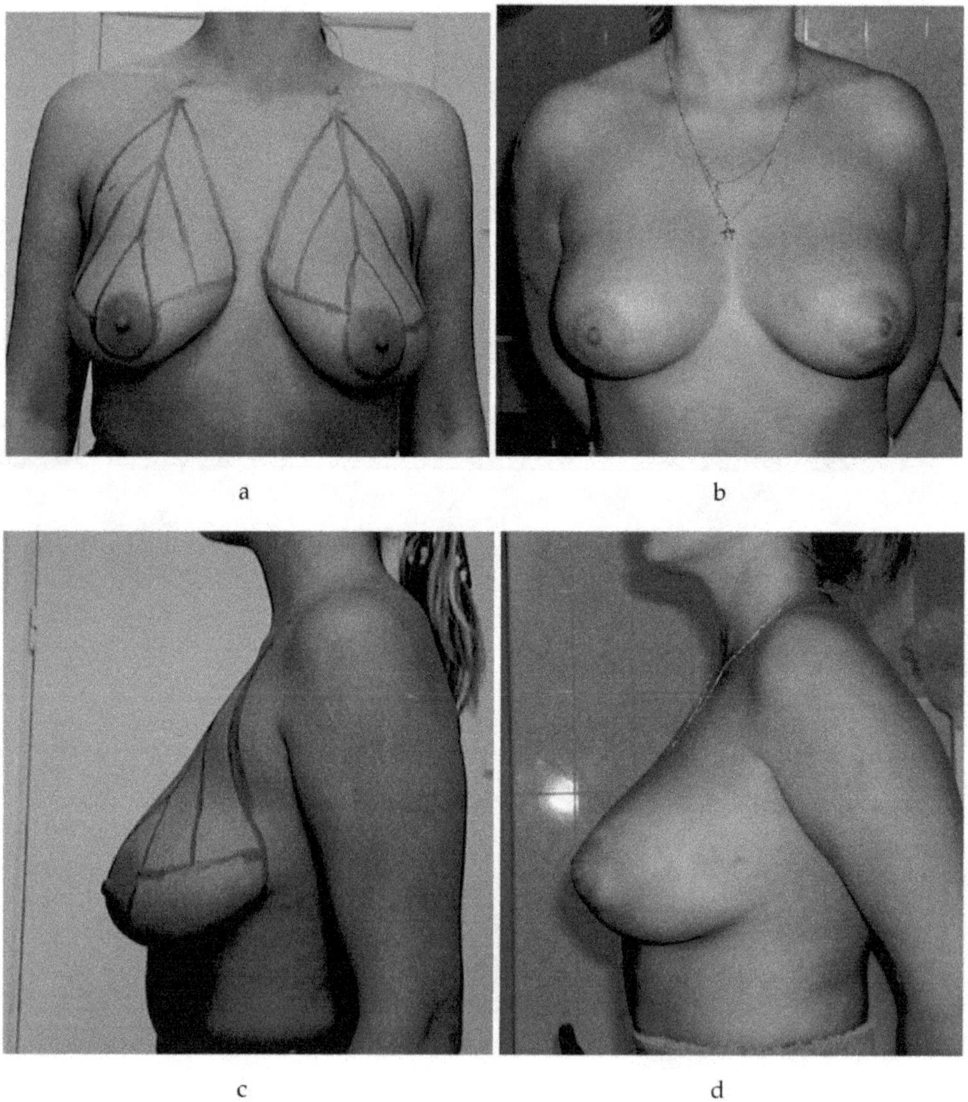

Figure 12. Patient E, 35 years old, before (a,b) and in 2.5 years (c,d) after the breasts lifting with a reticular implant.

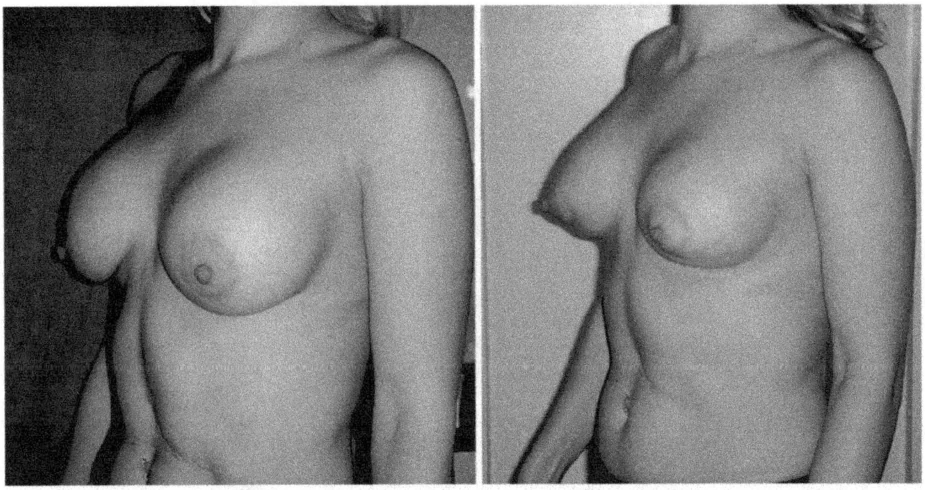

a b

Figure 13. Patient F, 30 years old. Some years ago the patient underwent augmentational mammoplastic in a different clinic. At the admission to our clinic she complained about the dissatisfying condition of her breasts. During the examination capsular contracture was observed. The implant remained in its place, while the tissue of the gland shifted down (glandulus ptosis). The patient underwent a thread breast lifting. Before (a) and in two months after the intervention (b).

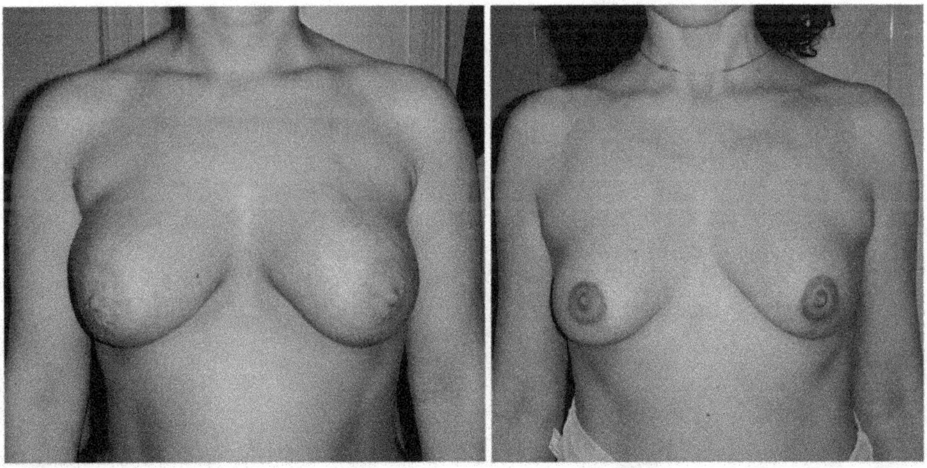

a b

Figure 14. Patient G, 38 years old. Complication – failure of the thread knot in three days after the thread lifting recurrence of the left breast ptosis. Before (a) and in a year after the re-operation (b).

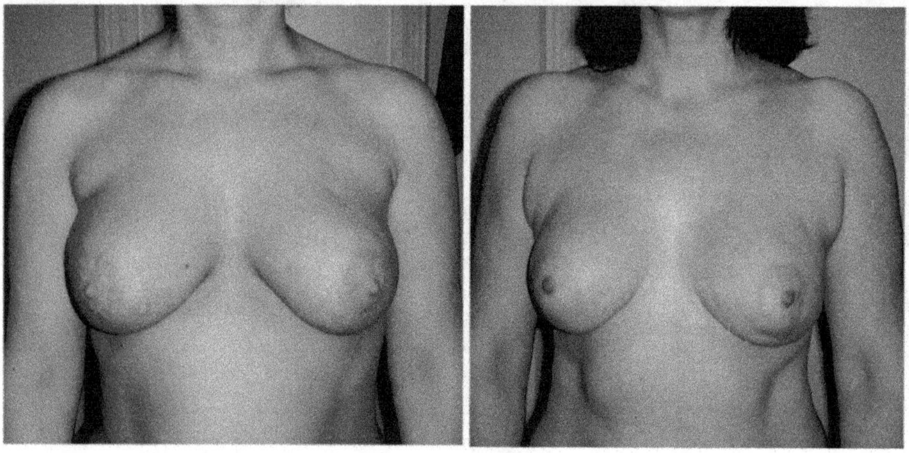

a b

Figure 15. Complication - atrophic scarring (a); visualization of the threads – indrawing of skin in the areas of the turns of the needle and skin-deep needle conduction (b).

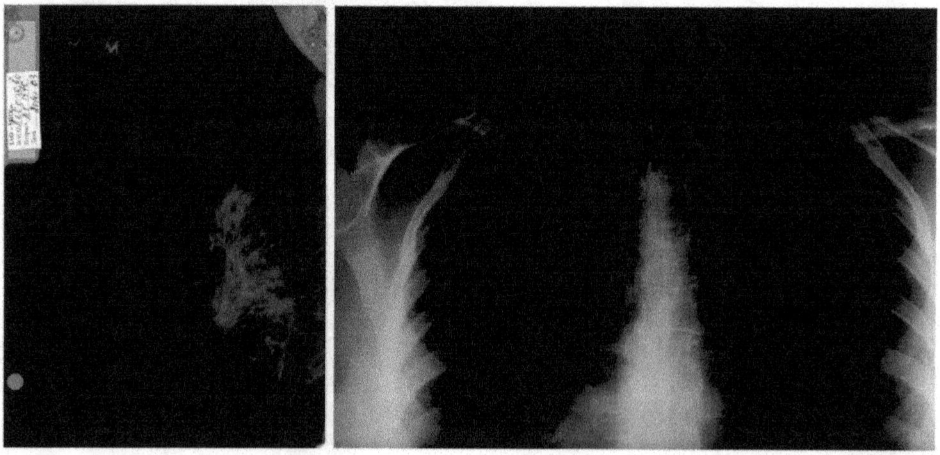

a b

Figure 16. Patient E. X-ray examination of the breasts (a,b) and the chest in two years after the breast lifting with installation of a reticular implant.

Besides, in our practice there have been two cases of pregnancy, delivery, and further lactation. No problems were observed (figure 17).

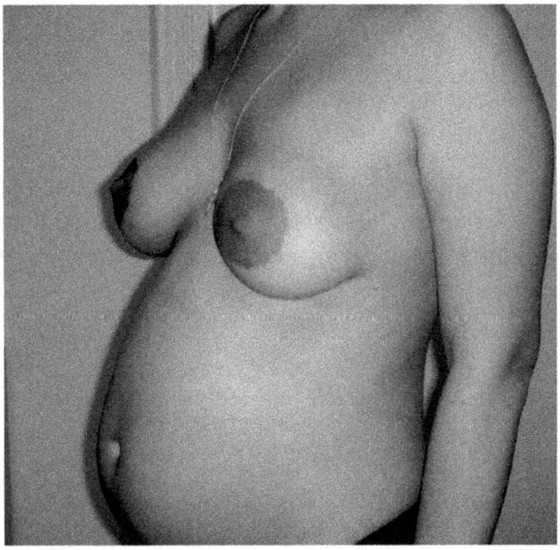

Figure 17. Patient K, 28 years old, in 2.5 years after the thread breast lifting, pregnancy period.

5. Conclusions

A group of surgeons of Total Charm clinic have presented the following methods and techniques, which serve to improve the results of mastopexy:

- suspension of the lifted breasts to the clavicle providing its stable attachment to the firm osteal structure, which does not allow the breast to move down gradually in the long run;
- insertion of a reticular implant in the hypodermic area of the lower and lateral segments of breasts, envelopment of these areas of the milk gland and its suspension to the clavicle, which leads to strengthening of the breasts and acquiring of the necessary aesthetically accepted form;
- thread sewing of the breasts through the cuts in the skin and its further suspension to the clavicle – girth of the milk gland from all the sides with solid surgical sutural material with application of hypodermic seams without incisions in order to create a resilient stroma of the gland with conical shape and to prevent its cephalic movement.

The first two methods are widely known in plastic surgery, but have been considerably modified by our group, the latter method is original and has been developed by the group.

Six-year period of performing mastopexy using "hypodermic bodice" method by underrunning of the breasts with Aptos threads, numerous examples and accumulated experience have shown that the method has justified the hopes. During the post-operation period, no patients have shown abnormal changes of milk glands, substructure, and the clavicle. No cases of dissatisfaction complaints have been reported.

Also attention should paid to the method of hypodermic dissection of the soft tissues (to create a cellulocutaneous flap) which is performed with the use of wire scalpel (Aptos Wire). The operation is easy, simple and minimally invasive, without significant hemorrhage. In comparison with the endoscopic method, it does not require costly equipment and special training of the surgeon, while the post-operational rehabilitation of the patient is reduced. The acquired cellulocutaneous flap has even thickness, good blood supply, and survives well in the donor wound.

The presented methods of milk gland ptosis correction in combination with the use of reticular endoprosthesis for mastoptosis correction are regarded as promising areas in aesthetic surgery of minimal invasion, and they require further examination and accumulation of experience.

Author details

M. Sulamanidze, G. Sulamanidze and K. Sulamanidze
Clinic of Anaplastic and Aesthetic Surgery Total Charm, Moscow, Russia - Tbilisi, Georgia

6. References

[1] Adamyan A. A., Romashov Y.V., Kopiltsov A.A. Mammoplast in postlactational involution. Annals of plastic, reparative, and aesthetic surgery, 1997; (4);47-54.

[2] Borovikov A.M. Ter-Nokogosiyan G.A. Aesthetic mamoplast. What we talk about. Annals of plastic, reparative, and aesthetic surgery, 2002; (3);41- 46.

[3] Borovikov A.M. Milk gland ptosis. Selected issues of plastic surgery, 2005; 1(12).

[4] Burdin V.V. Beliyaev M.V. To the question of the choice of operational intervention in the postlactational involution of the milk glands. Annals of plastic, reparative, and aesthetic surgery, 2001; (2); 16-20.

[5] Milanov N.O., Startseva O.I., Chausheva S.I. Analysis of experience in single-stage mastopexy and endoprosthesis replacement of milk glands. Annals of plastic, reparative, and aesthetic surgery, 2005; (1); 44-51.

[6] Frishberg I. A. Surgical correction of cosmetic deflection of women's breasts. – Moscow, 1997.

[7] Sulamanidze M.A., Savchenko S.V., Vozdvizhenskiy I.S., Sulamanidze G.M., Osipov A.G.. Horisontal mammoplast. Annals of plastic, reparative, and aesthetic surgery, 2002; (3); 40-46.

[8] Sulamanidze M.A., Vozdvizhenskiy I.S., Sulamanidze G.M., Sulamanidze K.M. Application of reticular endoprosthesis in mamoplast. Our experience. Thesis collection II Intermational Conference "Modern technologies and opportunities of reconstructive and reparative aesthetic surgery". October 19-20, 2010 – Moscow, 2010.

Section 2

Barbed Thread Lifts

Chapter 12

Morphological Foundations of Facelift Using APTOS Filaments

A.A. Adamyan, M.A. Sulamanidze, N.D. Skuba and Z.R. Khusnutdinova

Additional information is available at the end of the chapter

http://dx.doi.org/10.5772/56318

1. Introduction

Correction of earlier involutional changes of the face, in the first place facial skin ptosis, encounters some difficulties. On the one hand, these changes are not serious enough to serve as an indication for radical aesthetic surgery. On the other hand, traditional minor surgical interventions fail to ensure well-apparent beneficial effect.

Moreover, many women are reluctant to undergo extensive surgery since it entails prolonged rehabilitation which may sometimes take one and a half months to be completed.

No wonder, many plastic surgeons tend to resort to a combination of minor invasive interventions that are apt to significantly shorten the rehabilitation period and are possible to perform in an outpatient setting.

2. Materials and methods

Recent years witnessed wide implementation into clinical practice of aesthetic surgery of an effective, atraumatic method of treatment of facial involutional alterations – lifting of the soft tissues with the help of specially designed "APTOS" threads [1, 4, 5, 6, 7, 8].

The method is based on the use of specially designed polypropylene APTOS filaments and is recommended for managing moderate involutional changes in the facial soft tissues and local face lifting. One side of an APTOS thread bears barbs that extend forward in the direction of its movement through the tissue, on the other side the barbs extend backward, i.e. in the opposite direction. Barb length - 1 mm, barb angle thickness could vary from 30 to 50 degree depending on the barb resistance force. Such a design ensures that the filament gently glides through soft tissues in a desired direction but resists drawing in the opposite one, i.e. remains fixed as appropriate. As a result, subcutaneously implanted filaments keep in place the lifted facial tissues uniformly drawn into puckers, do not allow them to slip down, and thus maintain a new facial contour.

However, until now it remains unknown how the APTOS threads behave within the tissues in time and what are the local and morphological processes maintaining the tension and creating the rejuvenating effect.

In an attempt to clarify the mechanism of tissue reactions to subcutaneous implantation of APTOS filaments, an experimental study of the resulting morphological changes was undertaken at the A.V. Vishnevsky Institute of Surgery. A group of 20 white rats was used as a model from which 72 tissue samples were obtained for histological studies [3]. Morphological findings were compared with the results of examination of tissue samples following implantation of smooth polypropylene filaments to another group of animals that served as control.

The material for histological analysis included implants, their capsules, and the surrounding tissues.

Relative vascular bed density (RVBD) at different time intervals after implantation was estimated and compared with RVBD of intact rats to evaluate changes of blood supply to the tissues surrounding implanted polypropylene filaments [2].

Relative vascular bed density was calculated by the following standard formula

$$RVBD = \frac{\textit{Number of points in the blood vessel field}}{\textit{Total number of points in the examined field}} \times 100\%$$

3. Results and discussion

On day 3 after subcutaneous implantation, the filament was found to be isolated from the surrounding tissue mass by an immature connective tissue capsule (fig. 1a) the lateral sides of which gave rise to connective tissue bands. The capsule wall was much thicker close to the barbs than near the smooth thread portions. Also, the capsule wall facing epidermis was significantly thicker than its remaining part, probably due to mechanical pressure exerted by the integumentary tissues on the filament and the capsule developing around it. Such variability of the capsule wall thickness is considered to be beneficial for the final face lifting effect and improve its stability.

The histological study revealed marked hyperemia of the microvascular bed. It was especially pronounced where barbs rose from the shaft of the thread. The barbs looked braided with tissue cells. The inner capsule layer at the base of the barbs was composed of fibroblasts dominated by young cells. Connective tissue bands growing from the capsule wall were readily apparent as well as inflammatory reaction that resulted in fibroblast accumulation around the barbs and thickening of the capsule wall where it faced epidermis. There were practically no signs of inflammation in the form of infiltration around the implanted filaments.

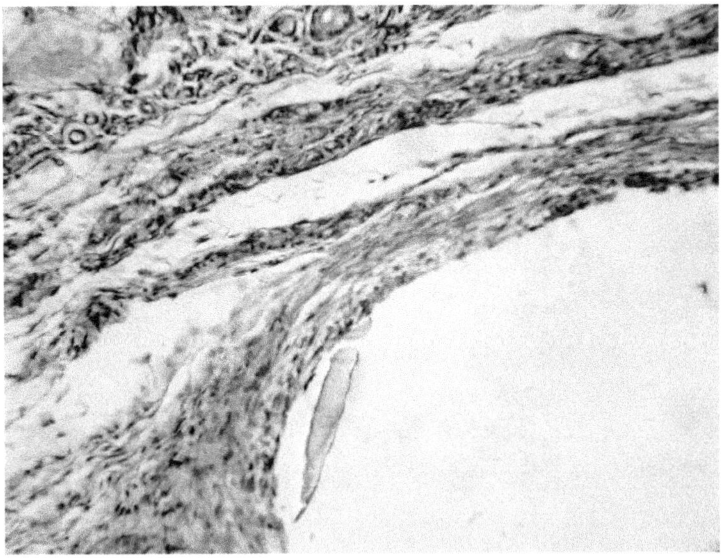

a

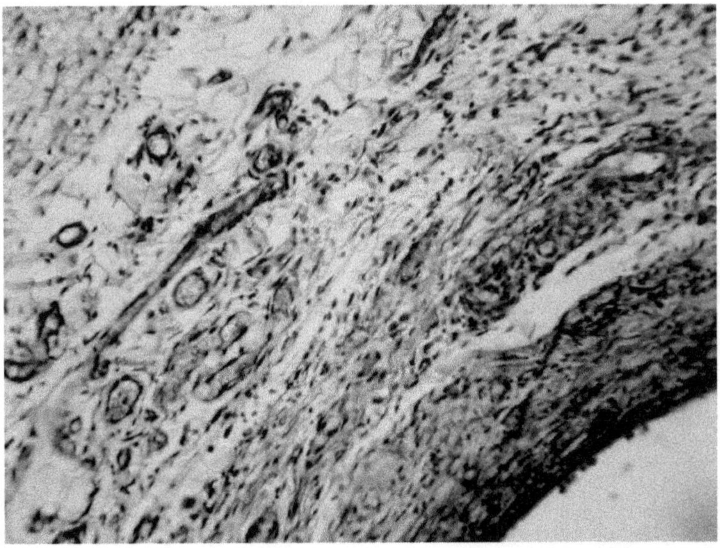

b

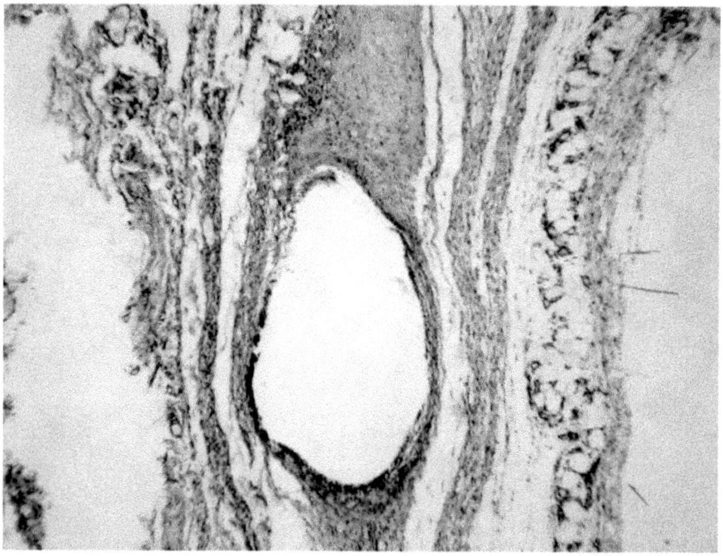

c

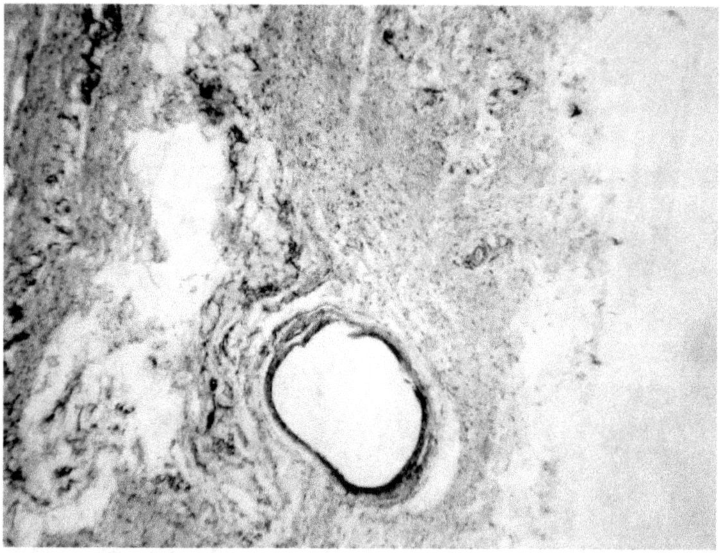

d

a - 3 days after implantation. Cellular elements predominate over fibrous ones, the number of microvessels increases (x100); b - 7 days after implantation. The capsule has a bilayer structure, persistent hyperemia develops due to marked vasodilation (x100); *c*-*7* days after implantation. Connective tissue bands can be seen arising from the upper poles of the capsule (x40); *d* - *7* days after implantation (x40)

Figure 1. Microphotographs of the capsule surrounding APTOS filament (a-c) and smooth polypropylene thread (d). Van-Gieson pyrofuchsin staining

The structure of the capsule surrounding a smooth polypropylene filament on day 3 after implantation was not substantially different from that formed around a barbed APTOS filament. Only the wall thickness was smaller, being 19.25 mem on the side facing epidermis and 23.5 mem on the side facing the subcutaneous fat layer. A thinner capsule around smooth filaments was due to the absence of barbs and the respective less injurious effect of the implanted material.

The shape of the capsule developing after the implantation of both APTOS and smooth filaments was that of a rhombus. However, the capsule around smooth filaments gave out no connective tissue bands arising from their lateral walls.

On day 7, the capsules around APTOS filaments became thicker due to a rise in the number of collagen fibres. Each capsule exhibited two distinct layers characterized by different cell to collagen fibre ratio (fig. 1b):

1. inner layer enclosing the filament and dominated by young cells and
2. outer layer in which collagen fibres predominated.

The capsules assumed the rhomboid shape while their lateral apices gave rise to connective tissue bands that became thinner as the distance from the capsule increased (fig. 1c). The total length of a band (the capsule wall inclusive) was 886 mem, the width ranged from 108 to 187 mem. The capsules remained well-vascularized despite a progressive rise in the number of collagen fibres within 7 days after filament implantation. The capsule walls were penetrated by a large number of capillary vessels, microvascular hyperemia persisted both in the immediate proximity to the filaments and at a certain distance from them. No signs of pyogenic inflammation could be seen.

The outer capsule layer, although rather thin, always contained a large number of capillary-type vessels.

Isolated lymphoid and plasma cells as well as swollen fibroblasts were readily apparent close to microvessels. The amount of blood congestion in the microvascular bed decreased with the distance from the filament.

The thickness of the capsule formed around a smooth polypropylene filament by day 7 after implantation was 17.75 mem on the side facing epidermis and 17.25 mem on the side facing the subcutaneous fatty layer. Lateral walls were as thick as 54.5 and 25 mem (fig. 1c).

On the whole, the major morphological characteristics of the tissues surrounding smooth filaments on day 7 after implantation underwent significantly smaller modification compared with the tissues responding to APTOS filaments.

On day 40, further thickening of the capsule wall around both the shaft and the barbs of APTOS filaments took place; however, the capsule development was not completed. The capsule wall facing epidermis was significantly thicker than that facing the subcutaneous fat layer (58 and 18.75 mem, respectively). Connective tissue bands arising from the capsule walls, shafts and barbs of APTOS filaments became thicker and longer than before. Simultaneously, the number of microvessels increased. Most of them underwent hyperemia, but no signs of exudation were documented.

A peculiar morphological finding on day 40 was parallel bands composed of connective tissue fibres and extending towards the subcutaneous fat layer. According to micrometric measurements, the bands were from 5,000 to 8,000 mem long and from 900 to 300 mem wide. They occupied a total area of 4,200 mem.

Characteristic changes in loose connective tissue close to the implanted filaments included:

- an increased number of vessels in the microcirculatory system (arterioles, venules, pre- and postcapillaries, and capillaries) compared with tissues located farther from the implants;
- microvessels looked overfilled with blood, i.e. had an open lumen, any time after the implantation of APTOS filaments; in other words, implantation induced persistent hyperemia and therefore stimulated blood supply to the tissues surrounding APTOS filaments;
- fibroblasts of loose connective tissue had enlarged nuclei and plasma volume and finely dispersed chromatin which suggested a functionally active state.

Staining with toluidine blue revealed an increased number of mast cells in the loose connective tissue layer surrounding APTOS filaments. These cells were concentrated in perivascular space of the microcirculatory system (fig. 2).

The tissue response to smooth polypropylene filaments on day 40 after their implantation was not significantly different from that to APTOS filament. However, the capsule

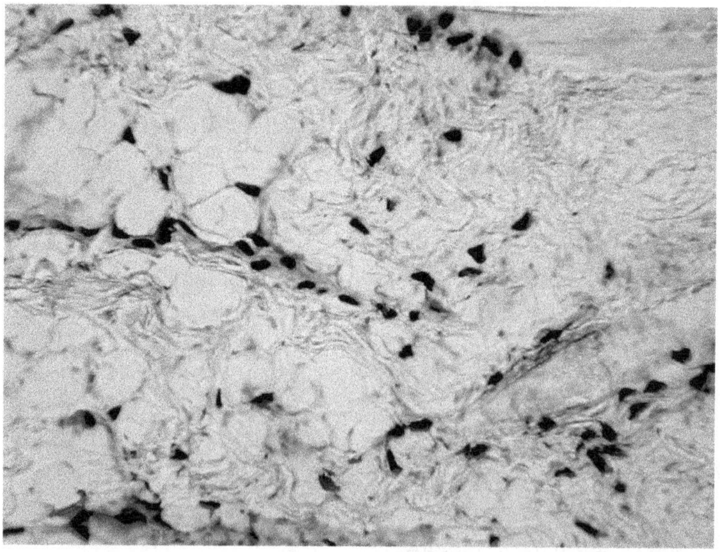

Figure 2. Microphotograph showing accumulation of mast cells around APTOS filament. Staining with toluidine blue (x 40)

developing around smooth polypropylene threads had thinner walls and matured quicker than around APTOS filaments, evidently due to less severe irritating effect on the tissues.

The capsule wall thickness varied from 52,5 mem on the side facing epidermis to 42.75 mem on the side facing the subcutaneous fat layer. The lateral walls of the capsule were approximately 400 mem thick. The width of the middle part of the lateral walls was around 136.75 mem. Tissues surrounding smooth filaments contained an increased number of microvessels, but hyperemia and vascularization were less pronounced than around APTOS filament.

On day 90 after the implantation of APTOS filaments, the inner capsule layer was composed of functionally active cells, each containing a large amount of cytoplasm. The outer layer consisted of collagen fibres and a small number of fibrocytes (fig. 3a).

Fibrous capsule structures and similar structures of the surrounding tissue merged into one another giving rise to a continuous network.

In the course of time, the fibrous capsule became more and more tightly integrated with the surrounding tissue which promoted solid fixation of the implanted filaments. Both the shaft and the barbs of the filaments were braided with fibrous tissue structures. The capsule wall near the barbs was thicker but less mature than around the shaft of the filaments; it contained more cellular elements than fibrous ones. Simultaneously, the number of mast cells increased. Giant cells close to the filaments were very rare and localized near the barbs.

Smooth polypropylene filaments had better developed capsules than APTOS filaments on 90 days after implantation. Fibrous elements in their walls predominated over cellular ones. The capsules displayed neither inflammatory reaction nor signs of resorption. Tissue vascularization in the immediate proximity to smooth polypropylene threads was less pronounced than around APTOS filaments.

The capsule had a rhomboid shape. However, unlike the capsule around APTOS filaments, it gave out no laterally extending connective tissue bands. This confirms that smooth polypropylene threads are unsuitable for facelift.

On day 210 after implantation, the connective tissue capsule around APTOS filaments continued to develop having the wall thickness of 39.6 and 35.4 mem on the sides facing epidermis and subcutaneous fat layer, respectively.

The capsule became thinner, fibroblasts underwent conversion into fibrocytes, collagen fibres predominated over cellular elements. Capsular fibrous structures merged with the fibrous structures of the surrounding tissue, i.e. their further integration occurred.

The capsule around filament barbs looked less mature than around the shaft (fig. 3b) due to irritating effect of the former on the adjacent tissue.

No giant cells indicative of resorptive macrophagal reaction could be seen in the capsule.

Prolonged period of capsule development around barbs ensured stronger adhesion between implanted filaments and the surrounding soft tissues (fig. 4a).

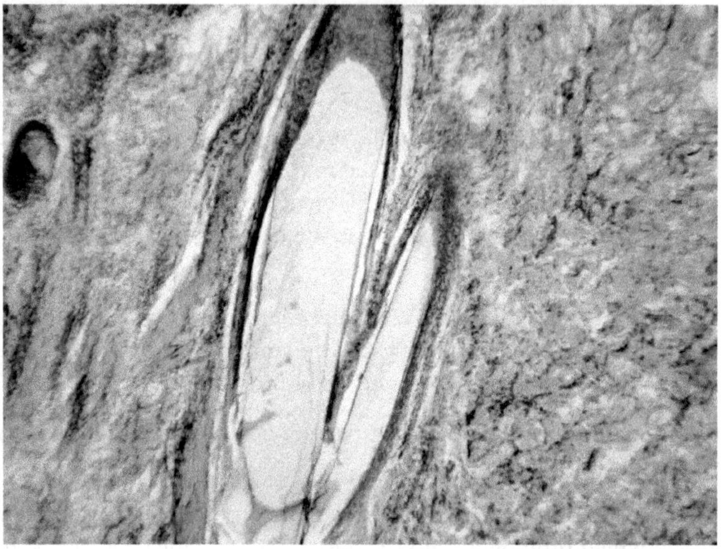

a

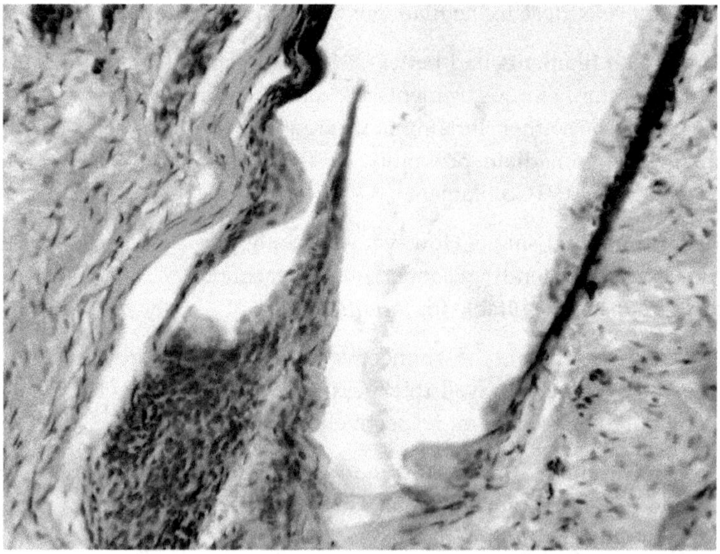

b

a - 90 days after implantation. The capsule wall around the barb is much thicker than around the shaft. Cellular elements predominate (x 40); *b* - 210 days after implantation. The capsule wall around the shaft is thin and contains few cells. The capsule around a barb contains many cellular elements (x 40)

Figure 3. Microphotographs of the capsule surrounding APTOS filament and its barb. Van-Gieson pyrofuchsin staining *(a-b)*

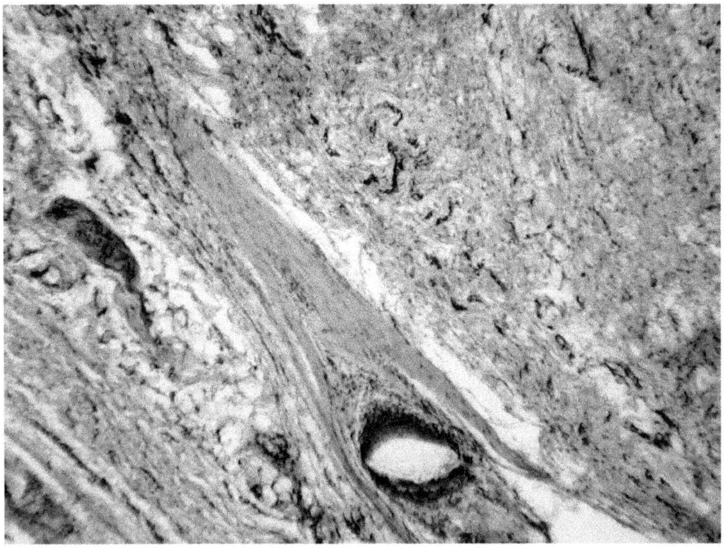

a

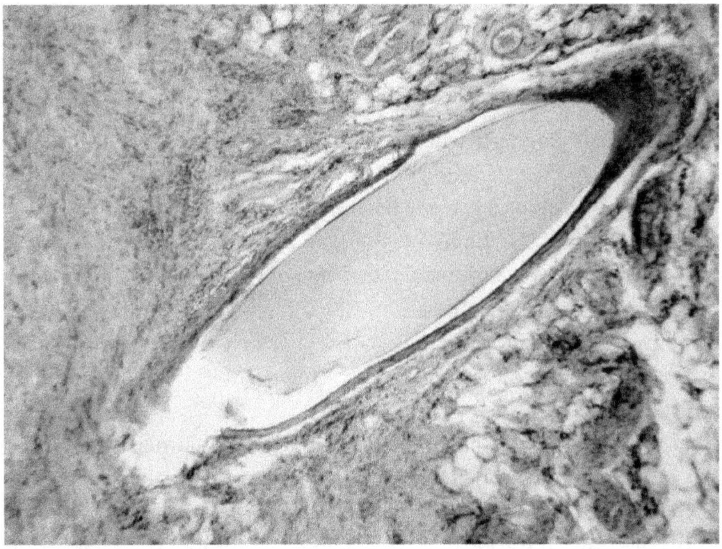

b

a - the capsule gives rise to well-apparent connective tissue bands. Collagen biosynthesis continues (x 40); b - the capsule contains few cellular elements throughout its length. Cellular elements in the right top corner show themselves as a result of oblique section across the filament and the surrounding capsule (x 40)

Figure 4. Microphotographs of the capsule surrounding a barb of APTOS filament (a) and a smooth polypropylene thread (b) 210 days after implantation. Van-Gieson pyrofuchsin staining

The capsule wall thickness around the barbs varied from 150 to 54.2 mem, the lateral walls were 220 mem long and 133 mem wide.

The structure of the capsule that developed around smooth polypropylene thread by day 210 after implantation was practically identical with that of the capsule around APTOS filament, but its maturation was about to be complete, and fibrous elements predominated over cellular ones (fig. 4b).

A study of blood supply to the tissues surrounding implanted filaments based on the estimation of relative vascular bed density has demonstrated its 20% increase on day 3 after implantation of APTOS filaments compared with only 6% in case of smooth polypropylene threads (a 8.1 and 7.9% rise, respectively from the baseline level in intact rats).

A maximum increase of the relative vascular bed density occurred on day 40 after implantation (11.0 and 9.1% in tissues surrounding barbed filament and smooth thread, respectively).

In the course of further follow-up, the relative vascular bed density remained constant in the tissues surrounding both APTOS filaments and smooth polypropylene threads.

4. Conclusions

To summarize the results of comparative histological study of the soft tissues surrounding implanted filaments, the following conclusions can be drawn:

- Collagen biosynthesis begins earlier and ends later after the implantation of APTOS filaments than after the implantation of smooth polypropylene threads; moreover, it is more extensive and involves a greater tissue volume in the former case.
- Fibrous capsule around the filament shaft and barbs gives rise to connective tissue bands that extend towards epidermis and subcutaneous fatty layer and merge with connective tissue fibres of these tissues.
- Tissues surrounding APTOS filaments contain much more microvessels than tissues enclosing smooth threads where the microcirculatory system extends but insignificantly.
- Microvessels formed after the implantation of APTOS filaments have an open lumen. This feature referred to as «phenomenon of persistent hyperemia» can be seen at any time after the implantation, unlike the case of smooth polypropylene threads when hyperemia occurs only in the early postimplantation period.
- Barbs of APTOS filaments are enclosed in their own connective tissue capsule having significantly thicker walls than the capsule around the shaft of the filament. This greatly contributes to solid fixation of APTOS filaments in the surrounding tissues.
- A capsule around the barbs is less mature than around the shaft of the filament. This suggests a stronger stimulatory effect of the barbs on the surrounding tissues which in

turn accounts for prolonged collagen biosynthesis and thus promotes fixation of both the filaments and the lifted tissues.

- Tissues surrounding APTOS filaments contain mast cells, the number of which remains virtually constant throughout the postimplantation period. These cells contribute to vasodilation in the microcirculatory system and transportation of hyaluronic acid to the tissues around the filaments. The number of mast cells in the tissues surrounding smooth polypropylene threads is signiicantly smaller.
- Implantation of APTOS filaments induces no phagocytic reaction.
- The relative microvascular bed area increases by 26% after the implantation of APTOS filaments leading to a marked improvement of local tissue oxygenaion and blood supply. Implantation of smooth polypropylene threads causes a much smaller increase of relative vascular bed density.

Author details

A.A. Adamyan, M.A. Sulamanidze, N.D. Skuba and Z.R. Khusnutdinova
Clinic of Anaplastic and Aesthetic Surgery Total Charm, Moscow, Russia - Tbilisi, Georgia

5. References

[1] Adamyan A.A., Skuba N.D., Sulamanidze M.A., Khusnutdinova Z.R. "Morphological substantiation of facial skin lifting with APTOS threads" International Congress on Plastic, Reconstructive and Aesthetic Surgery, Abstracts of Papers, Moscow., 2002, p. 9 – 10.

[2] Avtandilov G.G., Fundamentals of pathoanatomical practice, Moscow, «RMAPO», 1998, 505 p.

[3] Bykov V.L., Cell biology and general histology, St. Petersburg, - "Sotis", 1998, 364 p.

[4] Sulamanidze M.A., M.D., Fournier P.F., M.D., Paikidze T.G., M.D., Sulamanidze G.M., M.D. Removal of Facial Soft Tissue Ptosis With Special Threads. DERMATOLOGIC SURGERY, Vol. 28 No. 5, May 2002.

[5] Sulamanidze M., Paikidze T., Sulamanidze G., Utilisation du fil "APTOS" dans le lifting facial. La revue de chirurgie esthetique de langue Francaise. T. XXV, N103, May 2001, Pp. 17-22.

[6] Sulamanidze M., Paikidze T., Sulamanidze G., Lifting facial con hilos APTOS. International Journal of Cosmetic Medicine & Surgery. Volumen 3 Numero 3. Diciembre 2001, Pp. 139-142.

[7] Fournier F.P., Reflexions sur les fils tuteurs APTOS de Sulamanidze. La revue de chirurgie esthetique de langue Francaise. T. XXV, N104, septembre 2001, Pp. 23-27.

[8] Fournier F.P., Fils et fillings. La revue de chirurgie esthetique de langue Francaise. T. XXV, N105, decembre 2001, Pp. 3-6.

Chapter 13

Experience in Preventive Measures and Treatment of Complications at Face and Neck Thread Rejuvenation

M.A. Sulamanidze, I.S. Vozdvizhenskiy, G.M. Sulamanidze, K.M. Sulamanidze and E.G. Azizyan

Additional information is available at the end of the chapter

http://dx.doi.org/10.5772/56250

1. Introduction

Face and neck soft tissues lift with the use of special threads is a relatively new and not a thoroughly studied approach to aesthetic surgical and cosmetological correction. Aptos method (anti ptosis) occupies a special place here, because its subjacent conception differs crucially from other thread methods as well as classical surgical ones. Seeming simplicity of intrusion in Aptos method, availability and cheapness of necessary materials and instruments brought a lot of doctors to the point of start in using it, but, unfortunately, without special training. The fact that the doctors do not have special training in Aptos method practice is the main cause of complications and unpleasant aftereffects, the information about which has recently started to appear in literature.

After having studied all the available sources, we have predominantly found the reports about successful results with a minor number of complications and side effects. In the majority of articles both the indications and the intrusion technique are described incorrectly, as well as causes of complications (without considering the anatomical facial special features and kinetics of different groups of muscles), and consequently, this leads to incorrect results.

That is why we have decided to analyze the complications, side-effects and unpleasant aftereffects at face and neck soft tissues thread lift application using Aptos method in various ways. We have analyzed the long-term Aptos method correction experience gained by the surgeons of our clinics (by now there have been performed up to 7000 operations), complications after the application of Aptos among the patients that came from other clinics, and the data presented by doctors from different countries.

The aim of the conducted work is to diagnose the causes of complications and work out recommendations for the treatment and preventive measures.

2. Materials and methods

Out of 900 medical case records taken arbitrarily from the clinical archives of the period from 2002 to 2010 (100 histories per year) only those have been chosen that have data about different complications, problems, and patients' discontent (75 records). According to these documents and the voluminous photo archives of our clinics, a statistical inquiry has been conducted, the results of which are presented in this report along with the commentaries and conclusions. The main products and the corresponding strategies used in our clinics are the following: Aptos thread, Aptos Needle, Aptos Spring, Aptos Thread 2G, Aptos Needle 2G. The manufacturer (Aptos-pro company) usually produces threads from non-absorbable (Prolene) as well as from absorbable (Caprolactone) material. Description of the product, procedure and surgery techniques is given in our numerous publications and presentations [2-5, 10], that is why in this article we present short basic information about Aptos methods. This is necessary for understanding the causes of complications, different in nature and severity, and negative manifestations.

Aptos Thread – the first generation of Aptos products – is a thread, 12 cm long, with convergent angle-wise pins; the thread is fixed subcutaneously with the help of a special hollow needle (figure 1a).

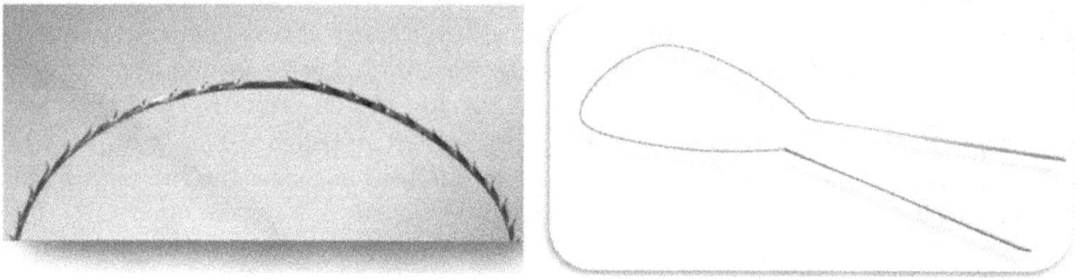

a b

Figure 1. a Aptos Thread, b Aptos Thread 2G

Aptos Thread 2G is the same kind of thread, but 25 cm long, the ends of which are connected with needles; the needles are sharpened in a special way, their points are joined and put together with temporary glue (figure 1b). This permits to stick the both needles with the jointed points subcutaneously, separate them at the required depth, and move each needle with the thread along the trajectory, marked beforehand.

Aptos Needle is a unit with a thread, without pins, which is connected with a double-edged needle in its middle part; such a construction permits to put a needle with a thread subcutaneously along the straight, arched or round (tobacco pouch shaped) contour without skin dimpling. The manufacturer produces three types of these needles (figure 2a).

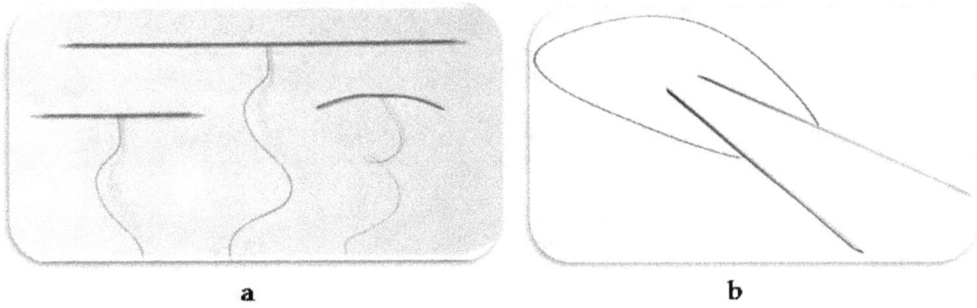

Figure 2. a Aptos Needle, Aptos Needle 2G

Aptos Needle 2G combines advantages of Aptos Thread 2G and Aptos Needle. The thread in this case is exactly the same as Aptos thread 2G, but up to 50 cm long and with convergent pins, connected with two double-edged needles in its middle part (like Aptos Needle), the points of which are put together with temporary glue. That is how the subcutaneous implementation of the thread with pins is performed, and notably, along any contour.

Aptos Spring is a helical elastic thread with "memory" which is used for the lift of the tissues with the most active facial movements.

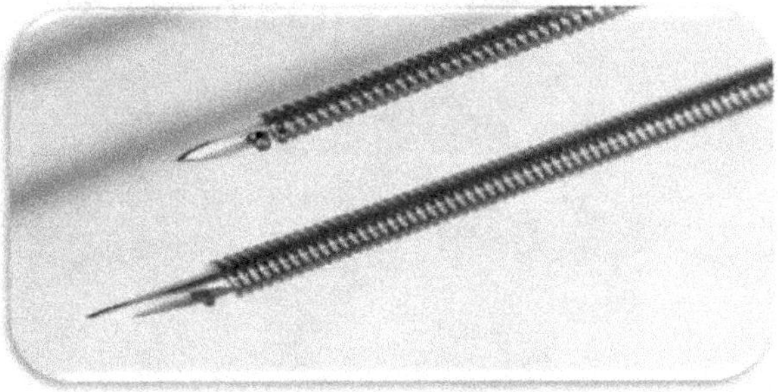

Figure 3. Aptos Springs

3. Research results and discussion

Carrying out the research, we have clearly decided on the definitions of complication and inevitable accompanying interference effect. Besides, it was important to understand which complications and disadvantages are characteristics for all aesthetic surgery interferences and which ones are characteristics only for thread lift methods (scheme 1).

For example, we do not regard light paraesthesia, pain, asymmetry and shallow indrawings in the needle puncture places to be complications. Overcorrection is a necessity, a mandatory operation attribute, we have tried to achieve it on purpose in order to stabilize the interference result and make it as long-term as possible (picture 4 a, b, c, d).

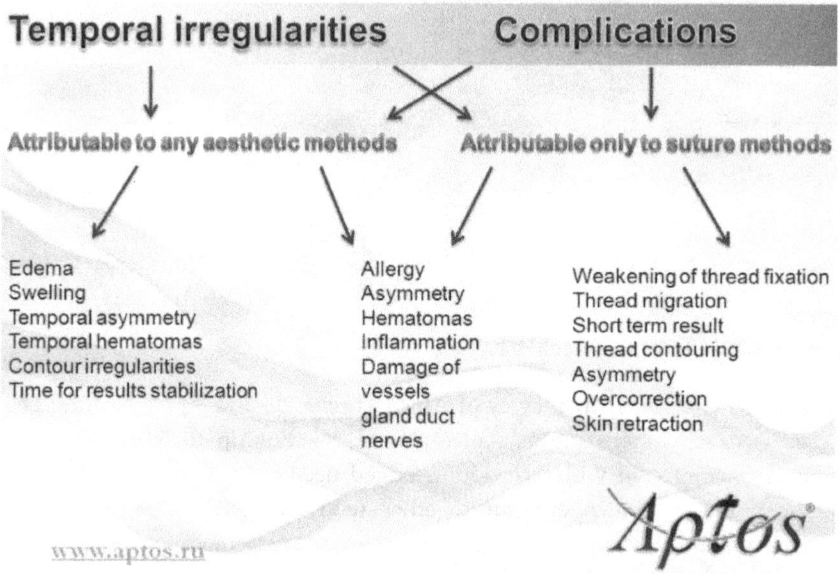

Scheme 1. Classification of Complications and Attendant Thread Lift Negative Factors

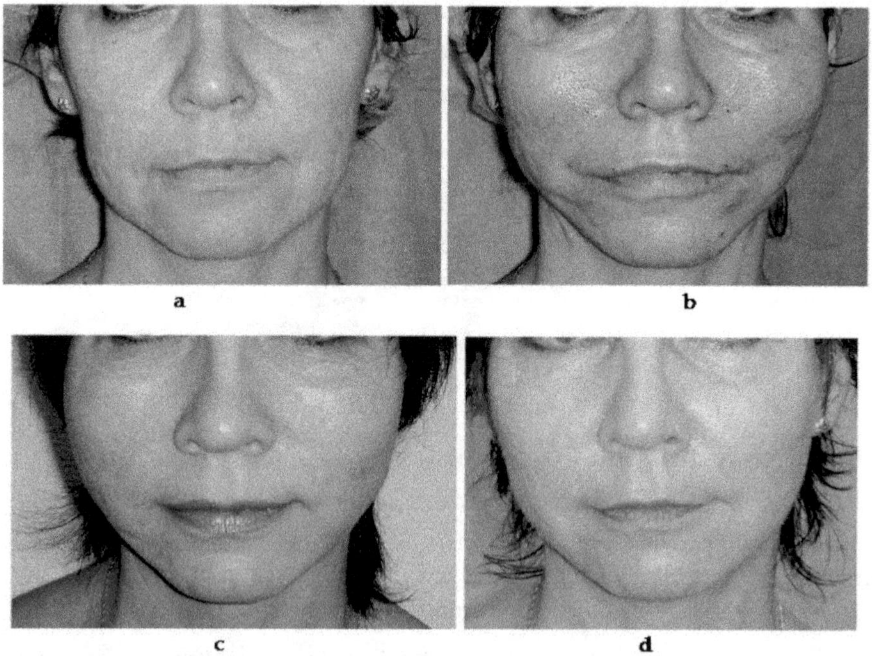

Figure 4. Patient N., 38 years old. Middle facial area lift – Aptos Needle 2G, mental area – Aptos Thread 2G, labiomental wrinkles – Aptos Springs: a – before; b – right after the correction; c – in 2 weeks; d – in 2 years after the interference

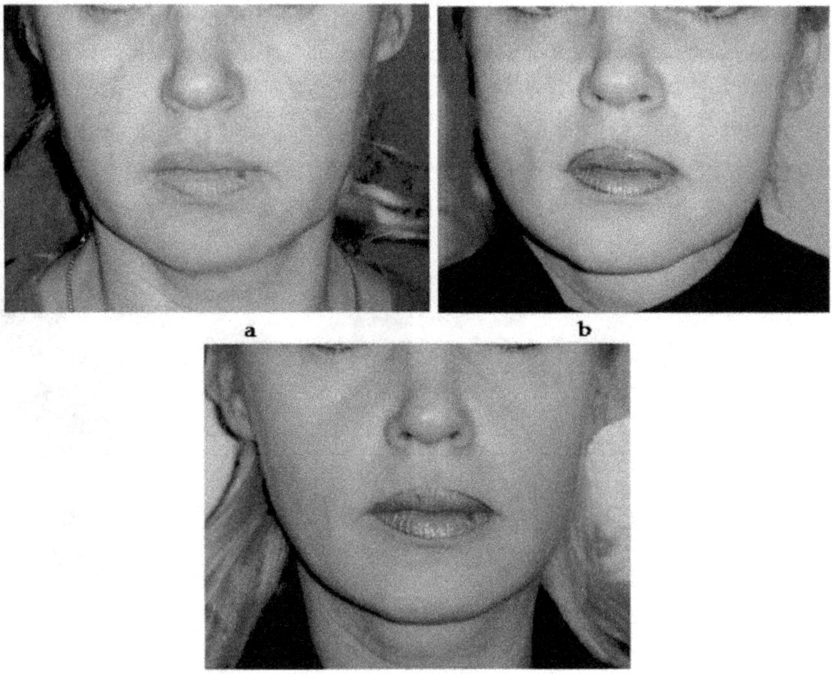

Figure 5. Patient A., 44 years old. Middle facial area and mental area lif – Aptos Thread 2G, labiomental wrinkles – Aptos Springs, submandibular and neck areas – Aptos Needle 2/0: a – before, b – in12 days, c – in 3 months after the interference

The interferences can be accompanied by moderate constraint of mimic, masticatory, swallowing and other facial movements, we do not regard these manifestations to be complications either. All the enumerated disadvantages usually go away on its own in dynamics, or you can use common resolving drug therapy or physiotherapy. We present a picture of a patient who had these unpleasant manifestations for 2 weeks, but subsequently the results stabilized and she was satisfied with the performed correction.

We regarded persistent edemata (more than 2-3 weeks), wrong contour, asymmetry, thread visualization, allergy, infection, bleeding along the thread trajectory, thread migration and thread protrusion onto the skin surface, early relapse of soft tissues ptosis, solution of vessels continuity, nerve trunks continuity, and other anatomical structures continuity to be complications.

We threat persistent edemata with additional general clinical methods. Probably, such cases were connected with patients' individual characteristics as it was not always possible to correlate long-term edemata with the severity of undergone surgeries.

In case of wrong contour, indrawn skin areas, if they were not corrected after massage we employed resolving drug therapy and physiotherapy, and eliminated the problem with the method of undercutting with the use of a wire scalpel, or corrected it with fillers. The asymmetry was corrected with additional thread lift or, on the contrary, with weakening excessively tight threads (figuree 6 a, b). It is most likely that the cause of asymmetry is the surgeon's work fault.

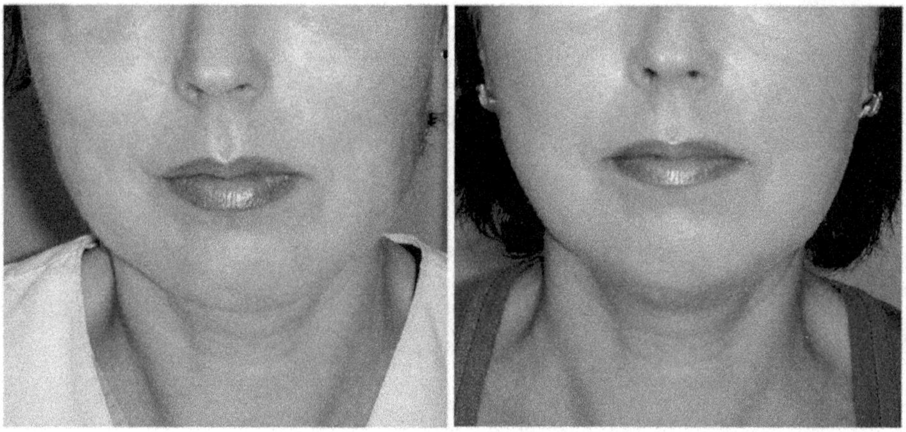

a b

Figure 6. Patient L., 47 years oldd. Middle facial area and chin area lift – Aptos Needle 4/0, mental area – Aptos thread 2G, labiomental wrinkles – Aptos Springs.

Two cases of late allergy to the intruded absorbable thread have been marked: the first one is in 10 days, the second one is in 2 months. In the first case the process was terminated with medications, in the second case the threads were removed. (figure 7).

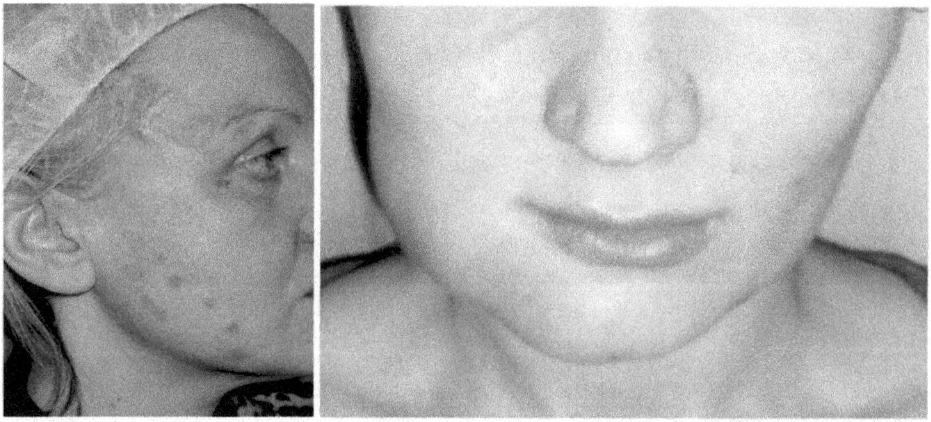

a b

Figure 7. a Allergic reaction to absorbable threads implementation in 10 days after the interference b. Allergic reaction to absorbable threads implementation in 2 months after the interference

Migration threads and threads with the end protruded onto the skin surface were also subject to removal (figure 8).

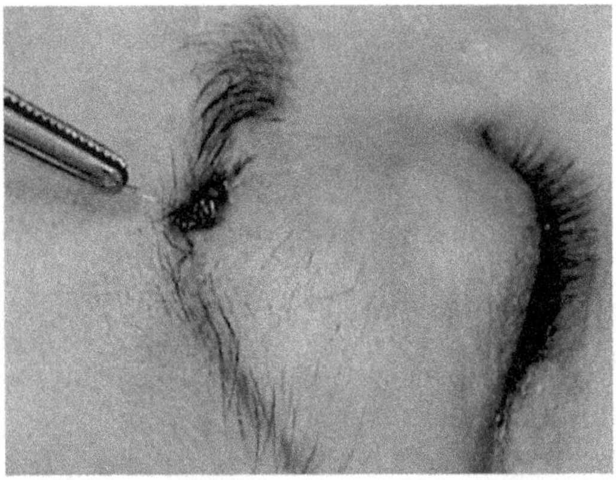

Figure 8. Thread migration case

Since 2008 the usage of prolene Aptos Thread has been stopped and replaced with more modern, second generation threads. And since that time we have not come across any similar unpleasant effects. Such a complication as thread vizualisation has always been connected with its shallow intrusion (except for the eyebrow lifting where this is a necessity). In most cases this problem was successfully eliminated by vigorous massage movements. In rare cases these threads were removed (figure 9).

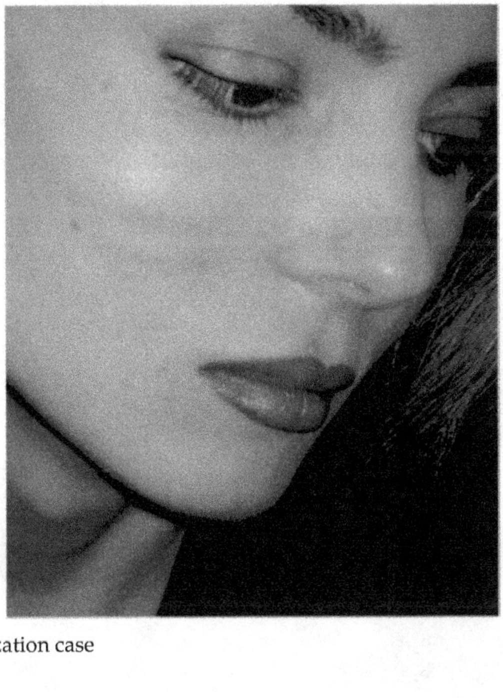

Figure 9. Thread visualization case

The appearance of complications of inflammatory nature is presumably connected with the infection intrusion into subcutaneous layers during the surgery or post-operative period (figure 10). Preventive measures for such complications involve observation of aseptic and antiseptic rules, following to the doctor's prescription in the post-operative period (taking antibiotics, proper skin care and other recommendations). The treatment is medicamental and general surgical; in case of indication the threads are removed. In our clinic we use noninvasive subcutaneous thread detection methods (US, bright main light visualization, diaphanoscopy) and its mini intrusive removal with the use of a special glover's needle (figure 11). This procedure does not present any technical difficulties for an experienced specialist.

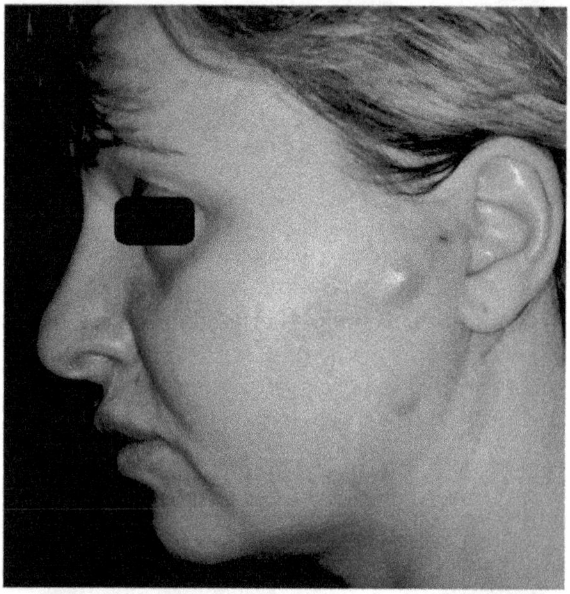

Figure 10. Pus abscess case around thread implementation

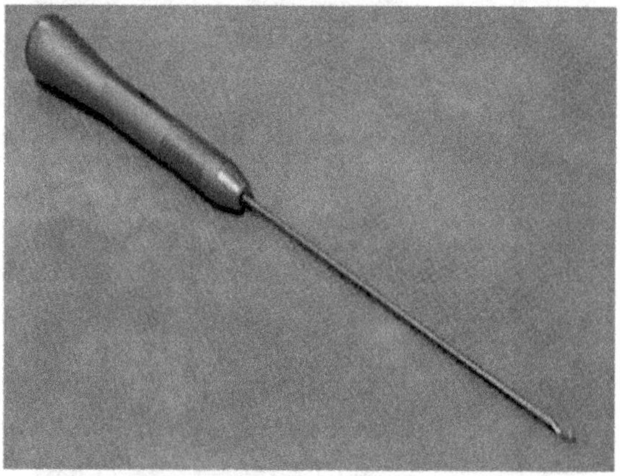

Figure 11. Glover's needle

In our clinical practice we have not come across the hematomas that needed emptying, macrovessel and nerve trunk continuity solution. However, there is a case of Stenon duct continuity solution described in literature that needed operative surgical intervention in order to be treated [13]. The cases of early soft tissues ptosis relapse are especially worth noticing.

The experience shows that sustainability and stability of thread lift results depend on the observation of a number of rules.

1. Strict selection of patients according to the indications

The best face tissues lift results in our clinics are achieved with patients under 50 years old with a slightly thick skin, without pronounced atrophy of subcutaneous fat, with moderate soft tissues ptosis manifestation (feebly marked nasolabial folds and soft-tissue bolsters above them; slightly wrong contour of infraorbital areas in the form of lacrimal grooves; presence of "jowls"), after the preliminary cosmetological deep skin cleansing procedure. For a variety of reasons these patients refused to do classical face lift operations and preferred light and medium face tissues lifts, imperceptible for the others. These were also the patients who were discontent with the previous results of rhytidoplasty, as the face tissues lift was feebly marked in the medial parts and the high volume of bucco-zygomatic areas was not reached.

2. **Preoperative Determination of the Interference Goal**_(tissue lift, tissue redistribution, creation of a new high volume or combination of these effects)

Aptos methods permit to reach the enumerated goals. For example, eyebrow tail lift and thread canthopexy are performed by Aptos Needle 2G method, while new high volume of the middle part of the face is performed by Aptos Needle 4/0 or Aptos Needle 2G. These methods permit to "border" the lifted tissues area and fix them rigidly to rigid structures.

3. Fixation of Threads With Pins is Effective Only in the Kinetically Inert Zones

Eyebrow, bucco-zygomatic, mental, and submandibular areas are among these zones, as they do not have active muscles and soft tissue layers can be easily shifted. That is why rigid lift methods are recommended only in the range of these zones. For the soft tissues lift of the kinetically active zones ("grief wrinkle" correction, mouth corners ptosis) we used an elastic lift – Aptos Springs method.

Simultaneous movement of soft tissue layers of two or more zones is a complicated action, as these zones are separated from each other by dense bands of fibrous tissue that do not allow a long-term lift of all the zones to be performed simultaneously [1, 8].

A number of colleagues in their practice ignore these circumstances and employ long threads from temporal or even parietal regions through the whole cheek down to the submandibular area (figure 10a). Of course, during masticatory and mimic movements parts of protuberances or the whole thread are easily destroyed and, consequently, the lift stability declines. Poor results of linear lifts performed by long threads from temporal areas down to the nasolabial triangle and "Marionette Line" can be explained in the same way (figure 10b).

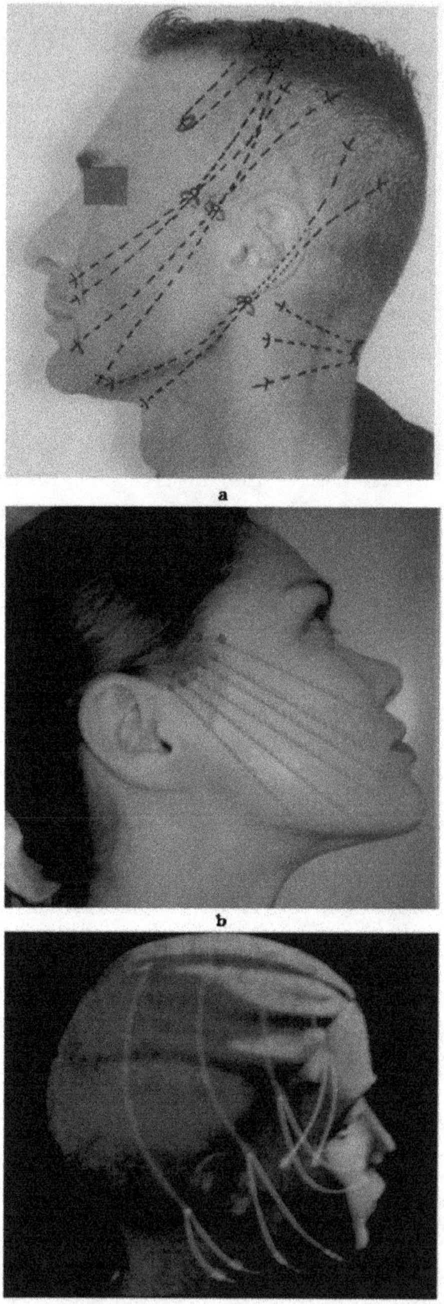

a

b

c

Figure 12. a. Marking before long threads implementatio, b. Linear thread direction for the middle facial zone lift, c. Whole face thread lift marking by the method of putting threads over the scalp

One of the doctors during the performance of the Aptos Thread surgery put long threads from one part of the face over the whole patient's scalp on the other in order to have the threads intruded on the right part of the face could support the threads on the left part of the face and vice versa (figure 10 c). It is not difficult to imagine the whole operation technology, the process of the practical thread implementation along such a long and difficult contour and the severity of the injury of the tissues along the thread implementation way. Of course, this is not a minimally-invasive intrusion any more [7, 14].

4. Thread Fixation Depth

It is determined by the stated objectives, the facial area, the skin depth and the chosen lift thread method. For example, in the case of eyebrow and "jowl" lift threads are fixed rather superficially, while in the bucco--zygomatic and infraorbital areas they are intruded rather deeply into the subcutaneous layer in order to create high volume of the middle facial zone.

Thereby it is possible to confirm that the preventive measures of complications and early relapse cases possible in applying Aptos method are based on the doctor's knowledge of the causes of age and contour facial deformations, the right understanding the idea of Aptos tissue lift, selection of patents according to the indications, the right method choice, irreproachable mastery of equipment, and the delicate intrusion performance. Complication and long-lasting side effects treatment include the achieved results correction (undercutting, implementation of absorbable fillers), elimination of eased and migrating threads, repeated thread or classical lift, physiotherapy, and massage [11, 12].

4. Conclusions

The absolute advantages of the Aptos thread method at the lift surgery performance are:

- Simplicity, easiness, efficiency;
- Minimal invasiveness and slight injuring procedures;
- Reliability, sufficient sustainability, and high quality lift;
- Possibility of combination with other interferences;
- Short rehabilitation period.

Complications and unpleasant side effects are not inherent in the very nature of the Aptos method; they are so rare, slight and easily corrected that aesthetic surgery specialists do not have to refuse the usage of lift thread methods.

Some authors present only negative results in their articles about thread lift [6, 9]. However, it must be emphasized that the results of our long-term work absolutely do not agree with the statistics of these publications (Diagrams 2 and 3). The unreasonably suspicious attitude towards the method does not assist the development and improvement of the thread lift methods, and minimally-invasive aesthetic surgery in whole like alternatives to classical lift methods and contour facial surgery.

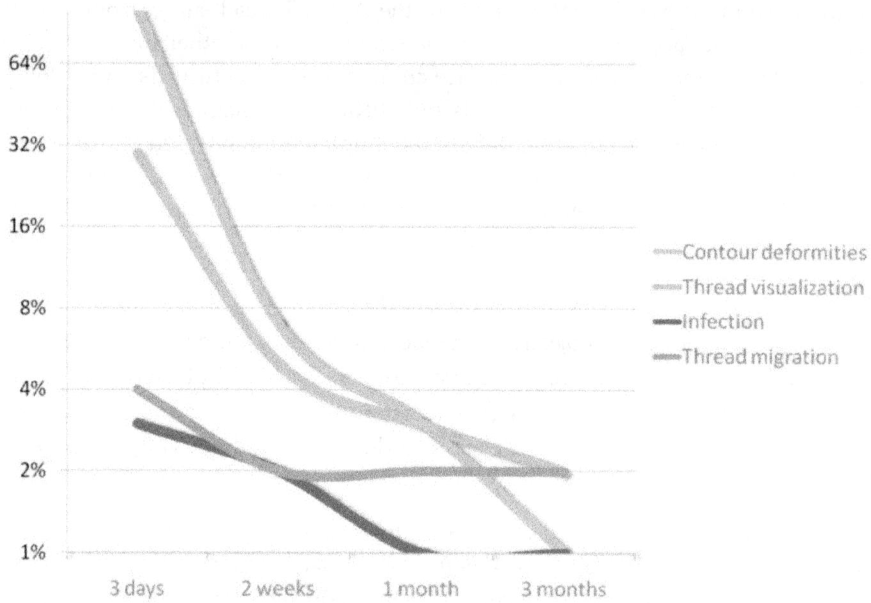

Scheme 2. Frequency and Appearance Dates of Complications in Thread Lift Case

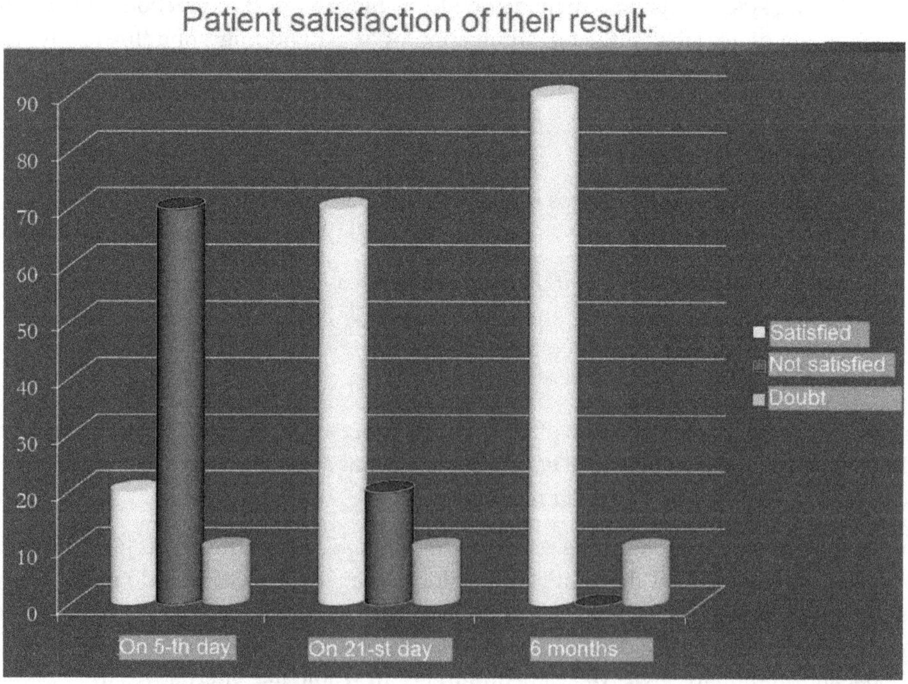

Scheme 3. Patients' Satisfaction with the Results of Thread Lift

Author details

M.A. Sulamanidze, I.S. Vozdvizhenskiy, G.M. Sulamanidze,
K.M. Sulamanidze and E.G. Azizyan
Clinic of plastic and Aesthetic Surgery and Dermatocosmetology TotalCharm, Moscow (Russia), Tbilisi, Georgia

5. References

[1] Kazinnikova O.G., Adamian A.A., Age specific changes in facial and cervical tissues // Annals of plastic, reparative, and aesthetic surgery, 2000, 1, 52-61.
[2] Sulamanidze M.A., Sulamanidze G.M. Flabby, ageing face. New approaches // II Congress on aesthetic and restorative surgery, Moscow, 1998:15
[3] Sulamanidze M.A., Sulamanidze G.M. Soft tissues lift: old philosophy, new approach - a method of internal stitching (Aptos Needle) // Annals of plastic, reparative, and aesthetic surgery, 2005, 1, 15-29.
[4] Sulamanidze M.A., Sulamanidze G.M. Aptos methods: past, present, future // Aesthetic Medicine Newsletter, 2007, 3, 23-32.
[5] Sulamanidze M.A., Sulamanidze G.M., Vozdvizhenskiy I.S., Sulamanidze K.M., Kadzhaya A.A. New Method of Elastic Thread Face Lift // Aesthetic Medicine, 2010, 3, 275-280.
[6] Aesthetic byers guide. – 2006
www.miinews.com
[7] Guillo D. Fils Aptos implantation en X. Surginevs 2005, 8, 10-13.
[8] Mendelson B.C., Muzaffar A.R., Adams W.P. Surgical Anatomy of the Midcheek and Malar Mounds // Plastic. And Reconstruct. Surgery. – 2002, September. – Vol. 110, №3. – P. 885-896.
[9] Rachel, J.D., Lack, E.B., Larson, B. Incidence of complications and early recurrence in 29 patients after facial rejuvenation with barbed suture lifting // Dermatol. Surgery. – 2010. - №36. – P. 348-354.
[10] Sulamanidze M.A., Fournier P.F., Paikidze T.G., Sulamanidze G.M. Removal of Facial Soft Tissue Ptosis With Special Threads// Dermatol. Surgery. – 2002, May. - №28. – P.367-371.
[11] Sulamanidze M.A., Sulamanidze G.M. Aptos Suture Lifting Methods. 10 Years of Experience // Clinics in Plast.Surgery. – 2009, April. – Vol.36, №2. – P.281-306.
[12] Sulamanidze M.A., Sulamanidze G.M., Sulamanidze C.M., Vozdvizhensky I.S. Lifting of Soft Tissues With Barbed Threads. Side Effects, Complications. // 11-th ESPRAS Congress Plastic, Restorative and Aesthetic Surgery, 20-26 September 2009, Rhodes, Greece. – Book of Abstracts. – P.25
[13] Winkler E., Goldan O., Regev E. Stenssen duct rupture (sialicele) and other complications of the Aptos thread technique // Plast. Reconstr. Surgery. – 2006. - №118. – P. 1468-71.

[14] Woffles Wu. Advances in Stitch Lift // 2-nd Regional Conference in Dermatological Laser and Facial Cosmetic Surgery. – 2006, 20-22 January, Hong Kong. – Programme Book. – P.30

Chapter 14

New Method of Face Elastic Thread Lift

M. Sulamanidze, G. Sulamanidze, I. Vozdvizhenskiy,
K. Sulamanidze and A. Kadzhaya

Additional information is available at the end of the chapter

http://dx.doi.org/10.5772/56316

1. Introduction

Within the last few decades the priorities for the treatment of facial ageing and sagging, especially in the paraoral area, have changed dramatically. Patients demand this interference to be performed with minimum risk to their health, minor injury, short postoperative rehabilitation period, and, above all, long-term aesthetic effect.

However, during the process of lifting operation on the mentioned facial zone mobilization and hypodermic soft tissues transfer (subcutaneous tissue, SMAS, muscles) into a new higher position and applying interrupted sutures through the soft tissues are regarded as key points of the long-term effect, that is impossible to achieve without a considerable operational trauma. Besides, the strongly pronounced mobility of this facial area brings the results of the interference to the relapse of the aesthetic deformation.

2. Classical methods of face lift and their disadvantages

It is known that traditional face lift methods are not effective enough to eliminate aesthetic age manifistations in the paraoral area, as these zones are at the maximum distance from the section and face lift line. That is why during face lift operations some surgeons make a wide separation of face skin up to the nasolabial folds and mouth corners, and then raise the skin fold upwards and laterally to the maximum possible extent, removing considerable skin surplus. Performance of such surgeries quite often leads to unnaturally stretched faces, alopecia in the temple area and hypertrophy of postoperative cicatrices, appearing deceitfully under auricula lobes and stretching them down (picture 1). Even deep plane lift methods (so called SMAS- and intraperiosteal lifts) do not always eliminate the aging face signs in its medial parts.

In picture 2 we can see a skin area with marking, in picture 2(b) – the same area after mobilization in the course of rhytidoplasty. It is clearly seen that the skin area that had been

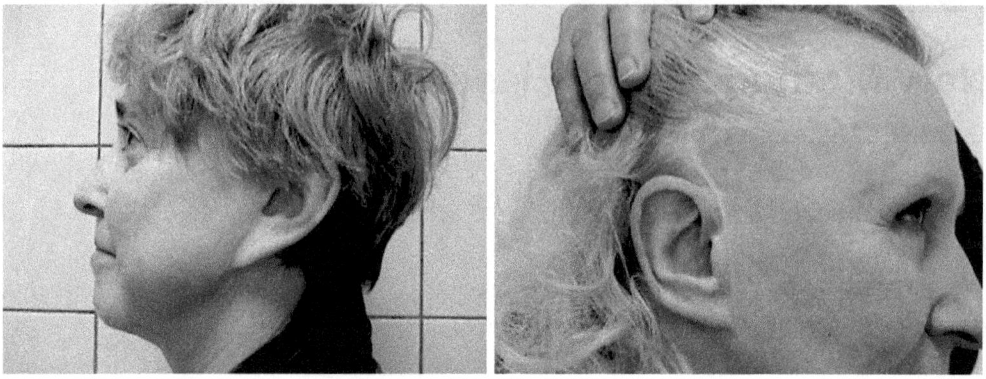

a b

Figure 1.

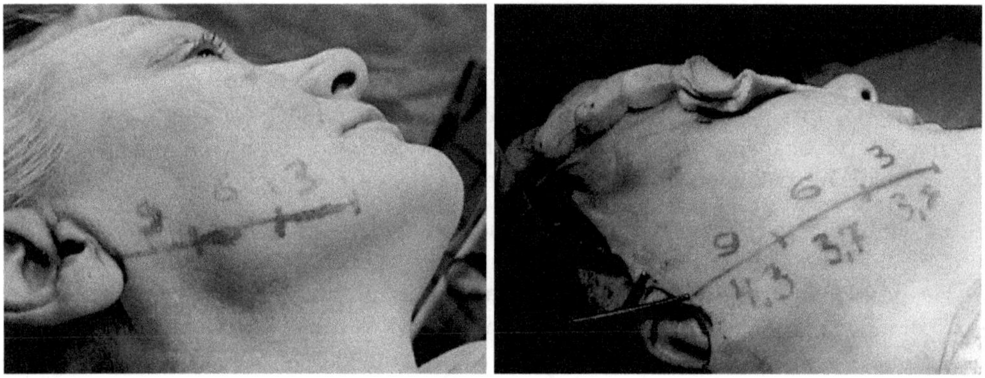

a b

Figure 2.

the furthest from the place of the force application stretched out insignificantly – only to 0.4 cm, while the nearest skin graft stretched considerably – it became 1.5 cm longer.

Furthermore, paraoral facial areas are in the zone of active influence of masticatory and mimic muscles, and in the nearest postoperative period the areas around the mouth corners, smoothed out as the result of the surgery, become sagged again. This factor also interferes with the stabilization of the face lift result [1].

In the last few years, despite the anatomic and functional features of the paraoral area, different methods of hard thread lifting have been used quite often for mouth corner soft tissue lift. Such an approach cannot give consistent long-term effect, as in this case the presence of highly developed and active masticatory and mimic muscles, which quickly destroy the achieved result (in 2-3 months a relapse is expected), is underrated.

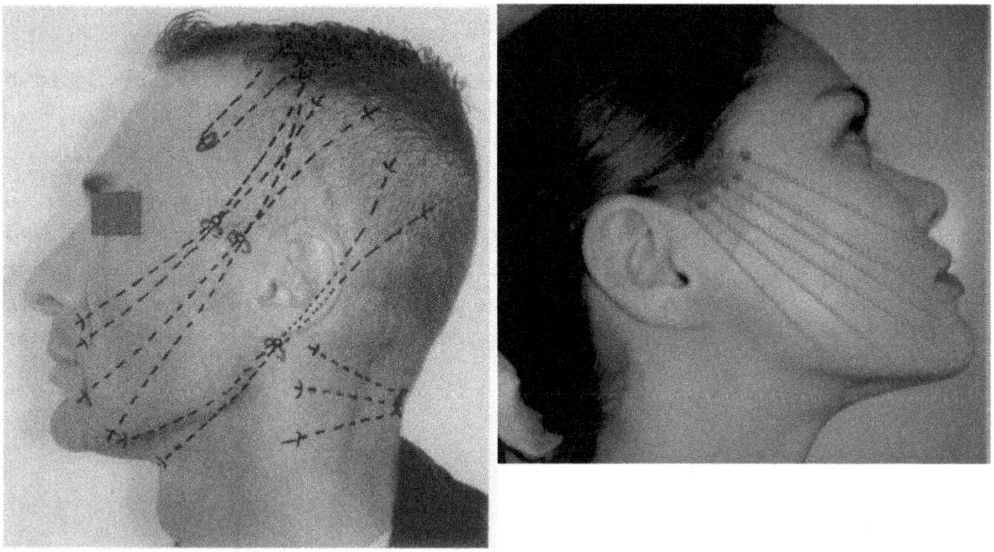

a b

Figure 3.

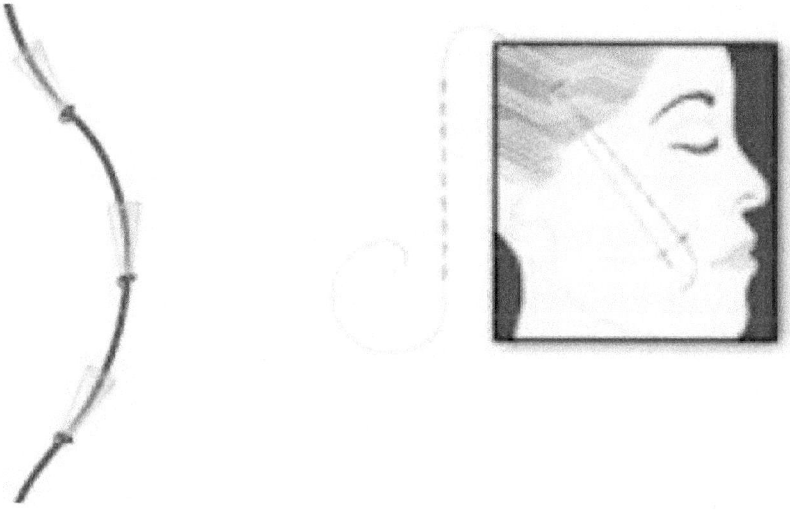

a b

Figure 4.

Even such powerful lift constructions as Silhouette Sutures, as they can seem at first glance, cannot resist kinetics of these muscles and cannot save lift results in such areas for a long period of time (picture 4), as the direction of threads' position resists muscle contraction and relaxation.

3. Elastic thread lift of the paraoral area. Aptos Springs Method

In 2004 elastic thread lift of the paraoral area – Aptos Springs Method – was developed in our clinic. Both the method and the threads developed for using in this technique have Russian and international patents [6, 7].

Aptos Springs thread is a special twisted in form of a spring polypropylene (non-absorbable) thread 2/0, which has a "memory". In the course of production this thread undergoes a special processing which provides it with spring type characteristics. A spring in a compressed position is wound around an injection needle of 1.1x100 or 0.9x90 mm (picture 5). There are two Aptos Springs threads of each size in one package, and one package usually is enough for one procedure.

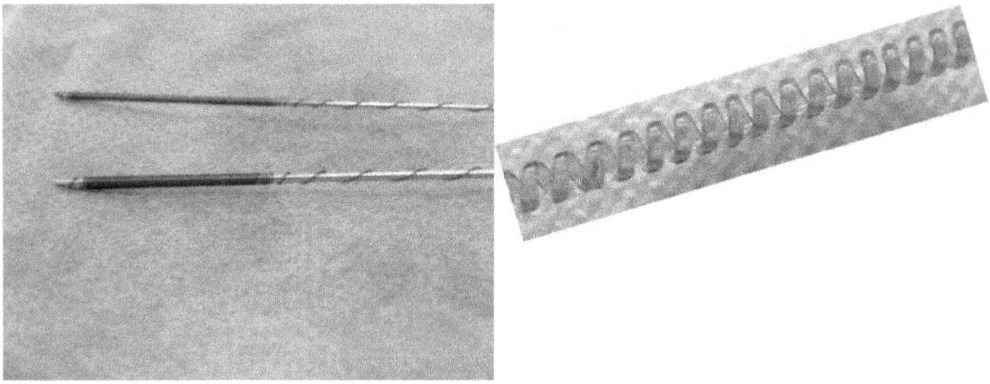

a b

Figure 5.

The manufacture produces Aptos Springs threads made from polypropylene (non-absorbable) as well as from absorbable Kaprolac threads (Light Lift), which gets fully absorbed in the tissues within a year, and the fibrosis, which appears in this place, keeps on "working".

In the clinical practice Aptos Springs threads are used for:

- labiomental fold elimination (Marionette Line) (variant I);
- mouth corners lift (variant II).

During the consultation the patient is informed about the method possibilities, details of the surgery performance, its duration, rehabilitation period special characteristics, and the duration of the lift effect. The patient decides on his/her own with the use of which product (absorbable or non-absorbable threads) the surgery is to be performed.

4. Variants of the surgery performance

4.1. Labiomental fold elimination (surgery technique, variant I)

The "marionette line" is marked and two parallel lines, 1 cm distant from each other, are drawn perpendicularly to the wrinkle (picture 6). The Aptos Springs thread of the bigger thickness is usually fixed above, and the one of the smaller size is fixed below.

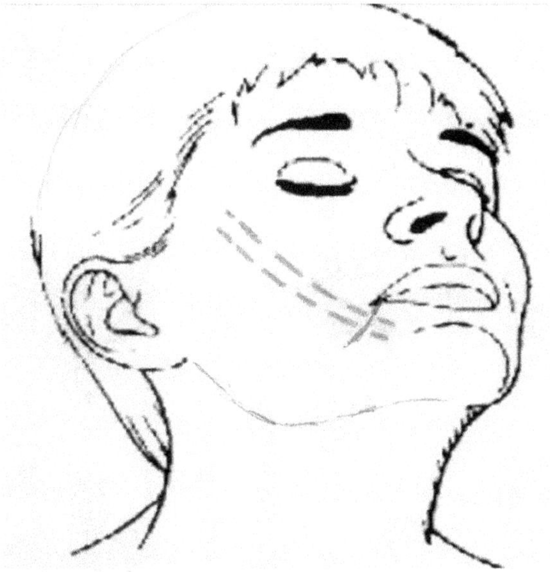

Figure 6.

Before it is fixed the spring is stretched along the length of the needle and is inserted subcutaneously in this position. The needle is inserted at the upper point and pushed towards the wrinkle; in the first half of the way it is deepened to the SMAS limits, in the second half it is shifted closer to the skin and crosses the fold at this depth. The needle is taken out from the skin 1.5 cm past the Marionette line, while the spring is left subcutaneously. After a slight lifting of the spring thread from the both sides, its surplus is cut off and the ends are buried under the derma. In this case there is no need to use any special thread ends' fixing as it is evenly and rigidly fixed in the tissues with the help of its coils.

Right after the fixation, on the operating table, you can see a lift effect and elimination of the labiomental folds and the soft tissue folds over them. By compressing Aptos Springs threads lift sagging soft tissues, and stretch and shrink in synchrony with facial muscles in the process of mimic, masticatory or other facial movements (picture 7).

Subsequently fibrous tissue appears around the thread, which in its turn provides strengthening of the lifting and spring type effect with a long-term consistent result (picture 8,9,10).

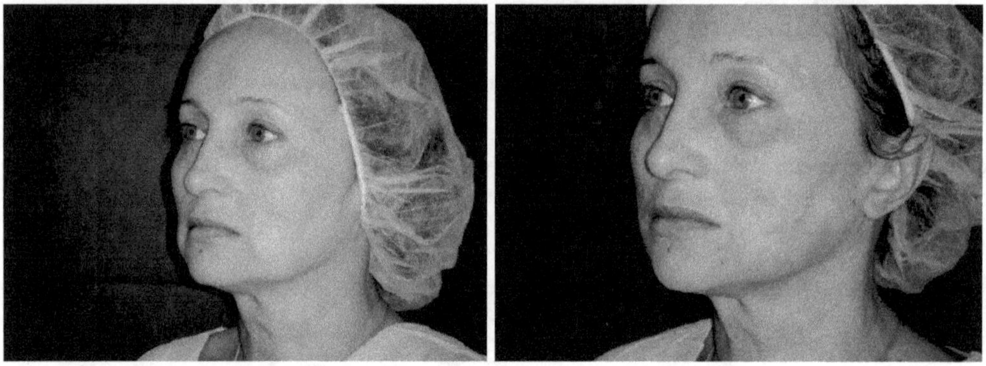

a b

Figure 7.

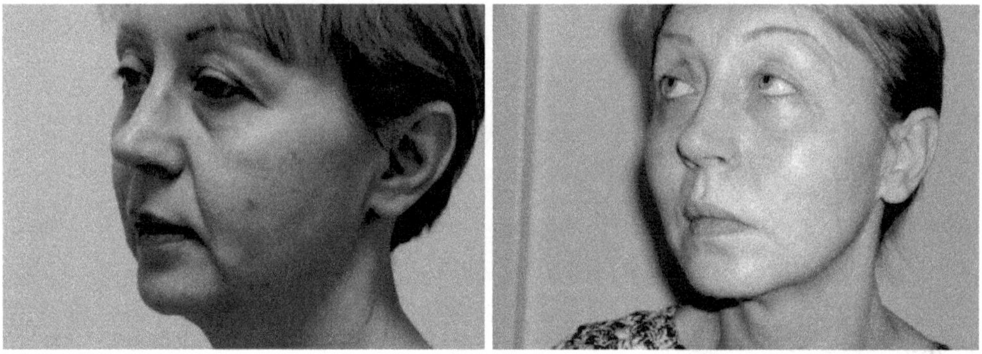

a b

Figure 8.

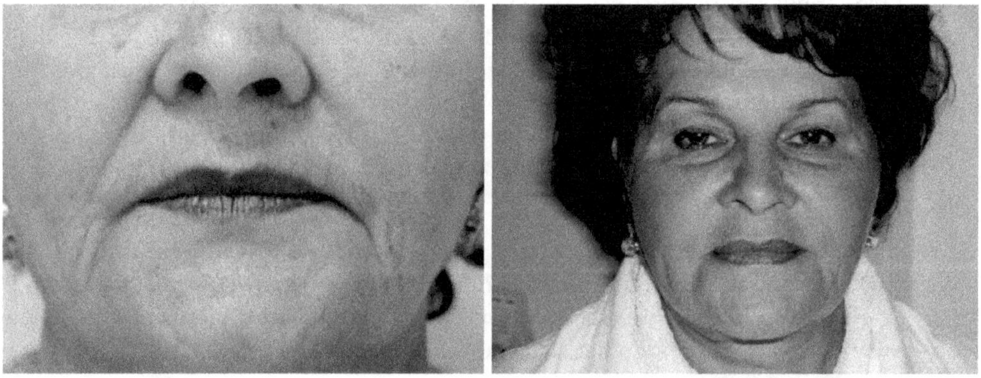

a b

Figure 9.

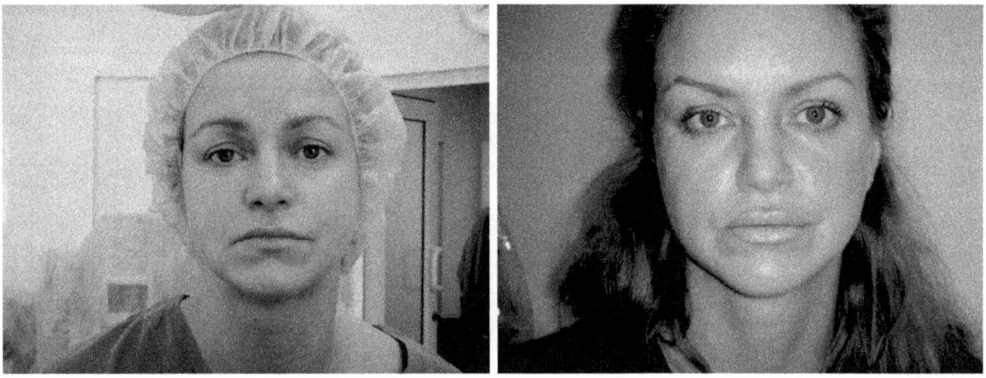

a b

Figure 10.

4.2. Mouth corners lift (surgery technique, variant II)

The marking used for the mouth corners lift surgery is made in the following way: one line is drawn perpendicularly to the "marionette line", just like in Variant I, while the second line is drawn parallelly up to the mouth corner, and then up and angle-wise, sideward the red border of the upper lip at a distance of 1.5-2.0 cm (picture 11).

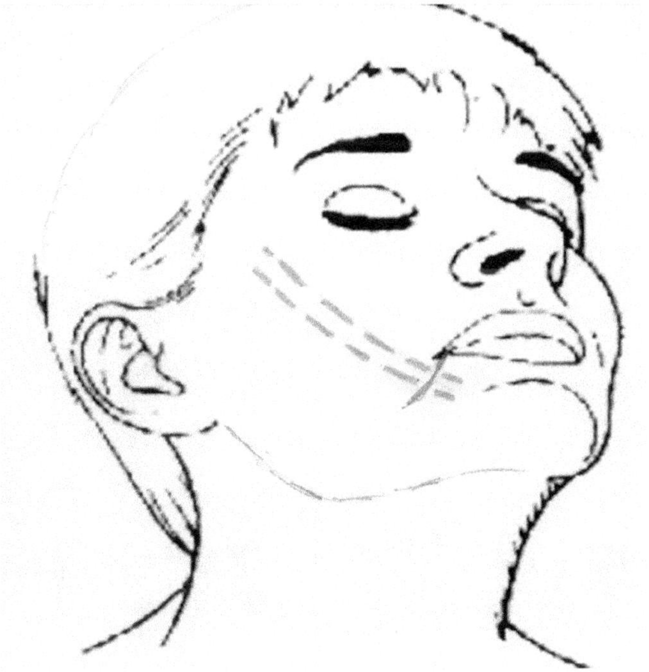

Figure 11.

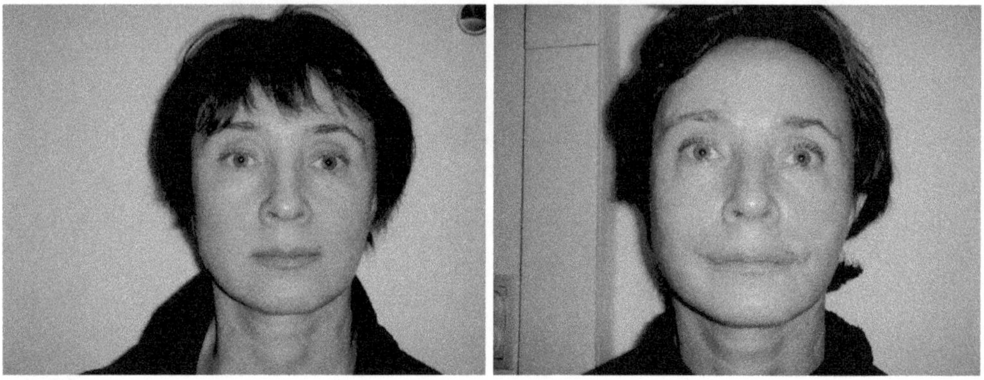

a b

Figure 12.

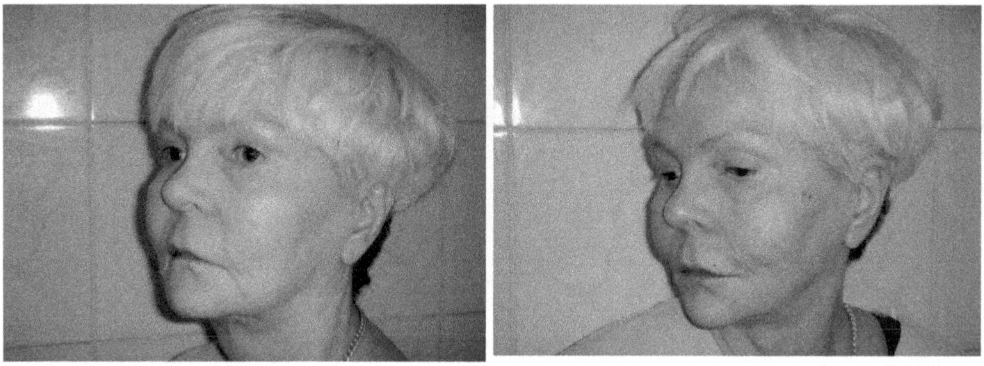

a b

Figure 13.

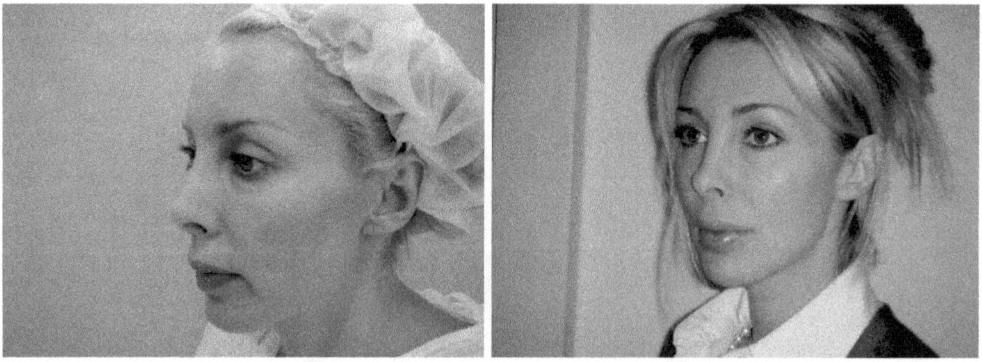

a b

Figure 14.

The Aptos Springs thread of the bigger thickness is fixed sideward the "marionette line", the thread of the smaller thickness is brought to the mouth corner and then inserted under the skin of the red lip border.

Right after the threads fixation (as early as on the operating table) we can see the mouth corner lift effect ("constant smile" effect), slight eversion of the lateral areas of the upper lip and labiomental folds elimination of slight expressiveness (picture 12, 13, 14).

5. Conclusions

Operations by Aptos Springs method are performed under local infiltration anaesthesia quickly, easily, without discissions, with a slight surgical trauma, little postoperative pains, and a short rehabilitation period. Since 2003 more than 2000 similar operations have been carried out in our clinic both in the form of monotherapy and simultaneously with other rejuvenation interference and always with good long-term results.

Author details

M. Sulamanidze, G. Sulamanidze, I. Vozdvizhenskiy,
K. Sulamanidze and A. Kadzhaya
*Clinic of Plastic, Aesthetic Surgery and Dermatocosmetology, Total Charm,
Moscow, Russia*

6. References

[1] Mendelson B.C., Muzaffar A.R., Adams W.P. Surgical Anatomy of the Midcheek and Malar Mounds // Plastic. And Reconstruct. Surgery. – 2002, September. – Vol. 110, №3. – P. 885-896.

[2] Guillo D. Fils Aptos implantation en X. Surginevs 2005, 8, 10-13.

[3] Matarasso A., Pfaifer T.M., The Use of Modified Sutures in Plastic Surgery. Plastic and Reconstructive Surgery, 2008; 122 (issue 2):652-658.

[4] Sasaki G.H., Komorovska-Timek E., Bennet D.C., Cabriel A. An Objective Comparison of Holding, Slippage and Pull-Out Tensions for Eight Suspension Sutures in the Malar Pads of Frech-Frosen Human Cadavers. Aesthetic Surgery Journal, 2008; 28 (4): 387-396.

[5] Sulamanidze M.A., Sulamanidze G.M., Sulamanidze C.M., Vozdvizhensky I.S. Lifting of Soft Tissues With Barbed Threads. Side Effects, Complications. // 11-th ESPRAS Congress Plastic, Restorative and Aesthetic Surgery, 20-26 September 2009, Rhodes, Greece. – Book of Abstracts. – P.25

[6] Sulamanidze M.A., Sulamanidze G.M. Aptos Springs – a new concept of lifting. Journal of the Japan Society of Aesthetic Surgery, 2005; 42(5):183.

[7] Sulamanidze M.A., Sulamanidze G.M. Surgical Thread and Cosmetic Surgery Method. WO, 2005/087283.

Section 3

Barbed Threads Sutured One Side

Chapter 15

Minimally Invasive Face and Neck Lift Using Silhouette Coned Sutures

Peter Prendergast

Additional information is available at the end of the chapter

http://dx.doi.org/10.5772/51677

1. Introduction

Over the last decade, the number of patients opting for minimally invasive procedures has increased [1]. In the US, noninvasive cosmetic procedures have increased by more than 350% since 1997, compared to about 70% for cosmetic surgical procedures. Although open facelift is still indicated for patients who have moderate or severe ptosis of the lower face and neck, younger patients with mild ptosis and patients who do not want to undergo open surgery or general anaesthesia are often suitable candidates for suture of thread lift techniques. Patients favour minimally invasive procedures because they are quick, relatively inexpensive, and do not require prolonged recovery time. Additionally, less invasive procedures typically produce less dramatic results compared to excisional surgery, so the result is subtle and natural looking (Fig.1). Although the story of barbed sutures probably began with Alcamo's design of a roughened suture in 1956, the concept of lifting the face or neck through minimal incisions or punctures using sutures or threads is relatively new. Buncke, a microsurgeon, referred to "facelifts and other cosmetic operations where the sutures would provide lines of tissue support beneath the skin" [2]. Following this, various sutures using different materials, morphologies, and designs were developed by surgeons in USA, Russia, Bulgaria, and elsewhere. Isse, an American surgeon, initially embraced the idea of using barbed sutures to lift soft tissues. He developed the Isse Endo Progressive Facelift Suture, a barbed suture similar to the sutures developed in Moscow by Sulamanidze, and Singapore by Wu. He later abandoned this design in favour of a novel approach—using cones instead of barbs to spear subcutaneous tissues. Isse designed these so-called Silhouette sutures for a number of reasons. He felt that the morphology of the cones or 'trumpets' along the suture would have superior holding power compared to barbs. He also believed that using cones made of an absorbable material (poly lactide) would incite an inflammatory reaction that would in turn stimulate neocollagenesis around the cones and potentially provide a longer lasting effect. Silhouette sutures are now FDA approved and distributed worldwide. The author utilizes these sutures for minimally invasive lifting of the brow, midface, and neck. The procedure is performed in an office setting under local anaesthesia without sedation. This chapter details the Silhouette suture morphology, important anatomy, indications, technique, and potential complications.

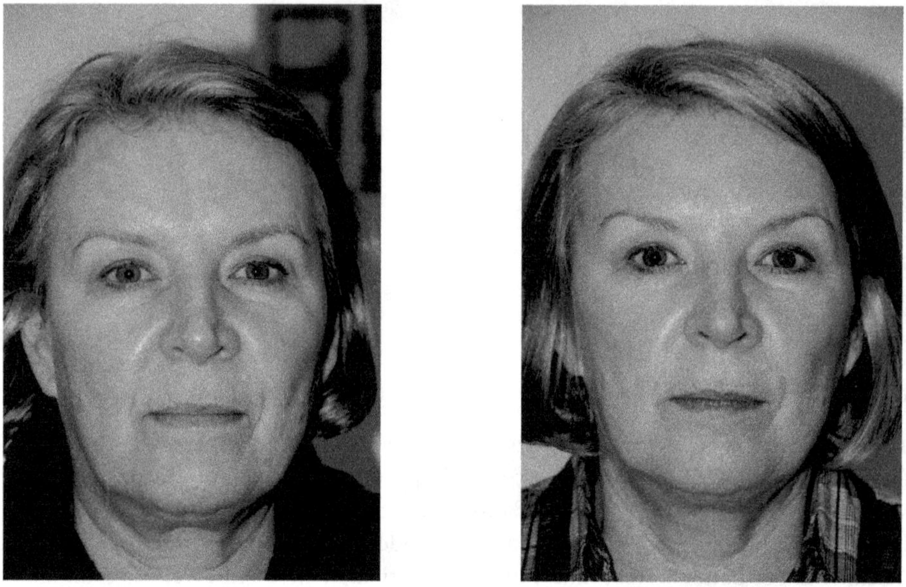

(a) (b)

Figure 1. a Before, b After Silhouette suture lift. With kind permission from Springer Science+Business Media: Aesthetic Medicine. Art and Techniques, Suture lifting techniques, 2011, p.413, P.M. Prendergast, fig. 34.15.

2. Silhouette suture morphology

The Silhouette suture consists of a dyed polypropylene suture with six regularly spaced transparent cones or trumpets along its length. There is a 20.3cm 20 gauge straight blunt-tipped needle swaged to the distal end of the suture and a 26mm half-circle needle to the proximal end. The cones are made of absorbable poly-L-lactic acid and are held on the suture by six regularly spaced knots (Fig. 2).

As the sutures are inserted the cones slide proximally and cover the knots. When the proximal end of the suture is retracted, the cones slide distally as they purchase on the tissues, and are held on the sutures by the more distally placed knots. Included with Silhouette sutures are 2 x 0.5cm polypropylene mesh patches for anchorage to deep fascia. The biomechanics of the cone morphology provides excellent lifting and holding ability and less propensity to "cheesewire" through friable or soft fatty tissues compared to barbed sutures [3]. The knotted suture means there has been no compromise to the structure of the main body of the suture, unlike barbed sutures where linear shredding can occur when

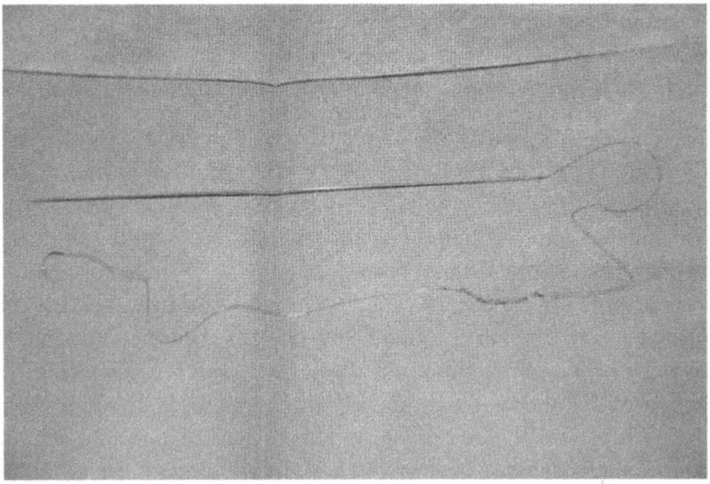

Figure 2. The Silhouette suture with blunt-tipped straight needle for placement

tensions are applied to the barbs. Coned sutures are somewhat bulkier than barbed ones, leading occasionally to irregularities or visibility in patients who have a thin soft tissue envelope. This softens out quickly without intervention. Although the original sharp straight needle is available for suture passage, a blunt one was recently introduced, presumably to reduce the chance of nerve or vascular injury during deployment of sutures. The disadvantage of the blunt-tipped needle is the need for an extra step: puncturing the skin with a needle prior to exiting the skin. Also, more force is required to pass the blunt needle through fibrous tissues such as the lateral neck area and temporal area. Haematoma is rare using either a sharp or blunt tipped needle provided the needle is passed through the correct plane, particularly when lidocaine with epinephrine is used for infiltrative anaesthesia.

3. Clinically oriented anatomy

A thorough knowledge of facial anatomy is essential for any surgeon who performs suture or thread lift techniques. The thread lift techniques described in this chapter require small incisions, and the passage of blunt-tipped needles blindly through the subcutaneous fatty and fibrofatty tissues of the face and neck. Care must be taken to avoid inadvertent injury to important structures, including vessels, sensory nerves, and motor nerves. Understanding the anatomy of the soft tissue planes is also important for Silhouette suture lift techniques since different planes are traversed with the sutures, and anchorage to deep fascia in the temporal area or neck is required to secure the lift and prevent slippage.

In the temple behind the hairline, the temporalis muscle is covered with a tough, shiny white, adherent deep temporal fascia (DTF). An anchor patch can easily be sutured to this fascia through a small (3cm) temporal incision. Loosely attached to the DTF lies the superficial temporal fascia (STF). This thin layer is continuous with the superficial musculoaponeurotic system (SMAS) in the face beyond the hairline and the galea aponeurotica medially over the forehead. At the hairline, the STF splits into two separate leaves that envelop branches of the temporal branch of the facial nerve. Close to the zygomatic arch, the DTF splits to envelop an intermediate fat pad and facial nerve branches.

The facial nerve emerges from the stylomastoid foramen 6-8mm medial to the tympanomastoid suture of the skull. The posterior auricular nerve and nerves to the posterior belly of digastric and stylohyoid branch from the main trunk before the facial nerve enters the substance of the parotid gland. Within the parotid gland, the facial nerve divides into its main branches: temporal branch, zygomatic branch, buccal branch, marginal mandibular branch, and cervical branch (Fig. 3). The temporal branch exists as 3-4 rami as it exits the superior part of the parotid gland and courses superficially over the zygomatic arch. From the zygomatic arch to the point where the nerve fascicles enter the orbicularis oculi above the brow, these nerve branches are susceptible to injury. Invariably, the temporal branch fibres cross the zygomatic arch between 0.8cm and 3.5cm anterior to the bony external acoustic meatus. They travel enveloped in two leaves of the superficial temporal fascia and enter fibres of frontalis and orbicularis oculi about 2cm superior to the brow. A danger zone exists in the plane of the superficial temporal fascia from the zygomatic arch to the temporal area where the temporal nerve branches are susceptible to injury by suture-passing needles [4].

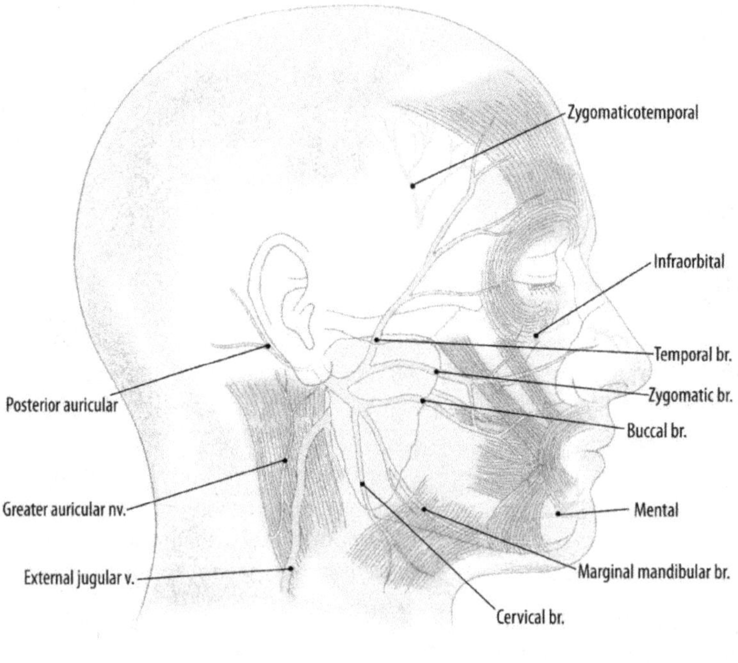

Figure 3. The five branches of the facial nerve: temporal, zygomatic, buccal, marginal mandibular, and cervical. With kind permission from Springer Science+Business Media: Advanced Surgical Facial Rejuvenation, Facial anatomy, 2012, p.11, P.M. Prendergast, fig. 1.11.

There may be up to three zygomatic branches of the facial nerve. One usually passes above the eye to innervate fibres of frontalis and orbicularis oculi. The lower branch passes under the origin of zygomaticus major and supplies this muscle, lip elevators, and the lower orbicularis oculi. Smaller branches also supply depressor supercilii and the superomedial orbicularis oculi. The buccal branch of the facial nerve is closely adherent to masseter within the parotidomasseteric fascia. It travels anteriorly over the buccal fat, below and parallel to the parotid duct. This nerve innervates the buccinators and muscles of the upper lip and nose. Injury to the buccal branches of the facial nerve during a Silhouette thread lift is unlikely since the needles pass in a more superficial plane to retract the superficial soft tissues and fat compartments.

The marginal mandibular nerve exits the inferior aspect of the parotid and travels anteriorly above the mandibular border, although it may drop to up to 4cm below the mandibular border. About 2cm posterior to the corner of the mouth, the nerve courses upward over the mandibular border, just deep to the wafer-thin platysma muscle. At this point, it is prone to injury during liposuction or surgical techniques in this area. Silhouette suture exit points are situated superiorly for midface lifting, although passage of the needles in the neck close to the mandible could theoretically injure this nerve.

Silhouette suture face lifting employs small absorbable cones to retract soft tissues of the midface. These soft tissues are essentially superficial fat compartments, separated from one another by condensations of connective tissue. The superficial fat compartments, as described by Rohrich [5] comprise the following: the nasolabial fat compartment, the medial, middle, and lateral temporal-cheek "malar" fat pads, the central, middle, and lateral temporal-cheek pads in the forehead, and the superior, inferior, and lateral orbital fat pads (Fig. 4). During midface elevation using Silhouette sutures, the nasolabial, medial, and middle cheek fat pads are retracted and elevated, compressing them somewhat against the inferior orbital and lateral orbital fat compartments. The result is volume restoration and softening of the nasolabial fold and tear trough deformity. Irregularities can occur where cones tether the ligaments that occur between these fat compartments. This is particularly true of the zygmoatic ligament, a true ligament that arises from the zygomatic periosteum and inserts into the dermis near the lateral canthus. As described later, cones should be excised from the suture to prevent irregularities in this area. False retaining ligaments are more diffuse condensations of connective tissue that connect superficial and deep facial fasciae [6]. The cones on Silhouette sutures also retract these ligaments, increasing the stability of the lift. The mild waviness or irregularity that occurs immediately following suture lifts is transient and softens out within a few days without intervention.

The sensory innervation of the face is via the three divisions of the trigeminal nerve (fifth cranial nerve) ophthalmic nerve, maxillary nerve, and mandibular nerve. The ophthalmic nerve supplies the forehead, upper eyelid, and dorsum of the nose via the supraorbital, supratrochlear, infratrochlear, lacrimal, and external nasal nerves. The maxillary nerve supplies the lower eyelid, cheek, upper lip, ala of the nose, and part of the temple, through the infraorbital, zygomaticofacial, and zygomaticotemporal nerves. The mandibular nerve has motor and sensory fibres. Its branches include the inferior alveolar nerve, lingual nerve, buccal nerve, and auriculotemporal nerve. These supply the skin over the mandible, lower cheek, part of the temple and ear, the lower teeth, gingival mucosa, and the lower lip (Fig. 5). The greater auricular nerve, derived from the anterior primary rami of the second and third cervical nerves, supplies the skin over the angle of the mandible.

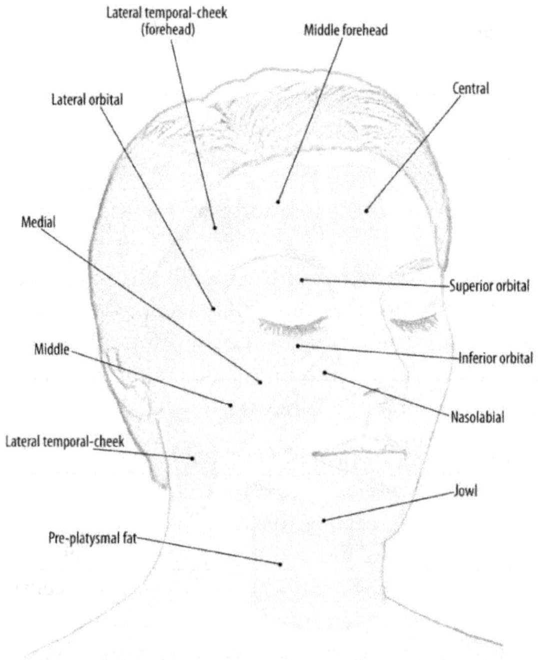

Figure 4. The superficial fat compartments of the face

Silhouette suture lifts are performed under local anaesthesia: infiltrative, regional, or a combination of both. Infiltrative anaesthesia provides a "hydrotomy" or fluid plane through which suture needles can easily pass. Infiltrative anaesthesia also provides local vasoconstriction, via epinephrine, and potentially reduces bruising and the risk of haematoma. Newer blunt-tipped needles are designed to reduce the likelihood of vascular (and neural) injury. Regional nerve blocks anaesthetize large areas of the face and cause less localised tissue distortion than infiltrative anaesthesia. Tissue filling and distortion with anaesthetic solution can make it difficult to assess the soft tissues intraoperatively and the degree of retraction required for a satisfactory lift. Regional blocks of the main nerves providing sensation to the temples and midface are described here.

The zygomaticotemporal nerve emerges from its foramen on the deep surface of the zygomatic bone and supplies the anterior temple. It is blocked by injecting 1-2ml anaesthetic behind the junction of the lateral orbital rim and the upper border of the zygomatic arch. The zygomaticofacial nerve arises from its foramen below and lateral to the inferolateral border of the orbital rim and supplies the soft tissues and skin over the malar eminence. To block this nerve, anaesthetic is injected over the periosteum at the site of the zygomaticofacial foramen.

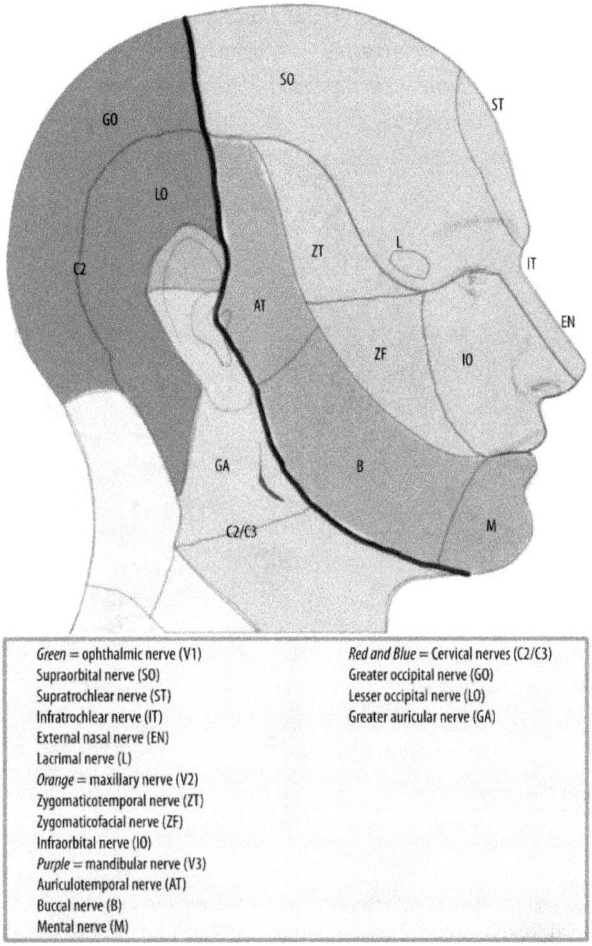

Figure 5. Sensory innervation of the face and neck. *With kind permission from Springer Science+Business Media: Advanced Surgical Facial Rejuvenation, Facial anatomy, 2012, p.12, P.M. Prendergast, fig. 1.12.*

The infraorbital nerve is the largest branch of the maxillary nerve. It enters the face through the infraorbital foramen 2.7-3 cm from the midline in men and 2.4-2.7 cm from the midline in women, about 7 and 6 mm inferior to the inferior orbital rim in men and women respectively. It supplies the lower eyelid, ala of the nose, medial cheek, nasolabial fold, and upper lip. To block the infraorbital nerve, about 2 ml anaesthetic solution is injected over the foramen. To reach the foramen, a transdermal or intraoral approach is used.

With proper placement of blunt-tipped Silhouette needles in the correct plane, bleeding is uncommon. Infiltrating small volumes of anaesthetic with epinephrine along the proposed suture paths provides a bloodless field and further reduces ecchymosis. It is important for the surgeon who performs suture lifting techniques to have a knowledge of the vascular supply to the face. The arterial supply is outlined here.

The skin and soft tissue of the face receive their arterial supply from branches of the facial, maxillary, and superficial temporal arteries—all branches of the external carotid artery. The ophthalmic arteries, arising from the internal carotid system, supply a masklike area including the central forehead, eyelids, and upper part of the nose (Fig. 6).

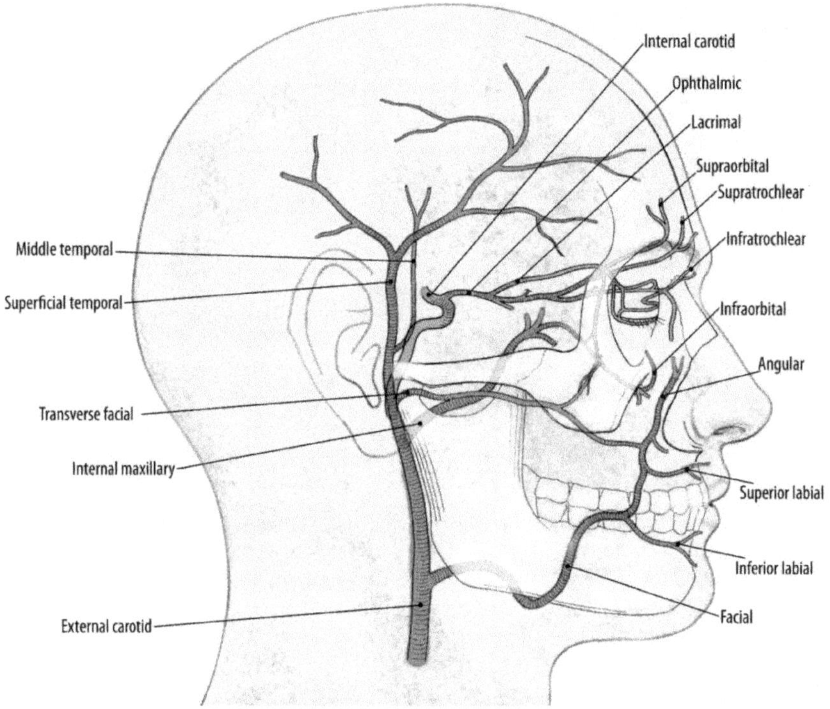

Figure 6. The arterial supply of the face. With kind permission from Springer Science+Business Media: Advanced Surgical Facial Rejuvenation, Facial anatomy, 2012, p.13, P.M. Prendergast, fig. 1.13.

The facial artery arises from the external carotid and loops around the inferior and anterior borders of the mandible, just anterior to masseter. It pierces the masseteric fascia and ascends upwards and medially toward the eye. It lies deep to the zygomatici and risorius muscles but superficial to buccinator and levator anguli oris [7]. At the level of the mouth the facial artery sends two labial arteries, inferior and superior, into the lips where they pass below orbicularis oris. The continuation of the facial artery near the medial canthus beside the nose is the angular artery.

The maxillary artery is a terminal branch of the external carotid with three main branches, mental, buccal, and infraorbital arteries. The mental artery is the terminal branch of the inferior alveolar artery that passes through the mental foramen to supply the chin and lower lip. The buccal artery crosses the buccinators to supply the cheek tissue. The infraorbital artery reaches the face through the infraorbital foramen and supplies the lower eyelid, cheek, and lateral nose. It anastomoses with branches of the transverse facial, ophthalmic, buccal, and facial arteries.

The superficial temporal artery is the terminal branch of the external carotid artery. In the substance of the parotid, just before reaching the zygomatic arch, it gives off the transverse facial artery which runs inferior and parallel to the arch and supplies the parotid, parotid duct, masseter, and skin of the lateral canthus. The superficial temporal artery crosses the zygomatic arch superficially within the superficial temporal fascia. Above the arch, it gives off a middle temporal artery that pierces the deep temporal fascia and supplies the temporalis muscle. Thereafter, about 2cm above the zygomatic arch, the superficial temporal artery divides into anterior and posterior branches. The anterior branch supplies the forehead and forms anastomoses with the supraorbital and supratrochlear vessels. The posterior part supplies the parietal scalp and periosteum.

The ophthalmic artery is a branch of the internal carotid system (Fig. 6). Its branches include the lacrimal, supraorbital, supratrochlear, infratrochlear, and external nasal arteries. There is significant communication between the external and internal carotid artery systems around the eye through several anastomoses.

4. Indications

Patients who may benefit from the Silhouette lift procedure include those with mild to moderate heaviness or ptosis of the face and neck. Typically, patients are 35 to 45 years old with normal or slightly excessive facial volume. The fat compartments in the midface have fallen slightly, accentuating the nasolabial crease. As the fat falls away from the lid-cheek junction, the tear trough deformity becomes apparent under the eyes. The anterior cheek flattens and the shape of the face changes from a youthful heart-shape to a more aging rectangular-shape. By elevating the midface fat compartments using the Silhouette sutures, all of these aging features can be improved. Repositioning the midface in a vector that is mostly superior improves the shape of the face, softens the nasolabial crease, and ameliorates the lid-cheek junction. It is important to remember that a Silhouette lift is not an excisional procedure, but one that merely repositions ptotic soft tissue. As such, if there is marked laxity of skin, a Silhouette lift is not indicated. Similarly, if the patient's face is very thin, Silhouette sutures are not appropriate. Where there is a very thin soft tissue envelope, lifting the fat with Silhouette sutures will simply bunch up the skin and create irregularities over the cones.

A Silhouette suture lift improves mild ptosis of the neck and helps restore an optimum mentocervical angle, which should be 80-95º. For more pronounced signs, including excessive laxity, heavy platysmal bands, and submental fat, other procedures may be more appropriate, including excisional surgery, platysmaplasty, liposuction, or chemodenervation.

Before any suture or thread lift procedure, the patient's expectations should be assessed. If the patient expects dramatic results, or a powerful lifting effect that could only be achieved through open surgery, the procedure should not be performed unless the patient can readjust their expectations. Suture lifting techniques do not replace open excisional surgery. The author explains to patients that suture lifts usually provide more lifting that external tissue tightening devices, but do not replace invasive surgery. They reposition tissue, but do not remove them. Once a patient has realistic expectations and appreciates that the aim is a natural-looking enhancement rather than a dramatic transformation, the likelihood of a successful outcome is high. Additionally, it should be explained to the patient that no intervention provides permanent results. Suture lifts can be repeated over time if necessary. The Silhouette sutures described here may be retightened during a secondary procedure.

5. Step-by-step technique

The author administers 1mg lorazepam and one solpadol (paracetamol 500mg, codeine 30mg) preoperatively for anxiolysis and moderate analgesia. Preoperative photographs should be taken in front, oblique, and side views.

5.1. Midface

Markings are made with skin markers with the patient in the sitting position. First, a guide line is marked from the corner of the mouth to the angle of the mandible. Exit points should not be made inferior to this line to prevent disruption of the sutures during facial animation. Next, the proposed exit points are marked. For midface lifting, the standard exit points are as follows: 1 cm lateral to the midpoint of the nasolabial fold, 1.5 cm inferior to the first point, 1.5 cm lateral to the previous point at or just above the guide line, and 1.5 cm lateral to this point (Fig. 7). Depending on the desired lifting vector, the suture paths are estimated using a dashed line from these exit points to a point where the lines converge behind the temporal hairline. A line is marked behind the hairline in the temporal scalp, measuring about 3 cm, where the incision is made.

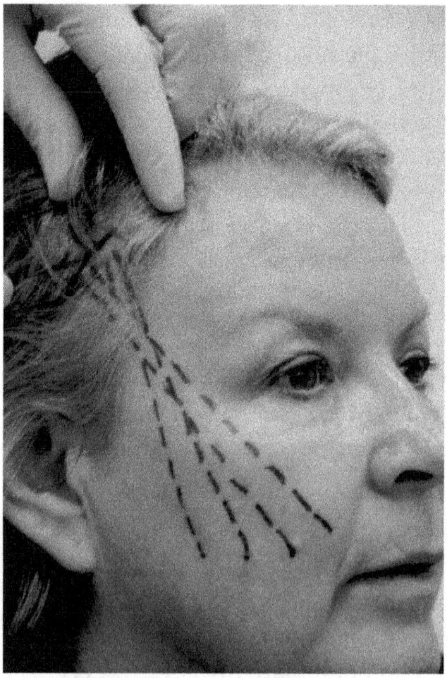

Figure 7. Preoperative markings for Silhouette midface lift

The patient is positioned supine for the procedure. Sterile technique is used, with formal skin preparation and surgical draping, exposing the operative field. The instruments and materials required for lifting using Silhouette sutures are shown in figure 8. A solution of 2% xylocaine (lidocaine 2% with epinephrine 1:200,000) and 0.9% sodium chloride is used for infiltrative anaesthesia. Using a combination of 30 gauge and 27 gauge short and long needles, the incision site and proposed suture paths are infiltrated. Adding sodium bicarbonate to the solution reduces discomfort on infiltration. A maximum of 7mg/kg lidocaine (with epinephrine) should not be exceeded to avoid lidocaine toxicity.

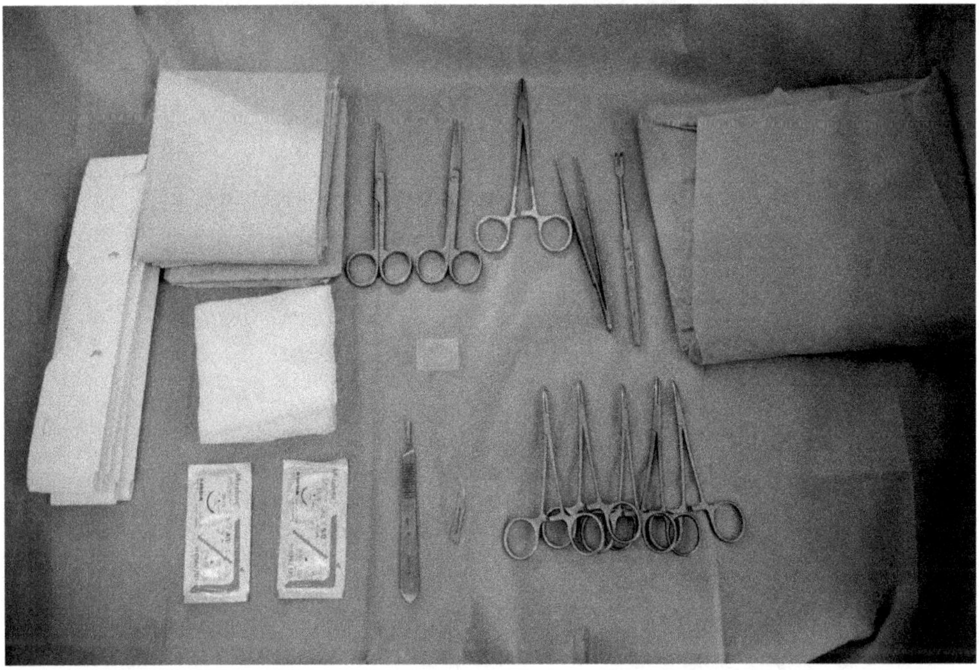

Figure 8. Instruments and materials required for Silhouette suture lift procedure

A 3 cm incision is made in the temporal area. Since this area is particularly vascular, diathermy is essential for adequate haemostasis. Once the skin is opened, the subcutaneous fat is gently retracted, exposing the superficial temporal fascia (STF). This thin layer is opened to expose the white, shiny deep temporal fascia (Fig. 9). A space is created by bluntly dissecting over the deep temporal fascia.

A small, 1 cm x 0.5 cm patch of polypropylene mesh (Suramesh) is placed on the deep temporal fascia and secured using a single vicryl suture. In order to delineate the planes before suture placement, sharp dissection above the superficial temporal fascia separates the subcutaneous fatty plane and the superficial temporal fascia (Fig.10). To avoid placing the needles close to the temporal branch of the facial nerve beyond the hairline, the needles are placed in the subcutaneous fat above the superficial temporal fascia. It is best to start in the correct plane, rather than start deep to superficial temporal fascia (STF) and then change course at the hairline to come superficial to the STF blindly.

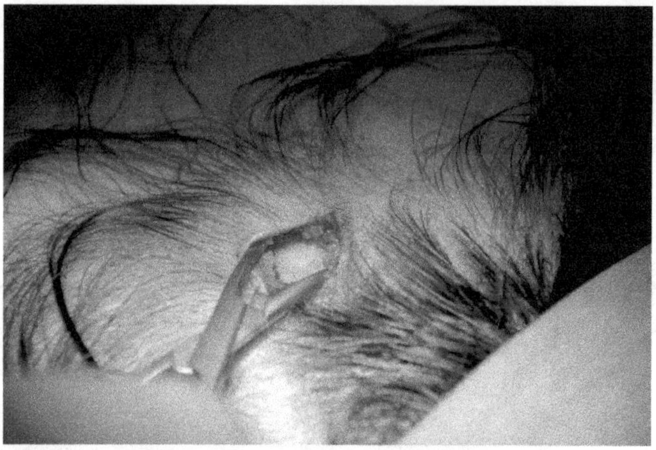

Figure 9. Temporal incision with exposed deep temporal fascia.

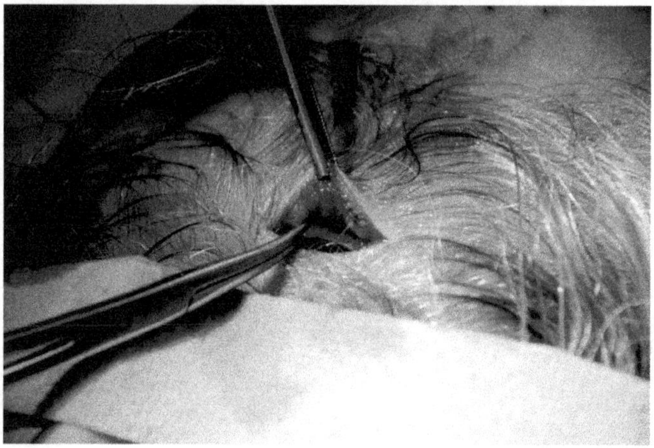

Figure 10. Superficial temporal fascia. The suture is placed just above the superficial temporal fascia in the subcutaneous plane.

Before passing the first Silhouette suture, the suture is placed over the face externally to determine how many cones should be left on the suture and how many (if any) should be excised. Once lifted, all cones should be positioned inferior to the zygomatic arch, to avoid tethering the zygomatic ligament, resulting in irregularities that can be difficult to correct. Usually, leaving 3-4 cones on the suture is sufficient, although this depends on the size of the patients face. The first suture is passed through the face by placing the blunt tip of the Silhouette needle subcutaneously, above STF, until the needle tip is ready to emerge through the dermis at the first exit point lateral to the nasolabial fold. The soft tissues should not be squeezed or compressed around the needle during passage to avoid irregularities. The malar fat can be lifted slightly to "present" it to the needle once the needle passes over the zygomatic arch. This maneuver also facilitates the needle to exit through the skin perpendicularly. A 16-gauge needle is used to puncture the skin over the exit point to allow the blunt-tipped needle to emerge (Fig. 11). The needle is pulled through gently. A characteristic clicking of cones is heard as they pass through the soft tissues. Care should be taken not to pull through too many cones; once they exit the skin they cannot be retracted back into the tissues. The predetermined number of cones is excised from the suture, and the suture is cut distal to the knot that lies proximal to the last cone being removed (Fig. 12). The proximal end of the suture is lifted to retract the knot back into the cheek and lift the tissues. The same process is repeated for the other sutures until all four sutures are placed in the fibrofatty malar fat pad. Although four sutures are usually placed for midface lifting, more or fewer sutures can be employed depending on the patient and indications. However, the lateral face region should be avoided since the soft tissue envelope in this region is thinner and the dermis is more adherent to the superficial musculoaponeurotic system.

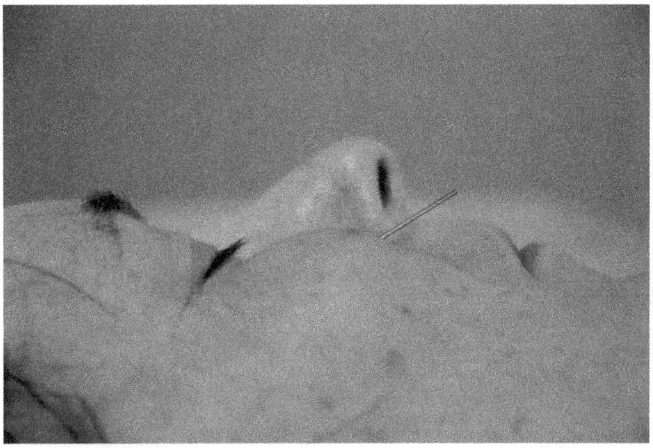

Figure 11. Blunt-tipped needle exits perpendicularly

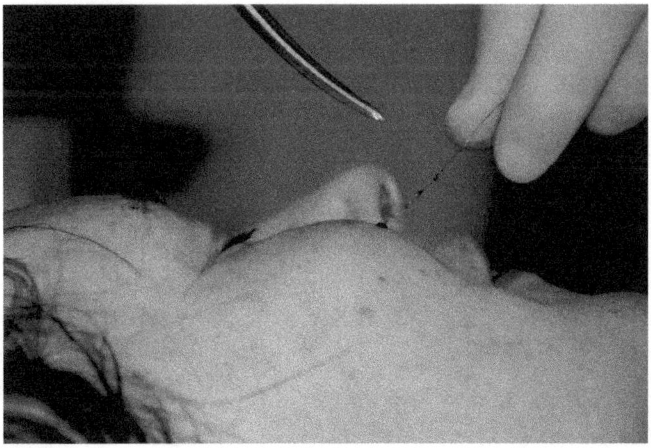

Figure 12. The suture is brought through and the predetermined number of cones is excised from the suture

The half-circle needle swaged to the proximal end of the Silhouette suture is passed first through the superficial temporal fascia. Then a bite of the deep temporal fascia is taken, emerging through the polypropylene mesh. Once all of the proximal needles are anchored to the deep temporal fascia and mesh in this way, the sutures are retracted gently to affect a lift on the midface (Fig. 13). The sutures are tied to one another in pairs over the polypropylene mesh. The superficial temporal fascia is closed with vicryl. Skin closure is performed with interrupted skin sutures or skin clips.

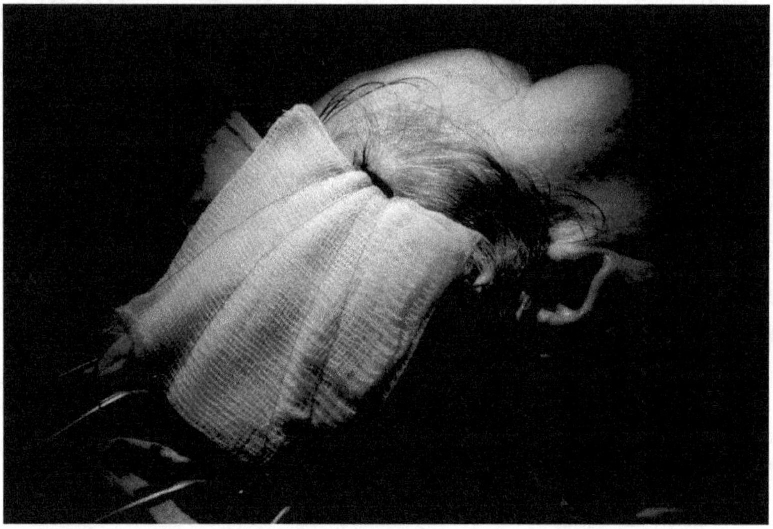

Figure 13. Four Silhouette sutures are used on each side to elevate the midface

5.2. Neck

Markings are made from an incision site at the hairline below the ear along the neck under the jawline toward the midline. Two exit points are marked on each side, before the midline (Fig. 14). Local anaesthetic is infiltrated subcutaneously along the suture paths. A 2 cm incision is made at the hairline and the cervical fascia is exposed with blunt dissection (Fig. 15). The first Silhouette needle is passed under the dermis toward the midline. Laterally, the dermis is adherent to the underlying fascia over sternocleidomastoid and more resistance is felt in this area using the blunt-tipped needle. More medially, less resistance is encountered as the needle glides through the preplatysmal fat. The dermis is punctured with a 20-gauge needle to allow the Silhouette needle exit. Most or all of the six cones on the Silhouette suture are left in place for neck lifting. In some cases, two cones are excised, leaving four on the suture to lift the tissues. Once both sutures are passed, the proximal ends are anchored by taking a bite of cervical fascia and tying the sutures down over a small pledget of polypropylene mesh. Care should be taken to avoid the mesh curling upward toward the dermis by seating it properly on the fascia. The skin is closed using 4/0 or 5/0 sutures. Moderate, transient bunching occurs laterally following Silhouette suture lifting of the neck.

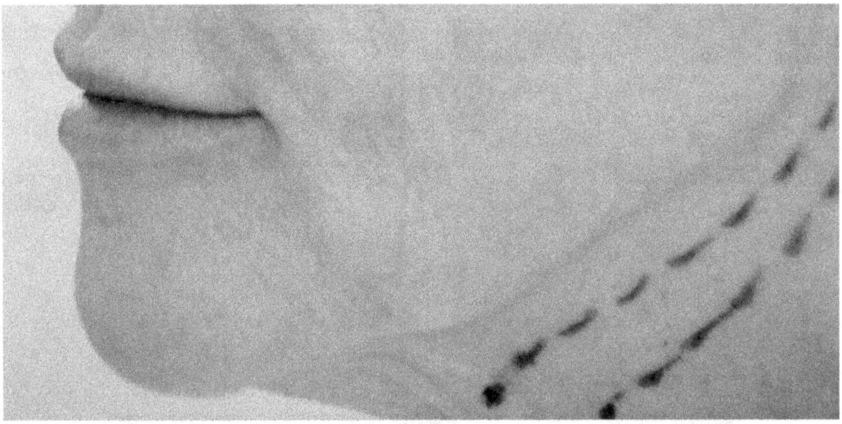

Figure 14. Preoperative marking for Silhouette suture neck lift. Two sutures are passed on each side from the hairline to a exit points near the midline.

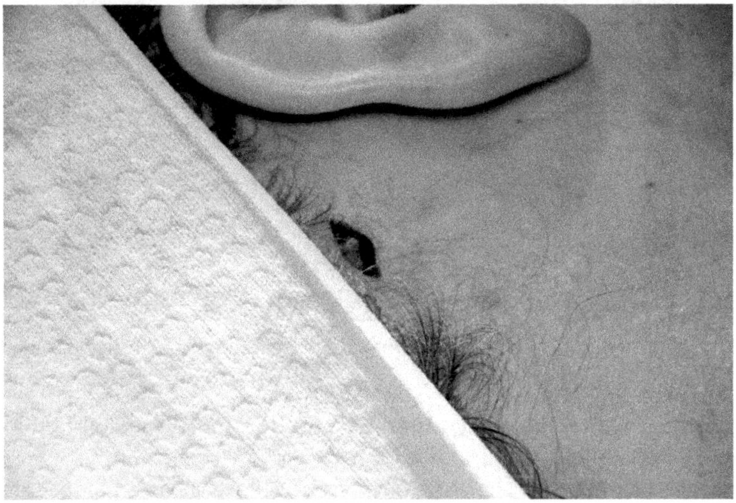

Figure 15. Incision for Silhouette suture lift of the neck

5.3. Brow

A Silhouette lift of the brow improves aesthetics by elevating the lateral aspect and tail of the eyebrow (Fig. 16). In heavy brows, elevation also reduces dermatochalasis. The author recommends chemodenervation of lateral fibres of orbicularis oculi with botulinum toxin at least two weeks prior to the suture lift to reduce downward movement on the cones.

The patient is carefully assessed to decide the best lifting points in the lateral brow (Fig. 17). The exit points and anchorage point will determine the ultimate lifting effect and shape of the brow.

Local anaesthesia is infiltrated along the suture paths, creating a hydrotomy that somewhat lifts the normally adherent dermis off the underlying frontalis. A 1 cm incision is made in the

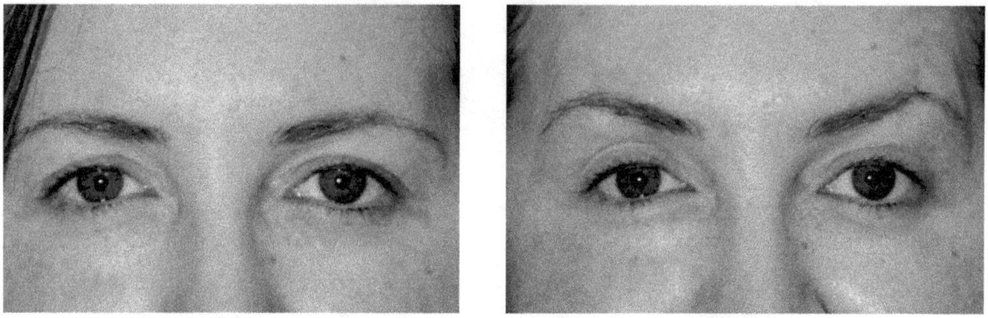

(a) (b)

Figure 16. a. Before, b. Immediately after Silhouette brow lift.

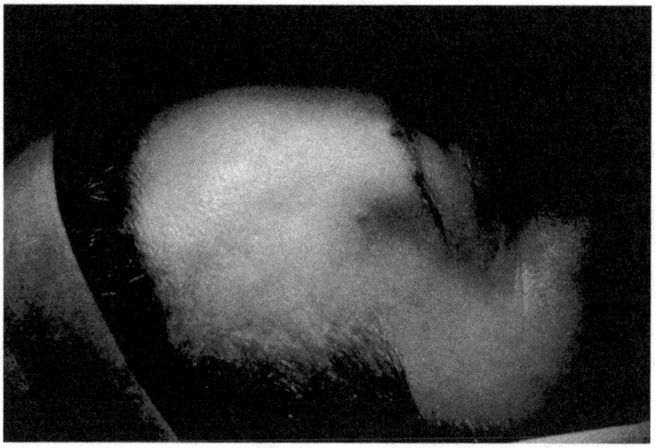

Figure 17. Preoperative markings for brow lift using Silhouette sutures. An incision is made at the hairline. There are two exit points at the brow.

skin at the hairline. The first Silhouette suture is passed from the incision to the exit point in the brow (Fig. 18). There is usually no need to excise any cones from the suture, leaving six cones to elevate the tissues above the brow. The second suture is passed in the same way. Each proximal end of the suture is anchored by passing the half circular needle deep to periosteum. The suture ends are tied to one another over a small pledget of polypropylene mesh, which sits on the galea. The pledget and suture ends are buried satisfactorily before the skin is closed.

Mild irregularities or bunching occur immediately following Silhouette brow lifting. This resolves and softens in a number of days.

6. Results

The Silhouette suture lift procedure elevates and suspends tissues providing immediate results. These minimally invasive techniques, performed under local anaesthesia, do not replace excisional surgery such as cervicofacial rhytidectomy, but are ideally suited for younger patients or those who do not want more invasive intervention. They can also be performed as a complementary procedure during open surgery.

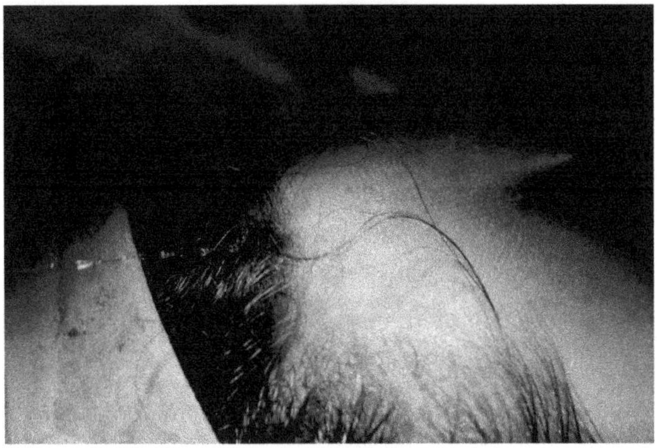

Figure 18. The first Silhouette suture is passed from the incision at the hairline to the brow.

Immediately after the procedure, there is usually mild swelling secondary to local anaesthesia, as well as some bunching or irregularities over the sutures. It should be explained to the patient preoperatively that it takes a few days for the tissues to smooth and soften and for the bunching to subside, particularly in the neck. The patient should not rub or massage the face or neck for several weeks. Gentle handling is important to avoid disruption of the sutures, and to allow fibrosis around the cones and knots on the sutures to occur.

After the poly-lactide cones on Silhouette sutures absorb over about 10 months, what remains are the polypropylene sutures, knots, and bundles of fibrous tissues that remain tethered to surrounding tissues. After 1-2 years, Silhouette sutures can be retightened by opening the old incision, re-suspending the proximal suture ends, and tying them down again to restore the desired lift. Alternatively, further sutures can be placed and anchored in a redo procedure.

7. Complications

Although complications associated with Silhouette suture lifts are uncommon, they can occur and the patient must be informed of all potential sequelae, side-effects, and risks. Normal after-effects include swelling, mild bunching and irregularities, ecchymosis, discomfort, and transient dysaesthesias. Complications are listed in table 1.

Infection should be treated with antibiotics initially. If there is evidence of infection along the suture, the sutures should be removed. Prophylactic antibiotics and sterile technique serve to minimise the risk of infection.

Whilst a small haematoma may resorb without intervention, if a large haematoma occurs, this may need to be evacuated. The presence of a haematoma also increases the risk of localized infection.

Non-absorbable sutures may extrude through the skin, even years following a suture lift. It is important to bury suture knots or seat the tied sutures or mesh deep where possible so that it is less likely to irritate the dermis. This is particularly important in the forehead with brow lifting and incision at the neck hairline with Silhouette neck lifts.

Persistent irregularities or dimples overlying sutures can usually be corrected with gentle manipulation of the tissues over the suture. If the dermis cannot be released using this maneuver, subcision may be used using a needle.

Infection	Facial nerve injury
Bleeding	Sensory impairment
Haematoma	Chronic pain
Suture extrusion	Palpability

Table 1. Complications associated with suture lifting

8. Conclusion

The Silhouette suture is a novel device used for minimally invasive face and neck lifting under local anaesthesia without the need for long incisions, tissue undermining, or skin excision. Retraction or suspension of soft tissues is achieved through absorbable cones distributed along the length of the suture. Silhouette sutures are most commonly employed for midface lifting, where the fibrofatty malar fat is elevated and anchored by suturing the proximal ends of the sutures to the deep temporal fascia behind the hairline. The non-absorbable polypropylene sutures allow secondary re-tightening at a later stage. Silhouette sutures are also suitable for lifting and improving ptosis in the neck and in the brows.

Author details

Peter Prendergast
Venus Medical, Dublin, Ireland

9. References

[1] The American Society for Aesthetic Plastic Surgery: Cosmetic surgery national database statistics 2011, ASAPS website, http://www.surgery.org (accessed 1 May 2012).

[2] Kress DW. The History of Barbed Suture Suspension: Applications, and Visions for the Future. In: Shiffman MA, Mirrafati SJ, Lam SM (eds.). Simplified Facial Rejuvenation. Berlin Heidelberg: Springer-Verlag; 2008. p247.

[3] Sasaki GH, Komorowska-Timek ED, Bennett DC, Gabriel A. An Objective Comparison of Holding, Slippage, and Pull-out Tensions for Eight Suspension Sutures in the Malar Fat Pads of Fresh-Frozen Human Cadavers. Aesthetic Surgery Journal 2008; 28(4) 387-96.

[4] Prendergast PM. Danger Zones in Surgical Facial Rejuvenation. In: Shiffman MA, Erian A (eds.). Advanced Surgical Facial Rejuvenation. Berlin Heidelberg: Springer-Verlag 2012. p24.

[5] Rohrich RJ, Pessa JE. The Fat Compartments of the Face: Anatomy and Clinical Implications for Cosmetic Surgery. Plastic and Reconstructive Surgery 2007; 119(7): 2219-27.

[6] Jones BM, Grover R. Anatomical Considerations. In: Jones BM, Grover R (eds.). Facial Rejuvenation Surgery. Philadelphia 2008. p18-22.

[7] Berkovitz BKB, Moxham BJ. Head and Neck Anatomy. A Clinical Reference. Philadelphia: Taylor and Francis; 2002. p118.

Section 4

Combined Techniques - Sutures and Barbed Threads

Chapter 16

T3 - Soft Face Lift by Suspension Surgery

Pier Antonio Bacci

Additional information is available at the end of the chapter

http://dx.doi.org/10.5772/56710

1. Introduction

Surgical strategy using barbed or not barbed threads is now an asserted truth with numerous and official follow-up and experiences. These strategies are named as "mini invasive aesthetic metholodologies" because provide for good results with little incisions and few complications

Today there are many different mini-invasive surgical techniques available, using different kinds of surgical suspension threads. All of these are due to four main authors: Guilleman, Sulamanidze, Serdev and Ruff.

2. The Guilleman technique

This is the basic technique known and published under the name of *"Curl Lift"* and is certainly the mother of all the other methods used.

It is the simplest and most intelligent method to lift the relaxed tissues with simple and everyday used surgical threads, absorbable or not. **(Fig. 1)**

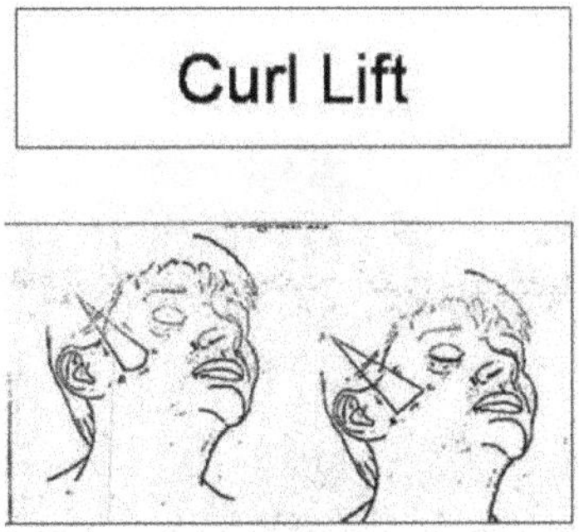

Figure 1. The initial idea of the Curl Lift

3. The Sulamanidze technique

This method uses a particular surgical thread with barbs, like opposing ears of wheat, thanks to which the threads support themselves in the tissue.

The criticism that can be made about this technique is the fact that the calibre of the needle-cannula used to introduce the thread into the tissue is greater than the thread itself, which can cause some difficulties in hooking the barbs and easy bruising. Finally, this method may be sometime as no long-lasting as the others. It can be very useful in some mini-invasive corrections of the face, such as of the eyebrows or neck. **(Fig. 2)**

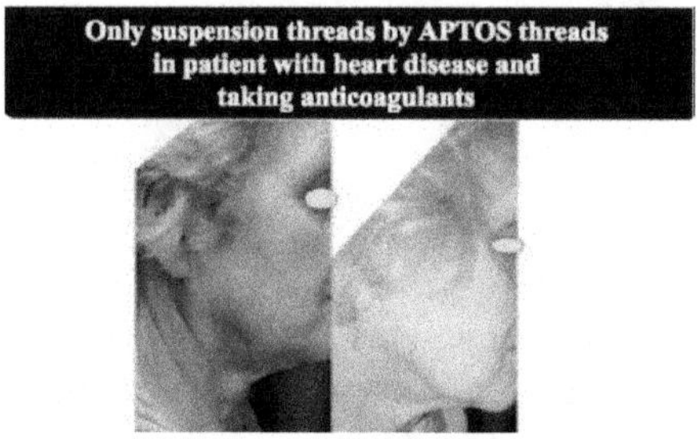

Figure 2. Mini invasive treatment of the neck with original Russian APTOS threads in a subject with heart disease taking Acenocumarol (*Bacci archive*)

4. The Serdev technique

Starting from French surgeons Galland and Clavier, the Bulgarian cosmetic surgeon Nikolay Serdev uses special semi-elastic threads with long-term absorption, along with special needles of his direct invention and preparation that are used to fix the tissues to solid or fixed structures.

In our experience this method has had almost always good results in various aesthetic pathologies, especially for outlining ill-defined cheekbones and the chin line, thanks to the possibility of creating tobacco-pouch sutures that allow us to define the outlines. **(Fig. 3-4)**

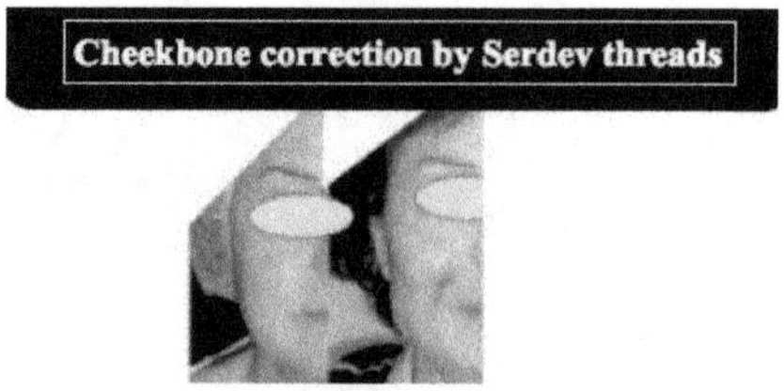

Figure 3. Definition of the cheekbones with Serdev threads (*Bacci archive*)

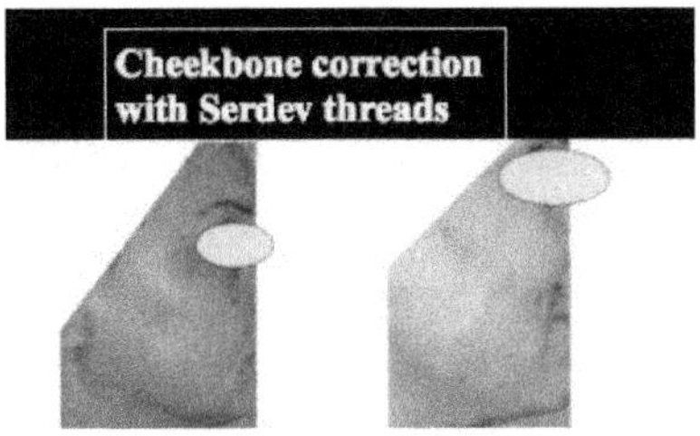

Figure 4. Definition of the cheekbones with Serdev threads (*Bacci archive*)

This is the ideal methodology for increasing volume and projecting the tissues without prostheses, for cheekbones, chin, breasts or buttocks, of course, in selected cases.

5. The Ruff method

This strategy has certainly represented a new era in cosmetic surgery as it is the first methodology officially approved by the FDA for rejuvenation of the face and neck using unidirectional barbed threads.

It is an effective mini-invasive strategy offer us good results. It uses barbed not-adsorbable one-directional threads introduced by special needles and a method that offers the concrete possibility of creating a true anchor point for the thread, thus becoming similar to a track upon which the skin slides and is anchored, thanks to the unidirectional barbs that are arranged in a spiral shape, guaranteeing its strong hold on the tissues. **(Fig. 5)**

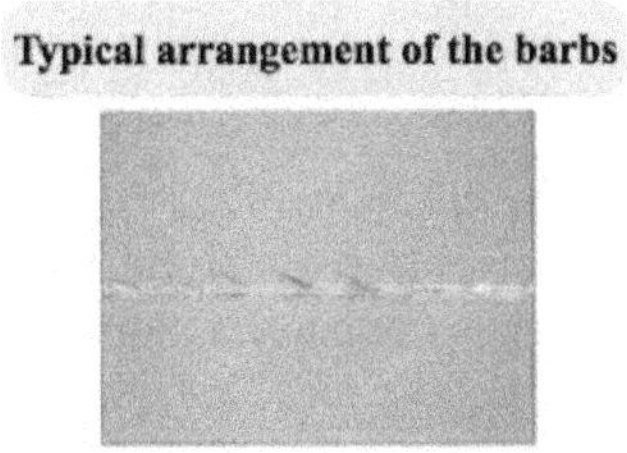

Figure 5. Typical spiral arrangement of the unidirectional barbs. (*Bacci Archive*)

Typical characteristic of these barbed surgical threads is the possibility to lift-up all part of the tissue, particurarly midface, neck and eyebrown, or the cutaneous layer that the adipose –muscular deep wraps.

To conclude, we have today four basical mini invasive strategy by threads, according to Guilleman, Sulamanidze, Serdev and Ruff, we can use different strategies, in integrate methodology too, on respect to different indications.

6. T3 - Soft Lift

In 2001 we began our first experiences with the integration of two methods, suspension threads and surgical soft lift.

We started with unidirectional, barbed absorbable surgical threads we made by hand in the operating room using a simple method with a monofilament. Our experience then developed particularly while observing their capacity to form a temporary tissue fibrosis along the thread's path in 8-12 weeks' time.

This is how we started the mini-invasive method we call *"T3-Soft Face Lifting"*, meaning *"Traction Threads Treatment"*, or a treatment that uses the traction on surgical threads to lift the tissues, avoiding more extensive dissection, in one or more sessions.

Basically, this strategy consists of two mini-invasive surgical sessions done with local anaesthesia.

- *1st session* - The purpose of this procedure is to introduce the barbed unidirectional "polypropylene" suspension threads using particular carriers that adapt to the various positioning needs of the different suspension threads. **(Fig. 6)**

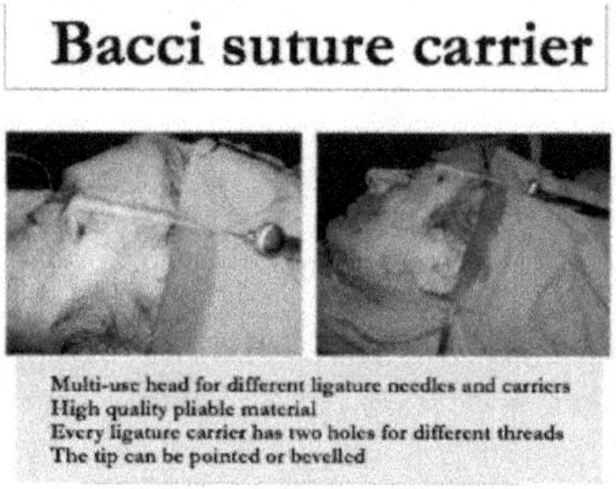

Figure 6. Bacci's instrument for introducing threads – (*Bacci Archive*)

Depending on need or the skin to be eliminated, an incision can also be made (as small as possible) along the classical lines in front of or behind the ear, in the frontotemporal area, then the smallest dissection necessary is done to traction the SMAS, doubling it or creating a small flap.

Then a typical vertical mini-lift is done, but using the traction of the threads, therefore avoiding tissue dissection and complications. **(Fig. 7)**

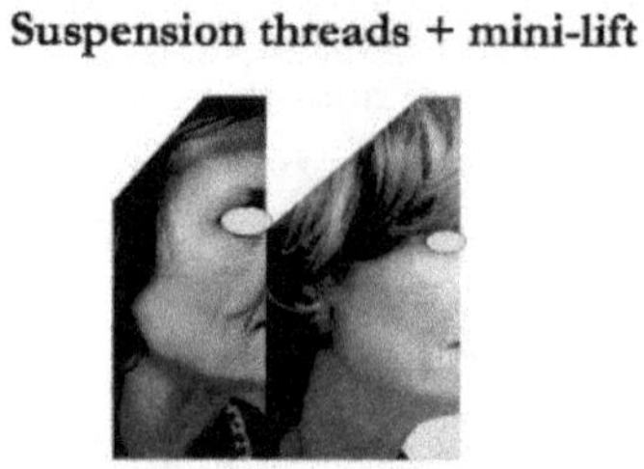

Figure 7. Suspension threads and mini-face lift (*Bacci Archive*)

In patients requesting or needing greater traction or greater excision of skin tissue we can also associate a more ample lift, lifting both the temporal region and the midface and neck, thus reconstructing a better triangle of youth, and still limiting dissection thanks to the use of unidirectional barbed threads or of Serdev's circular method. **(Fig. 8)**

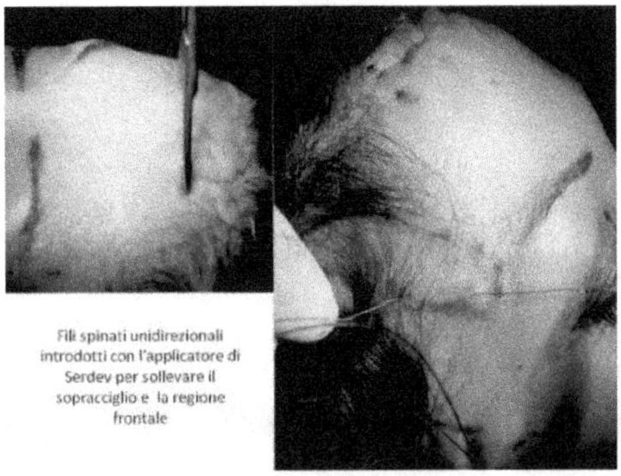

Figure 8. Suspension threads and superior blepharoplasty using Serdev Methodology *(Archive Bacci)*

Normally, in this first session lipofilling is associated with the suspension threads, allowing the tissue metabolism to activate thanks to the hormonal impulse given by the autologous fat tissue inserted into the tissue.

The suspension thread and fatty tissue association (*T3-Fat Lift*, or *stabilised lipofilling*) has a particular importance since it favours metabolic recovery of the tissues and vascularization of the cells of the fatty tissue injected, thus prolonging its life and active stay in the tissue.

Sometimes we also perform a superior blepharoplasty in this first session in order to increase eye brightness.

-2nd session -_When it is necessary, the second session is as a rule done after 2-3 years, it allows stabilization of the results and offers new traction without dissection. A small incision with local anaesthesia is sufficient to pick up, by Muller's hook for microvarices, the old thread which will be pulled and sutured to the fascia with a 5/0 nylon thread, in a new position.

Method

Usually, four or six non-absorbable unidirectional barbed threads are applied for side. They allow traction of the tissues, thus limiting dissection. Then a semi-circular or "S" incision is done, separating the layer as little as possible and locating the threads in place we traction on them and work the SMAS which is duplicated with suture, when it's necessary. **(Figs. 9-10)**

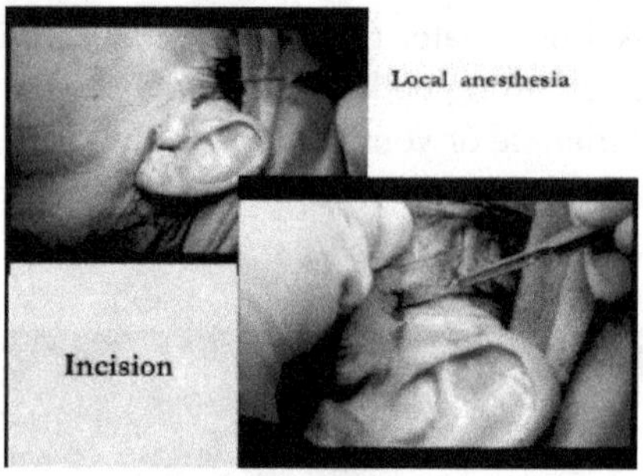

Figure 9. After a little local anaesthesia we traction the tissue and SMAS pulling the threads that hook onto the tissue, and then we suture. (*Bacci Archive*)

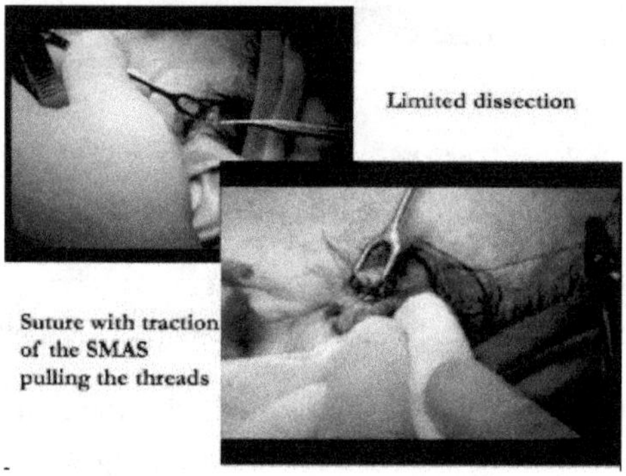

Figure 10. After a little local anaesthesia we traction the tissue and SMAS pulling the threads that hook onto the tissue, and then we suture. (*Bacci Archive*)

After this phase the excess skin is cut and then sutured, following the same traction path of the threads if possible and doubling the tissue for better harmony of the neck, within the same amount of operating time. **(Fig. 11)**

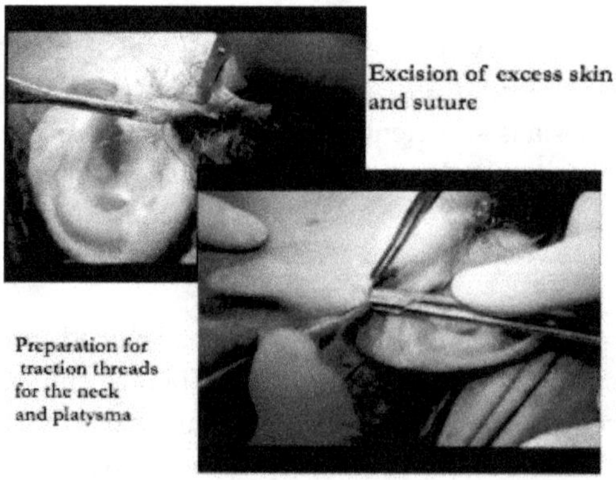

Figure 11. Skin excision and traction on the tissues of the neck. (*Bacci Archive*)

We then move on to reshaping the outlines and volumes of the face in the naso-labial, zygomatic areas, of the cheeks and chin with "rice grain" lipofilling, after taking fatty tissue from the abdomen and periumbilical area, where it guarantees greater resistance to possible initial deficits in vascularization. Usually this fatty tissue is reinserted directly without altering it or traumatizing it. **(Fig. 12)**

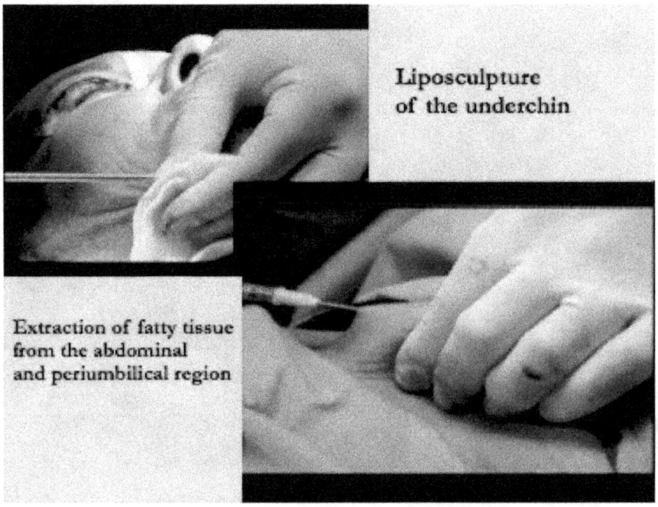

Figure 12. Our micro-cannulae for mini-liposculpture and for extracting fatty tissue, which can also be done with a simple needle, even if more traumatic. (*Bacci Archive*)

Fill - traction

Today, we have more than twenty years of experience with Sulamanidze and Serdev's methods, and we have ten years of experience with unidirectional absorbable or not-absorbable barbed threads, which are used to have a new position of the tissues and to activate processes of bio-stimulation, in particular with surgical threads absorbables by hydrolytic way, such as polydioxanone (PDO). **(Fig.13)**

Currently, thanks to the changing demands of patients seeking rejuvenation of the face even before the age of 40, methodologies are greatly reduced and they are absolutely minimally invasive.

We have reduced the incisions with small lines between the tragus or hidden in the hair or behind the ear. Were reduced detachments of the skin, as results have been virtually eliminated hematoma and major complications. **(Fig.14 - 15)**

The words "Fill-Traction" means a mini-invasive strategy that uses in the same session a Prolene 2/0 not-absorbable unidirectional barbed threads for side, both in the temporal region that in the midface.

In the same session we can apply unidirectional absorbable barbed threads to maintain the position of the skin and improve the contours in the same time.

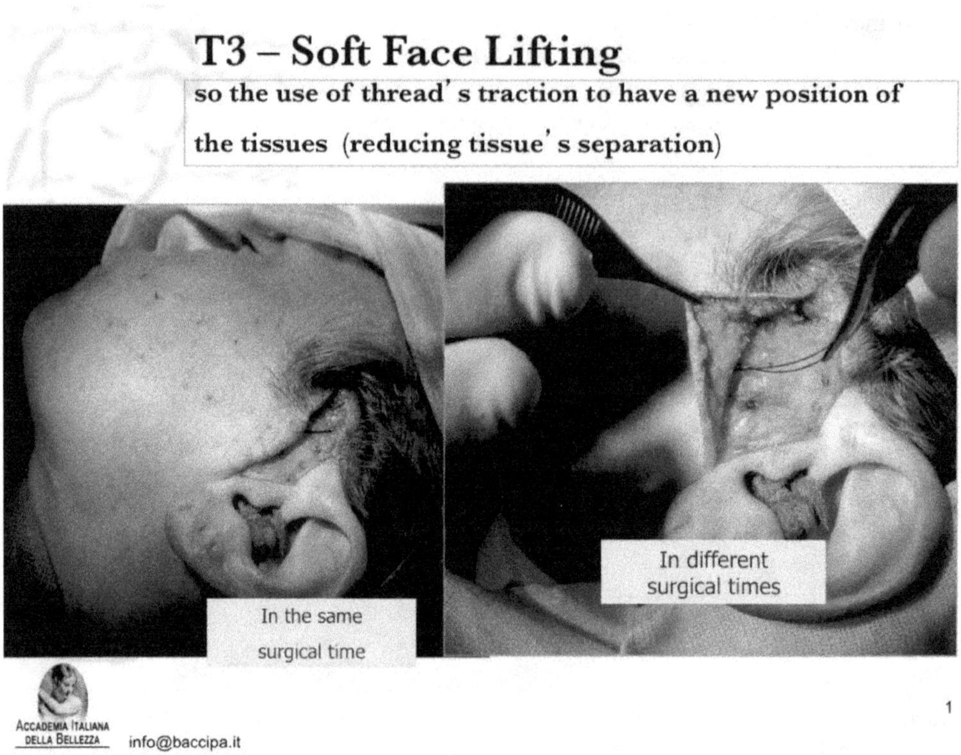

Figure 13. T3 –soft face lift (*Bacci Archive*)

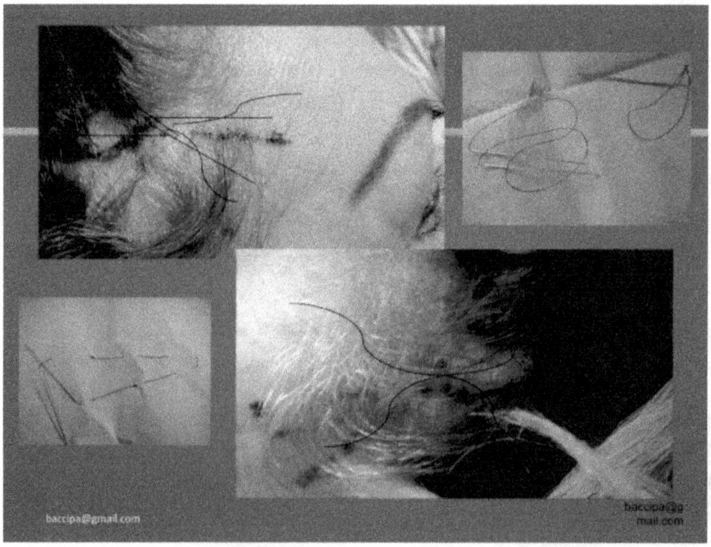

Figure 14. Mini invasive strategy using suspension barbed threads and skin stimulation using absorbable PDO minithreads. (*Bacci Archive*)

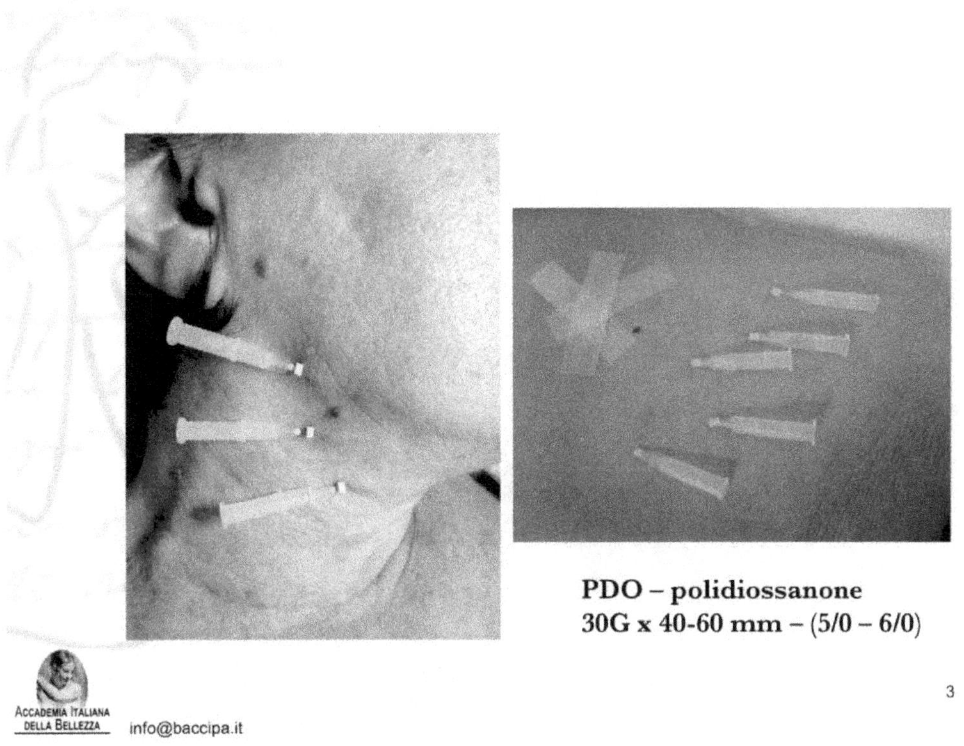

Figure 15. Mini invasive strategy using suspension barbed threads and skin stimulation using absorbable PDO minithreads. (*Bacci Archive*)

Also in the same session, we can use botulinum toxin or lipofiling when it is necessary.

Currently, to stimulate the tissues, we use less frequently fillers with hyaluronic acid, in fact today we can also use small threads in PDO - polydioxanone - according to the korean technique that allows us an interesting skin stimulation, in particular in the neck and in midface.

This small absorbable suture may be repeated after 6-8 months, demonstrating that we have good results with fast recovery and few complications using an integration of minimally invasive methodologies. **(Fig. 16-17)**

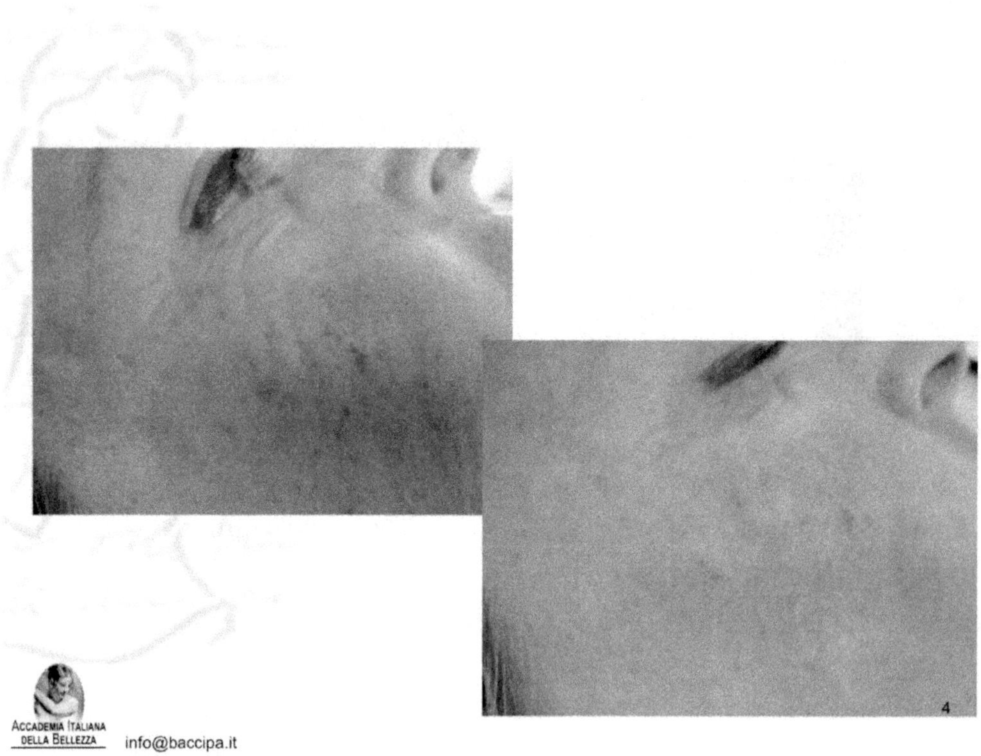

Figure 16. Interesting results using Fill-Traction. (*Bacci Archive*)

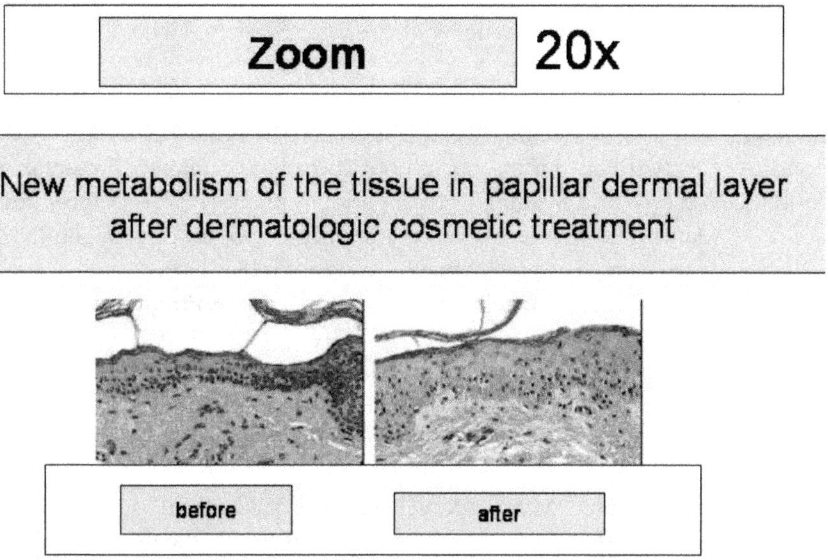

Figure 17. Interesting results using Fill-Traction. (*Bacci Archive*)

7. Conclusion

Certainly, today suspension surgery, as mini invasive aesthetic surgery by threads, is an official surgical strategy, but the best results are always lie to the precise diagnosis and in the rapport between doctor and patient, without never to have miracles or eternal results.

Author details

Pier Antonio Bacci
Mini invasive Aesthetic Surgery Italian Centre, Arezzo, Italy

8. References

[1] Abraham R.F., De Fatta R.J., Williams III E.F.: "Thread-lift for facial rejuvenation. Assessment of long-term results". Arch. Facial Plast. Surg. 11(3):178-183; 2009.

[2] Bacci P.A.: "T3 soft face lifting and bioresurfacing". Paper presented at the Cosmetic Surgery congress, Varna, June 2003

[3] Bacci P.A.: "T3-soft face lifting". Paper presented at the Aesthetic Medicine Congress AGORA, Milan, October 2004

[4] Bacci P.A.: "T3-soft face lifting". Paper presented at the 29th World Congress of Cosmetic and dermatology surgery, Manila, February 2004

[5] Bacci P.A.: "Soft face lifting and reposition threads". Presentazione al 49th World Meeting of the International Academy of Cosmetic Surgery, Lisbona, September 17-18th; 2004.
[6] Bacci P.A.: "T3-Biolifting using absorbable fillers with a few quantity of proteins". Presentazione al World Meeting AACS, Tokyo, 2005, February 24th; 2005.
[7] Bacci P.A.: "T3 Soft Face Lifting using new Threads and fillers". Presentazione al49th World Meeting of World Meeting EMAA, Parigi, September 30th – October 2rd; 2005.
[8] Bacci P.A., Mancini S.: "Chirurgia estetica mini-invasiva: fili di sostegno (Not invasive aesthetic surgery using threads)". Minelli, Arezzo; 45–180; 2006.
[9] Botti G.: "Chirurgia estetica dell'invecchiamento facciale". Piccin Editore, Padova, 521-540; 1995.
[10] Capurro S: "The Double-Tipped Needle". Plast. Reconst. Surg. 79 n°6: 1006-7, 1987
[11] Capurro S. Jr.: "The double tipped needle". Plast. Reconst. Surg., June 1987.
[12] De Lorenzi C.L.: "Barbed sutures: rationale and technique". Aesth. Surg J. 26:223-229; 2006.
[13] Eremia S., Willoughby M.A.: "Novel face-lift suspension suture and inserting instrument: use of large anchors knotted into the suture with attached needle and inserting device allowing for single entry point placement of suspension suture. Preliminary report of 20 cases with 6- to 12-month follow-up". Dermatol. Surg. 32:335–45; 2006.
[14] Fournier P., Flores M.: "Le lifting invisible". Rev. Chir. Esthet. Langue Fr. 27(113):9–20; 2003.
[15] Fournier P.: "Historie de l'aguille a deux pointes". Rev. Chir. Esthet. Langue Fr. 28(115):19–27; 2004.
[16] Goldman M., Bacci P.A., Hexsel D., & Coll.,: "Cellulite: diagnosis and therapy". Taylor & Francis Ed., New York, : 28-74; 2006
[17] Hernandez Perez E., Abbar K.: "A percutaneous approach to eyebrow lift: the Salvadorian option". Dermatol. Surg. 29(8):852–855; 2003.
[18] Hochman M.: " Mid-face barbed suture lift". Facial Plast. Surg. Clin. North Am.15(2):201-207, 2007.
[19] Horne D.F., Kaminer M.S.: "Reduction of face and neck laxity with anchored, barbed polypropylene sutures (Contour Threads). Skin Therapy Lett. 11(1):5-7; 2006.
[20] Hudson D.A., Fernandes D.B.: "Caveats for the use of suspension sutures". Aesth. Plastic Surg. 28:170-173; 2004.
[21] Ingle N.P., King M.W., Leung J.C., Batchelor S.: "Barbed suture anchoring applicability to dissimilar polymeric materials, society for biomaterials". 29th annual meeting transactions, 26:100; 2003.
[22] Kazinnikova O.G., Adamian A.A.: "Age specific changes in facial and cervical tissue: a review". Ann. Plast. Reconstr. Surg.1:52–61; 2000.

[23] Khawaja H.A., Hernandez-Perez E.: "The Delta Lift : a modification of S-Lift for facial rejuvenation". Inter. J. of Cosmetic Surgery and Aesthetic Dermatology, Glendale USA, Mary Ann Liebert Ed., Vol.4, N.4:309-315; 2002.

[24] Lee S., Isse N.: "Barbed polypropylene sutures for mid-face elevation: early results". Arch. Facial Plast. Surg. 7: 55, 2005.

[25] Leung J.C., Ruff G.L., Megaro M.A.: "Barbed bi-directional medical sutures: biomechanical properties and wound closure efficacy study". Society For Biomaterials 28th annual Meeting Transactions 25:724, 2002.

[26] Lycka B., Bazan C., Poletti E., Treen B.: "The emerging technique of the antiptosis subdermal suspension thread". Dermatol. Surg. 30: 41, 2004.

[27] Mc Kenzie A. R.: " An experimental multiple barbed suture for the long flexor tendons of the palm and fingers". J. Bone Joint Surg.49:440-47; 1967.

[28] Rashid R.M., Sartori M., White L.E et Alii: "Breaking strength of barbed polypropylene sutures: rater-blinded, controlled comparison with non-barbed sutures of various calibers". Arch. Dermatol. 143:869–72; 2007.

[29] Serdev N.: "Own method scarless breast lift by suture and needles perforations only". Int. J. Cosmet. Surg. 1(1):1–41; 2001.

[30] Serdev N.: "Scarless Serdev suture methods in brow and face lifts". Int. J. Cosmet. Med. Surg. 3(1):9–15; 2001.

[31] Serdev N.: "Serdev suture for scarless buttock and ultrasonic liposculpture of the buttocks". Int. J. Cosmet. Med. Surg. 5(1):27–34; 2003.

[32] Serdev N.: "Scarless buttock lift using Serdev suture". International Journal of Cosmetic Surgery, Vol.3 N.3: 294-329; 2003.

[33] Serdev N.: "Scarless APTOS versus SERDEV suture lifting methods". Int. Journal of Cosmetic Surgery, vol. 4 – N. 2: 1-10; 2004.

[34] Sulamanidze M. A., Salti G., Mascetti M., Sulamanidze G. M.: "Wire scalpel for surgical correction of soft tissue contour defects by subcutaneous dissection". Dermatol. Surg. 26:146, 2000.

[35] Sulamanidze M. A., Fournier P. F., Paikidze T. G., Sulamanidze G.: "Removal of facial soft tissue ptosis with special threads". Dermatol. Surg. 28: 367, 2000.

[36] Sulamanidze M. A., Shiffman M. A., Paikidze T. G., SulamanidzeG. M., Gavasheli L. G.: "Facial lifting with Aptos threads". Int. J. Cosmet. Surg. Aesth. Dermatol. 4: 275, 2001.

[37] Sulamanidze M.A., Fournier P.F., Paikidze T.G., Sulamanidze G.M.: "Removal of facial soft tissue ptosis with special threads". Dermatol. Surg. 28:367-371; 2002.

[38] Stark G.B., Bannasch H.: "The 'Golden Thread Lift': radiologic findings". Aesth. Plast Surg. 31(2):206-208; 2007.

[39] Helling E.R., Okpaku A., Wang P.T. H., Levine R. A.: "Complications of facial suspension sutures". Aesth. Surg J.27:155–161; 2007.

[40] Lee C. J., Park J.H., You S.H., Hwang J.H. et Alii: " Dysesthesia and fasciculation: unusual complications following face-lift with Cog Thread". Dermatol. Surg. 33:253–255; 2007.

[41] Silva-Siwady J.G., Diaz-Garza C., Ocampo-Candiani J.: "A case of Aptos thread migration and partial expulsion". Dermatol. Surg. 31:356-358; 2005.

[42] Winkler E., Goldan O., Regev E. Mendes D., Orenstein A., Haik J.: "Stensen duct rupture (sialocele) and other complications of the Aptos Thread Technique". Plast. Reconstr. Surg. 118: 1468, 2006.

Chapter 17

Correction of Face Involutional Changes by Method of Light Lift Elegance Thread Reinforcement

O. Gaziullina, O. Zhukova and S. Shostak

Additional information is available at the end of the chapter

http://dx.doi.org/10.5772/50742

1. Introduction

The technology of face rejuvenation with the use of polylactic acid absorbable threads, which appeared a few years ago, has become a follow-up of Aptos polypropylene threads face lift. The techniques of fixation of threads made from absorbable and nonabsorbable material were identical. The only difference was the expected duration of the thread lift effect. [1,2,3,4] It has been histologically confirmed that it is already within the first month that there comes a delicate fibrous capsule around the implanted threads. It coats the threads as a small soft connective tissue cover, creating artificial ligaments which occur to be those face-lift agents that strengthen the effect achieved after the thread introduction. The effect remains for years. [2] Light Lift Elegance threads are absorbed completely within some time by way of hydrolysis. Due to the polylactic acid, they stimulate the activity of fibroblasts, thus activating the mechanism of neocollagenesis. As the result, there has been noted a double effect of absorbable threads usage – consistent mechanical lift effect and tissue revitalization. [6]

These observations have resulted in creation of a special thread reinforcement technique - Light Lift Elegance. It is indeed an elegant method of atonic skin transfer which leads to consistent skin graft lifting. This technique can also be used by dermatologists and cosmetologists who would like to offer their patients more effective procedures.

2. Materials

Light Lift Elegance threads are thin threads with micro cogs throughout the length which directed towards each other. It allows to fix the skin graft using a special fixation technique and to hold the tissue in this position until a new collagen framework is formed. Thus, the main feature of these threads is their structure. It is the cogs directed to the middle part of the threads that allow to lift the overstretched atonic skin and to achieve the effect of consistent skin graft lift.

3. Methods

The method of Light Lift Elegance thread fixation, i.e. reinforcement, is used for correction of the involutional changes of the middle third and lower third of the face, submandibular area, neck, low neck, inner shoulder surface, thighs, abdomen, and patellar areas. Since our main task is to strengthen the surface tissues of the body, the threads should be placed along the lines of the natural skin stretching. Possible schemes of Aptos Elegans thread fixation coincide with the lines of Langer (C.R. Langer, 1819-1887, German anatomist) – relative lines on the skin surface, indicating the direction of its maximum distensibility and corresponding to the location of fascicles of collagen fibers.

Fixation depth, the degree of thread tension and tissue transfer criterion

Thin and delicate threads LL Elegance perform two functions – creation of subdermal frame and skin revitalization. Therefore, the depth of the threads plantation should correspond to their main purpose. It should be done subdermally but contouring is to be avoided. The threads have small cogs from the end of the thread to its middle, which allows to shrink the tissue a little, thus making the skin graft smaller. If one retracts the skin a little at the moment of the thread plantation, the cogs will help to fix it in this position and create a strong connective frame around the thread. The skin surface tends to become plicated after the thread fixation. This effect wears off within a week. It is undesirable to create strong overstretchings and visible tucks. [1]

4. Fixation technique

Infiltration anesthesia is used after taking pictures, marking, skin aseptic cleaning, and draping. It contains 2% Lidocaine, Marcaine or Ultracaine 1:2000000, adrenaline 0.1% -0.1 ml and 5% NaCO2 as a buffered solution used for relieving pain during anesthetics administration, equal infiltration and hydro undermining of tissues. The threads are fixed in sequence in accordance with the marking. While inserting a thread one can be guided by the Arcus zygomaticus projection and while taking it out – by the Corpus mandibular projection. [1]

The ends of the threads are cut off after their fixation. The remaining ends are being placed subdermally and massaged gently. The skin over the place of the thread plantation can be stretched a little to eliminate the excessive folding. [1]

5. The selection of patients

What categories of patients fit for this delicate method of thread lift?

First of all, it is patients with initial manifestations of age-related changes that cannot be corrected with the help of modern hardware-based and injection techniques. LL Elegance can be applied both as a mono-method and also in a combination with a wide range of modern cosmetic treatment.

Patients with atonic, rugulose skin with manifestations of photoaging can also improve their appearance using this method. L.L. Elegance works perfectly in combination with hyaluronic acid fillers, peelings, and botulinum toxin.

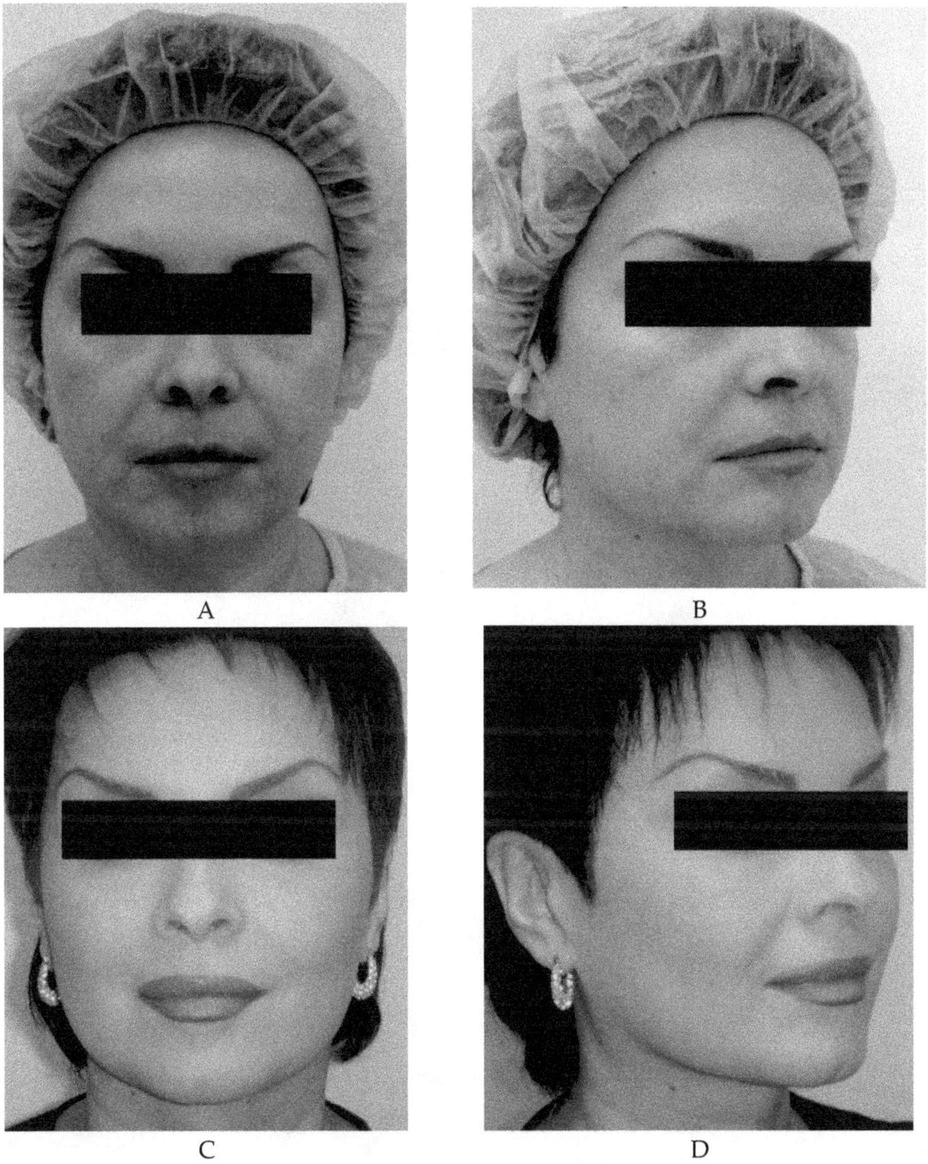

Figure 1. Patient N. 49 years old. Photo (A;B.) Before threads plantation.
Photo (C;D.) Here is a correction of the middle third and lower third of the face. 1 month later.

Patients with face sebaceus disproportion, gravitational ptosis of subcutaneous fat, hyperextension of the collagen fibers and the formation of deep wrinkles should use a combination of several methods of thread correction. In this case, it is recommended to use a combination of methods of zone, deep lift by Thread 2 G, Needle2G, Spring threads, and methods of the surface subdermal plantation of LL Elegance threads.

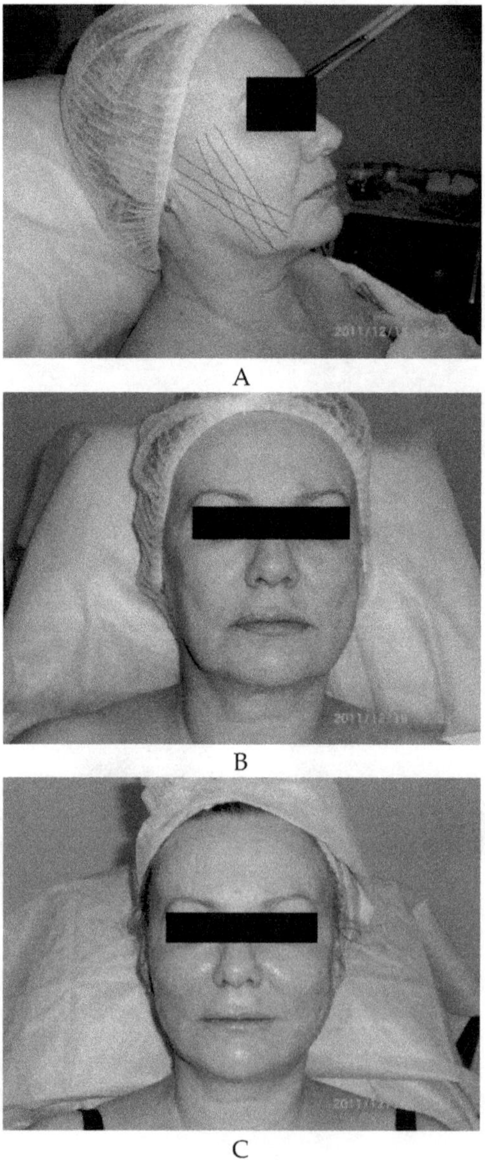

Figure 2. Patient K. 58 years old. Photo (A;B.) Before threads plantation. Photo (C.) Here is a correction of the middle third and lower third of the face. This is a result just after operation.

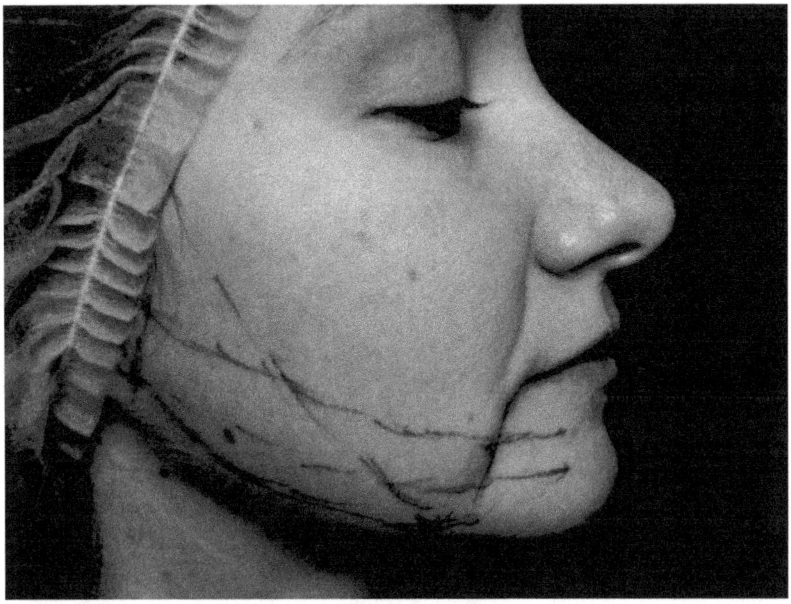

A

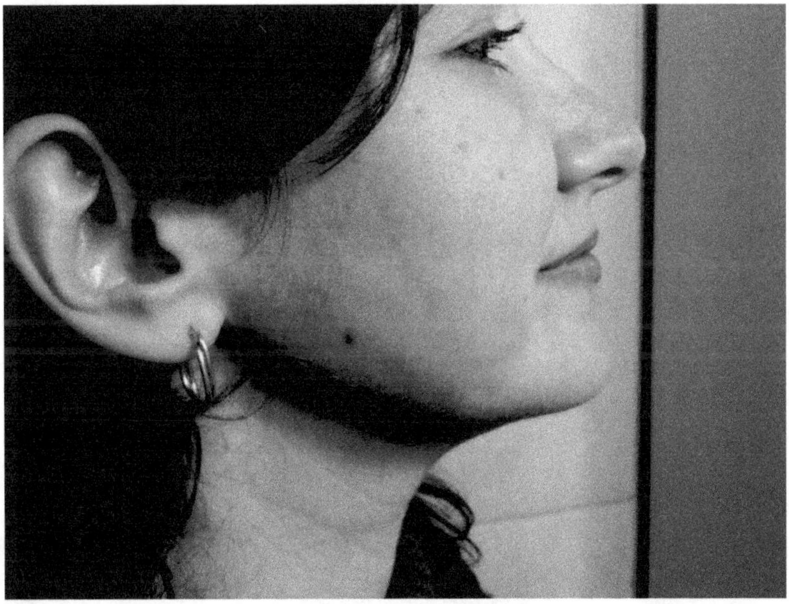

B

Figure 3. Patient M. 45 years old.
Photo (A.) Before threads plantation.
Photo (B.) Here is a correction of the lower third of the face 3 weeks after plantation.

It would be good to focus on the method of complex correction of submandibular and neck areas with an excess of soft tissues in these areas. It is recommended to reduce fatty tissue using a mechanical or chemical (mesolipolisis) way. Then follows the insertion of a hammock in the submandibular area and the use of reinforcement of the neck area for a simultaneous fixation of tissues in these areas.

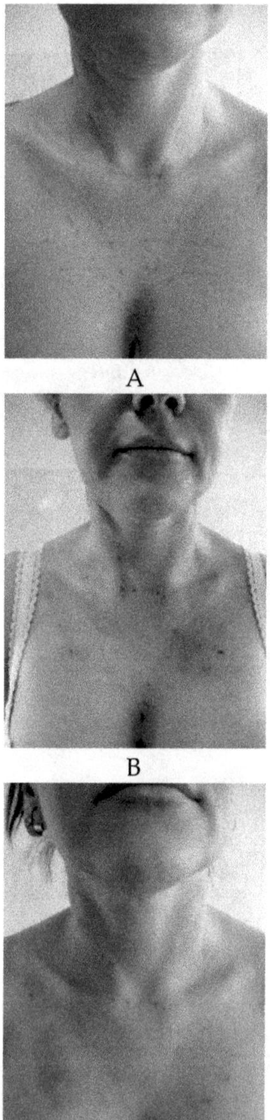

A

B

C

Figure 4. Patient S. 48 years old. Photo (A.) Before threads plantation.
Photo (B.) Here is a correction of the neck and lower neck area. The result is just after operation.
Photo (C.) This is a result of threads plantation 6 days later.

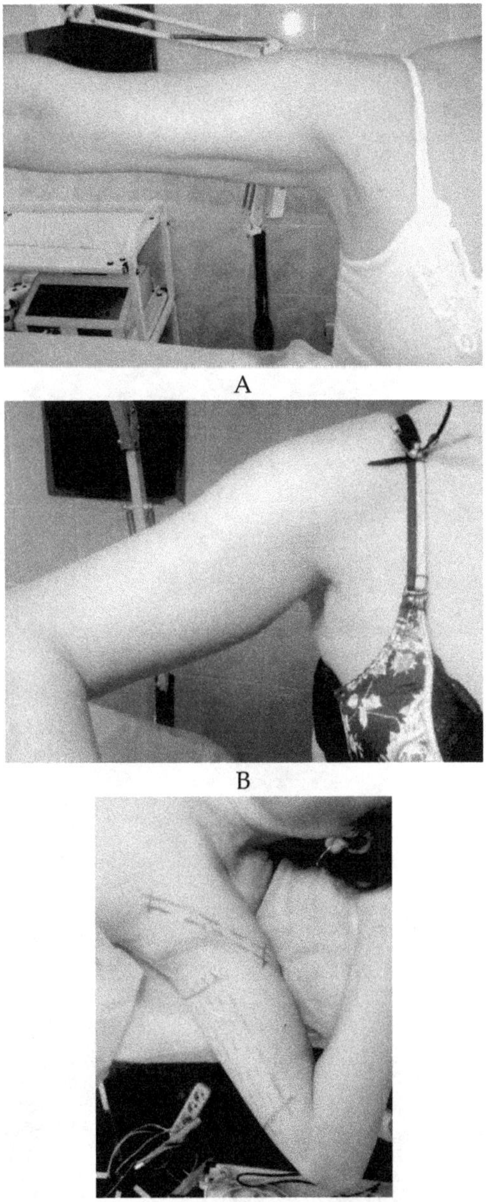

Figure 5. Patient S. 48 years old. Photo (A; B.) Before threads plantation. Photo (C.)The sketch of threads plantation in inner shoulder surface.

When using Light Lift Elegance method, the patients should be selected among those with signs of sclerosis and skin and subdermal tissue sagging. It is recommended to consider all the variants of lipodystrophy (especially in the initial phase) because thinning of the surface investing tissues (and consequently the flabbiness) is always the main symptom.

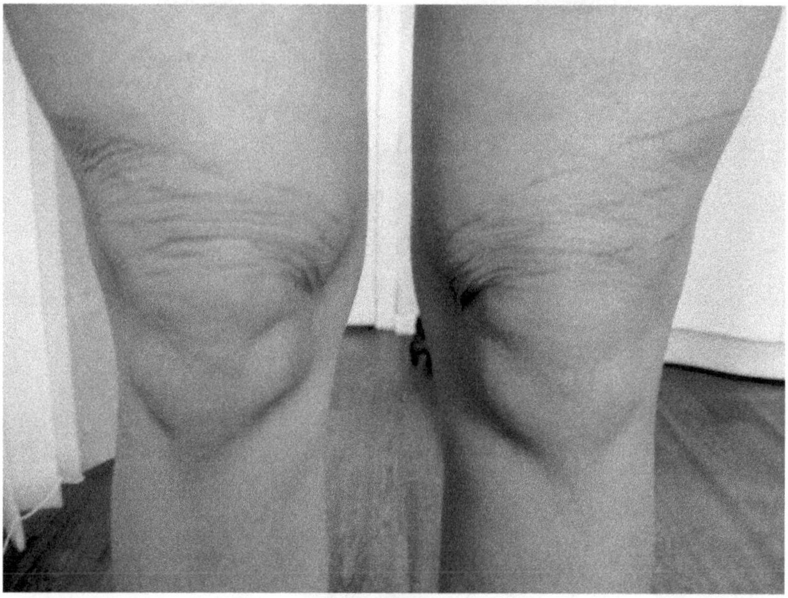

A

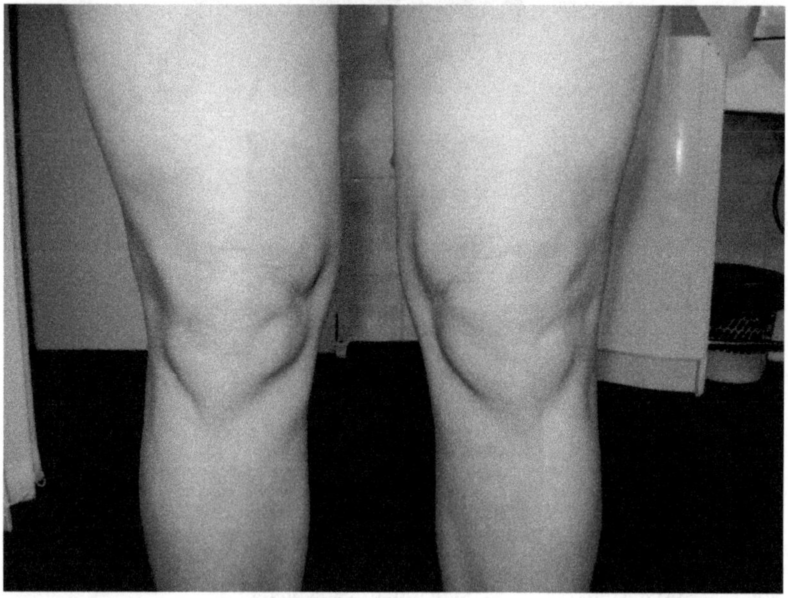

B

Figure 6. Patient B. 42 years old.
Photo (A.) Before threads plantation.
Photo (B.) Patient 2 months after correction of patellar areas.

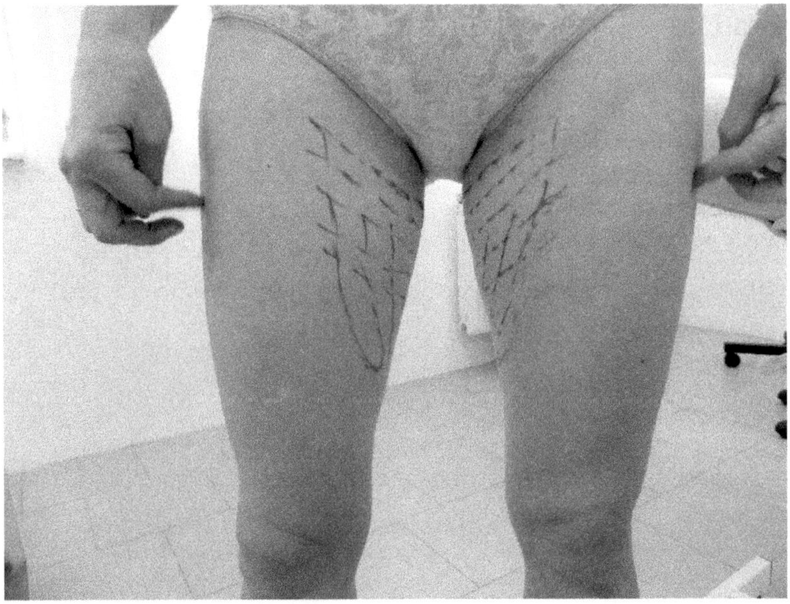

A

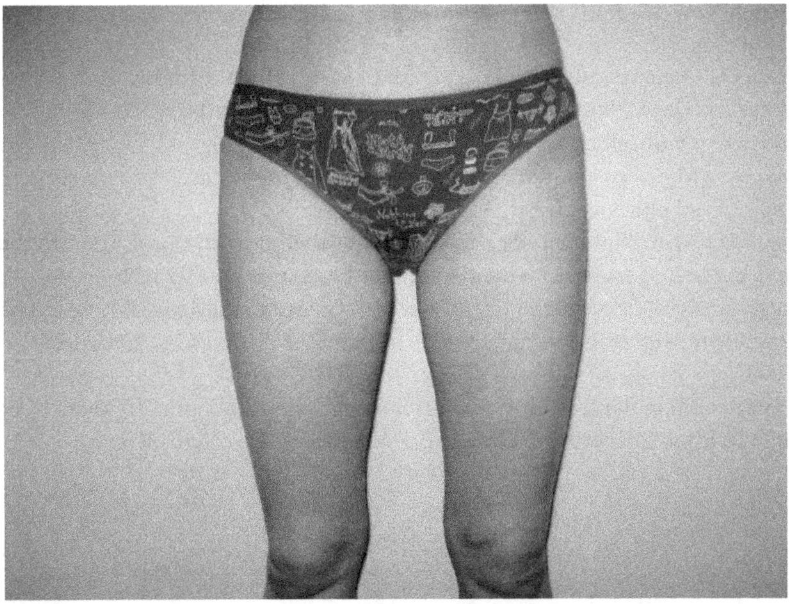

B

Figure 7. Patient L. 49 years old.
Photo (A.) Before threads plantation.
Photo (B.) Patient 2 months after correction of thighs areas.

6. Complications

- Hematoma, swellings, painfulness;
- Threads contouring connected with the surface plantation;
- Inflammation around the thread;
- Disruption of the threads;
- Thread exposure on the skin surface;
- Temporary paresthesia.

All complications are to be treated in accordance with the cause of their formation.

Author details

O. Gaziullina, O. Zhukova and S. Shostak
Clinic of Aesthetic Medicine and Laser Cosmetology "Time of Beauty",
People's Friendship University of Russia, Clinic of Aesthetic Medicine "Total Charm",
Ufa, Moscow, Russia

7. References

[1] M.A.Sulamanidze, G.M.Sulamanidze, I.S.Vozdvizhenskiy, K.M.Sulamanidze, A.A. Kadzhaya. New Method of Elastic Thread Face Lift // Aesthetic Medicine. – Volume IX-N3, October 2, 2010.

[2] Skuba N.D., Adamyan A.A., Sulamanidze M.A., Husnutdinova Z.R. Morphological foundation of face skin reinforcement by «Aptos» threads. // The annals of plastic, reconstructive and esthetic surgery. – 2002. - №3. – P. 19-26.

[3] Sulamanidze M.A., Sulamanidze G.M. Hyposthenic, aged face. New treatment // Thes.II Congress of esthetic and plastic surgery. – M., 1998. – P.15.

[4] Sulamanidze M.A., Sulamanidze G.M «Aptos» methods: the past, the present and the future // Vestnik of esthetic medicine. – 2007. – Vol.6, №3. – P. 23-32

[5] Sulamanidze M.A., Fournier P.F., Paikidze T.G., Sulamanidze G.M. Removal of facial soft tissue phtosis with special threads.//Dermatol. Surgery. – 2002, May. - № 28. – P.367-371.

[6] Sulamanidze M., Sulamanidze G. Aptos Suture Lifting Methods. 10 Years of Experience // Clinics in Plast. Surgery. – 2009, April. – Vol. 36, № 2. – P. 281-306.

Chapter 18

Experience in the Use of Barbed Threads and Non-Barbed Serdev Sutures in Face and Body Lift – Comparison and Combination

Vilma L. Padín

Additional information is available at the end of the chapter

http://dx.doi.org/10.5772/51399

1. Introduction

1.1. Barbed threads

This technique created by George Sulamanidze uses barbed non sutured monofilament polypropylene threads called APTOS (Polypropylene sutures were modified by designing many dents along their lengths. These "APTOS" threads hold tissue firmly because of the sharp edges to the dents) [1] and allows to relieve facial soft tissue ptosis when it is light or moderate. With this method is possible to lift different areas of the three thirds of the face. This is a simple technique with simple instrumentarium. We use a modification of barbed Aptos threads called Fiberlift® (Firming threads, Multifix threads, and Fiberlift threads). These threads have bidirectional cogs and multidirectional cogs to get the lifting effect of the tissue and a new collagen generation. Barbed polypropylene threads are inserted through the fat tissue with only a long and thin (21 Gx2 or 21 Gx3.5) needle as a guide. These polypropylene barbed threads may be used in face, neck and body lift. This simple and non recovery time procedure, without incisions or scars, achieves to lift and gives new volume and contour with few complications and long lasting results. They get an adequate position of the soft tissue which decreases lymphatic stasis, improves oxygenation, provides energy and stimulates the muscles recovering the normal tissue metabolism and slowing the aging process [2]

1.2. Serdev sutures

The use of Serdev sutures in face lift treatments allows us to lift one mobile tissue, the SMAS, and carry it to a non movable point, stable fibrotic and fascia structures, using polycaproamide Serdev sutures and a Serdev special flexible, curved and semi elastic needle. [3] These methods may be done to lift several areas of the face, neck and body. We have experience in temporal face lift, medial face lift, brow lift, chin enhancement and buttock lift with Serdev sutures. These procedures are simple without scars and uncomplicated in the postoperative time and they get aesthetic proportions, aesthetics angles and aesthetic volumes avoiding the "operated look."

Since the year 2000, we have been practicing with the procedures of mini-invasive lifting with Aptos barbed *threads* (George Sulamanidze) and *sutures* (Nikolay Serdev). In the past it was believed that such techniques were only fashionable in the field of cosmetic surgery. After using these methods for 12 years and seeing the positive results in our patients not only within my country but in foreign countries as well, it has come to my attention that "threads" are not something in vogue but are here to stay for good as an important feature in mini-invasive cosmetic surgery. Proof of clinic results, photo images, dermatological examinations and patients' approval after 5 years should establish that lifting with threads and sutures are highly effective; no surgery marks or scars, natural results without undergoing an operation or post operative. It enables the patient to return to work immediately. Through the simple method of "barbed or anchorage threads" the results that are obtained show that reaching beauty may be a simple medical procedure, non invasive, responsible, ethical, in accordance with the physical and spiritual integrity of the patient. The facial softness treatment with the application of both barbed threads or Serdev sutures or their combination allows us to fulfill the requirements that nowadays the patients ask for daily in our clinic.

1.3. Materials

1. Polypropylene 2.0 Barbed threads are used with converging cogs called "FIRMING THREADS" (by Fiberlift®)

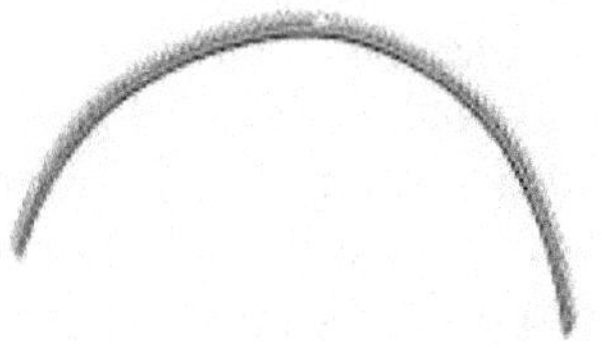

- Monofilament polypropylene 2.0
- Convergent cogs
- 6cm, 8cm, 10cm long
- 4 or 6 units pack

Source: Proesteticamed, 2003

Figure 1. Firming thread

2. Polypropylene 2.0 Barbed threads with multi-directional cogs, 2cm right section, and 2 cm left section called "MULTIFIX." (by Fiberlift®)

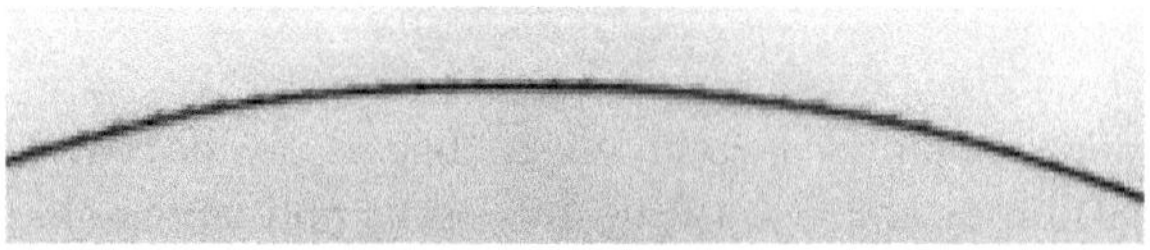

- Monofilament polypropylene 2.0
- Multi-directional cogs
- 12 cm long
- 4 units pack

Source: Proesteticamed, 2006

Figure 2. Multifix thread

3. Polypropylene 3.0 with diverging cogs in 2 stages, 3cm each one with one free central piece and 2 long plain ends, called "FIBERLIFT." (by Fiberlift®)

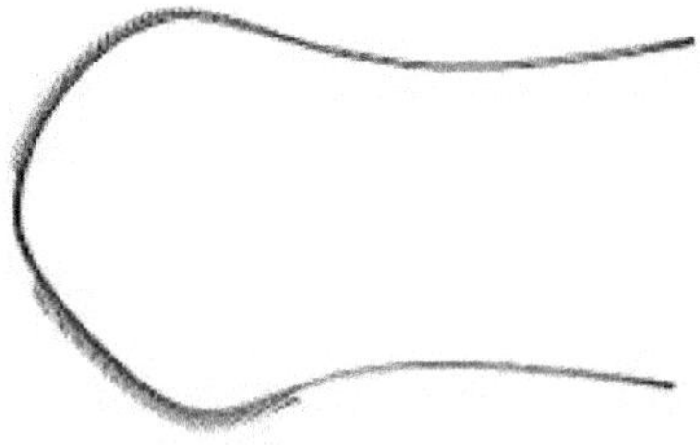

- Monofilament polypropylene 3.0
- Divergent cogs
- Center and ends without cogs
- 30 cm long
- 2 units pack

Source: Proesteticamed, 2004

Figure 3. Fiberlift® thread

All these barbed threads are made in Argentina as a modification of Aptos Threads, and they are sterilized abiding by the ISO regulations.

4. Serdev Sutures (Semi elastic, braided, yellow polycaproamide non barbed sutures)

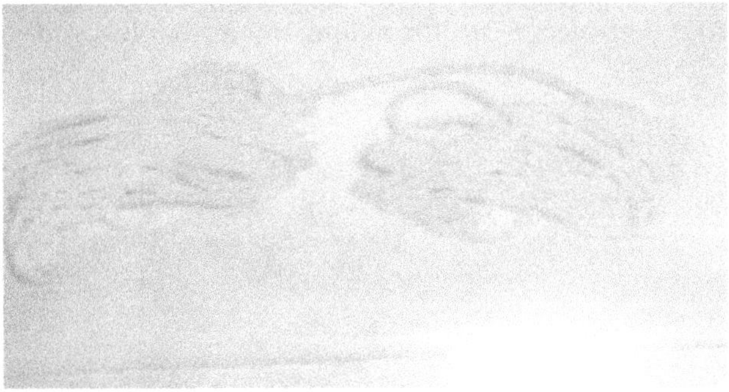

Source: Ambulatory temporal SMAS lift by sutures with or without incisions IJCS 2001; 1(4):97-106

Figure 4. Serdev sutures

1.4. Surgical instruments

- Halstead claw.
- Iris scissor.
- 21 Gx2 or 21 Gx3 needles.
- Syringe and 30 Gx½ needle for anesthesia.
- Lidocaine 2% with epinephrine.
- Special Serdev flexible needles in different sizes from a large to a mini- mini needle.

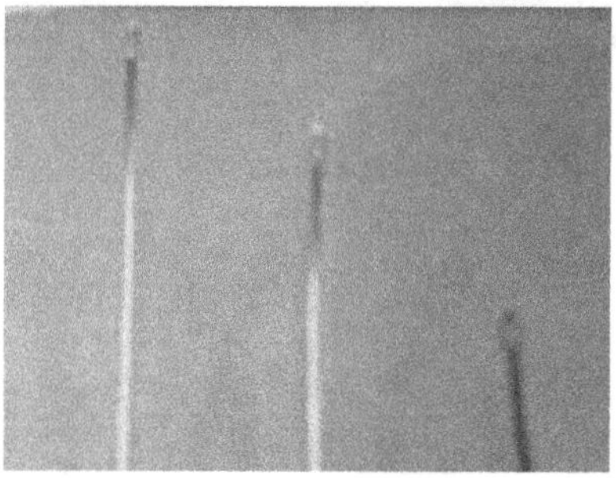

Source: Ambulatory temporal SMAS lift by sutures with or without incisions IJCS 2001; 1(4):97-106

Figure 5. Special Serdev elastic needles.

2. Procedures

2.1. Barbed threads in face and body lift -

2.1.1. Face lift

2.1.1.1. Lower third and jawline

The aim of this technique is to lift and improve the contour of the lower third of the face and jawlines. We insert eight polypropylene barbed (4 on each side) FIBERLIFT® FIRMING THREADS between 8 to 10cm long in a simple procedure and without recovery time.[4]

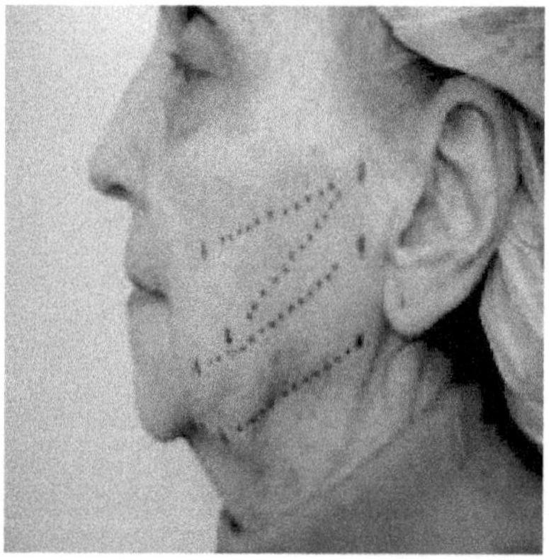

Source: Personal archive

Figure 6. Patient's marcation for operation

2.1.1.1.1. Materials

FIRMING THREADS: Polypropylene 2.0 barbed threads with convergent cogs.

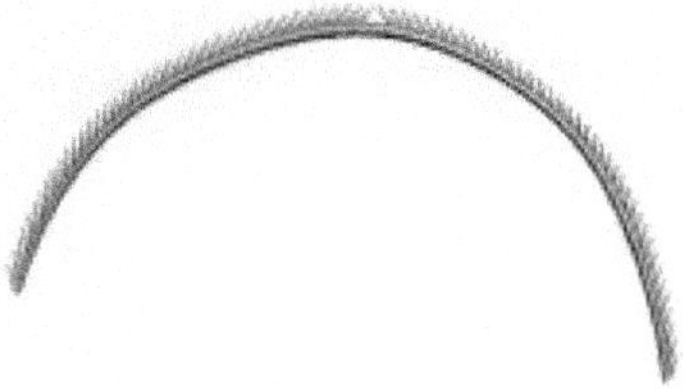

Source: Proesteticamed, 2003

Figure 7. Firming thread with convergent cogs

2.1.1.1.2. Description of technique

Step 1 First, we must take frontal and profile photographs	
Step 2 Feel along the patient's face with our fingers and mark it. With this, an individual sketch is obtained.	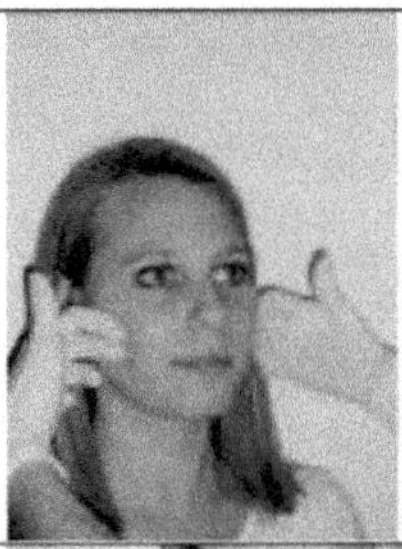
Step 3 Mark on the face of the patient the course of the thread drawing the shape of a "Z" on the lower third of the face, in the aim of inserting 2 barbed convergent parallel threads with a third one crossed in the form of an open Z. 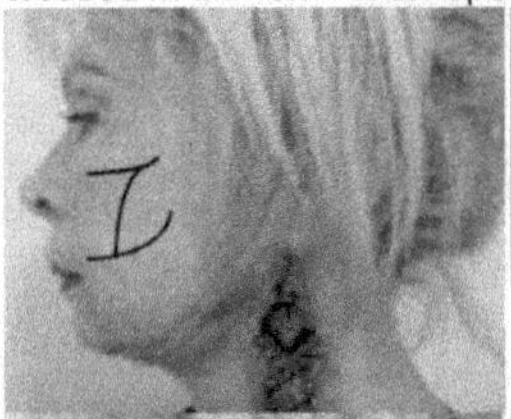 CORRECT "OPEN Z" In this way we avoid deformation of the mouth 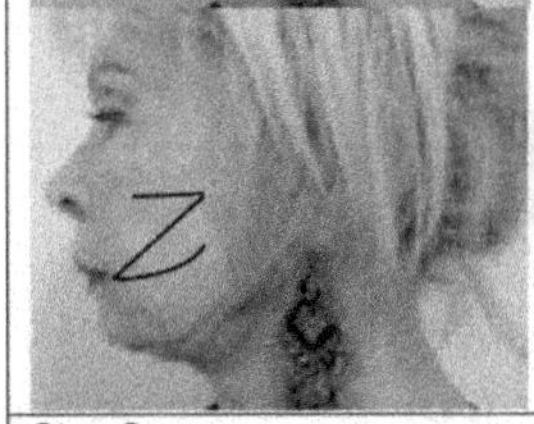 INCORRECT "CLOSED Z" In this way the mouth may be deformed	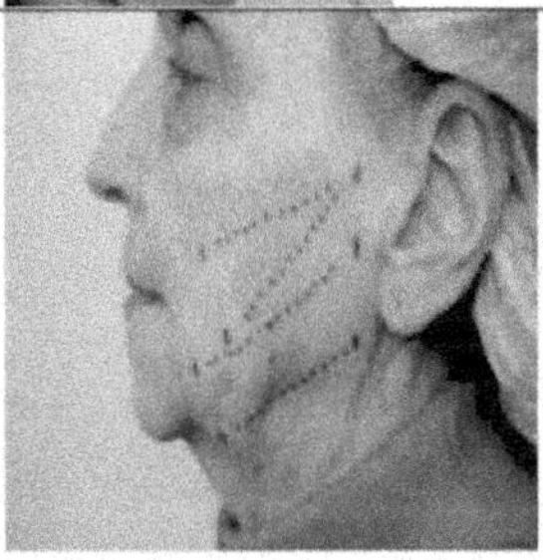
Step 2 Paint the face with povidone.	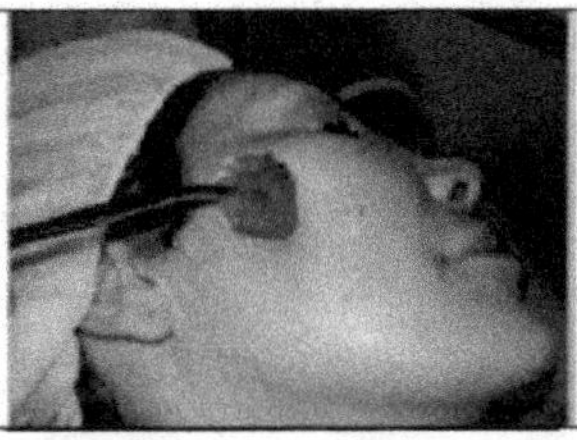

Step 3 Inject the anesthesia only at the entrance and exit points. Use lidocaine 2% with epinephrine 0,5 c.c per point.	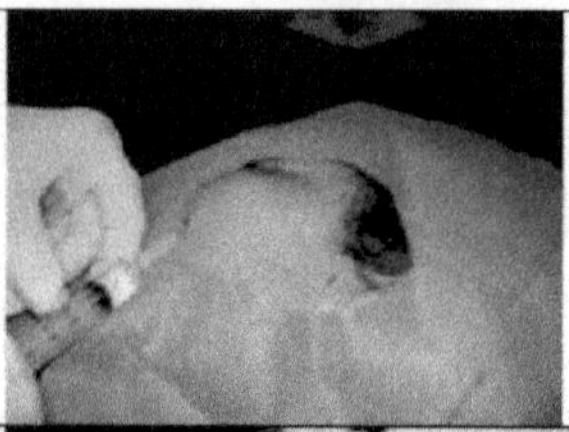
Step 4 Tunnel from the external point to the internal one, with a 21 Gx2 needle. Parallel threads must be inserted 1 cm away from the nasolabial fold to preserve the natural form of the face.	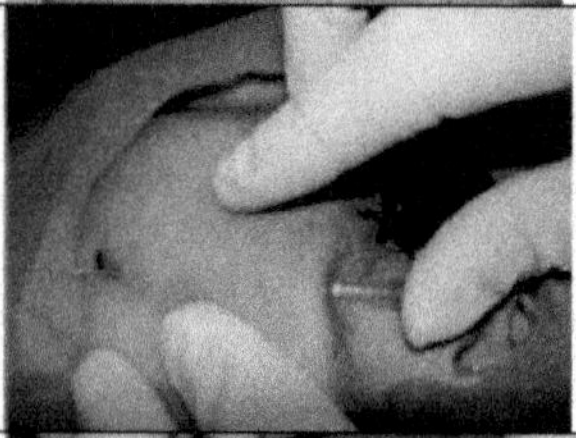
Step 5 Thread the barbed polypropylene thread, being careful with the cogs because they are convergent, so it's very easy to thread the first half but it is a little more complicated to pass the second half because the cogs are opposite to the sense of the needle. This situation is very easy to overcome by, with the use of a thicker needle. But using a 21 Gx2 needle we assured that the aesthetic results will be excellent and without scars.	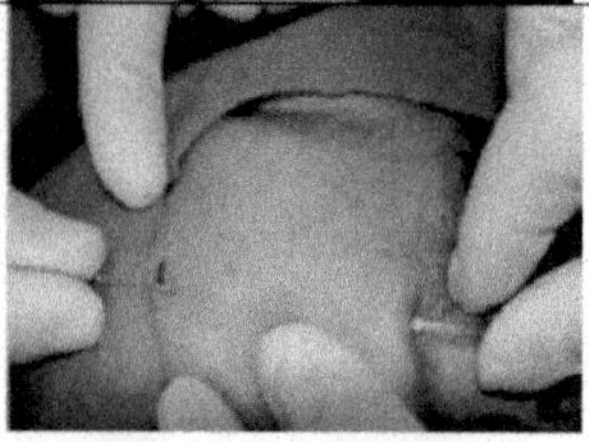
Step 6 Check that the thread is firm.	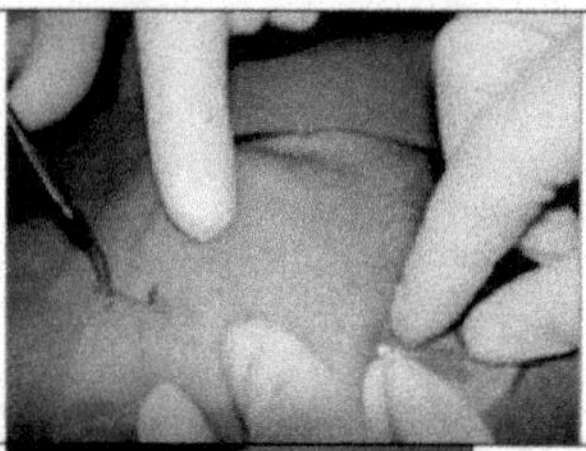
Step 7 Remove the needle and the ends of the thread will be found outside the surface of the skin.	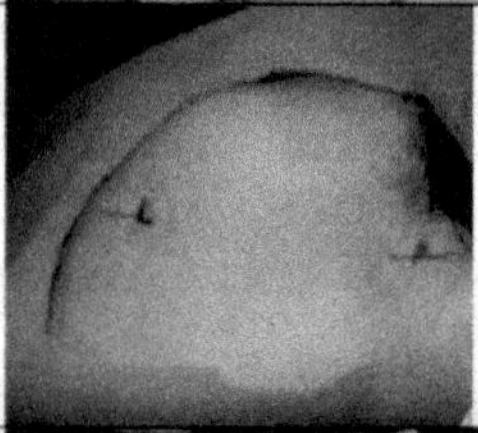
Step 8 Cutting the thread. We must be very careful cutting the thread. The skin should be pushed down with the scissors. This simple switching enables us to cut the thread at a good position avoiding it getting long.	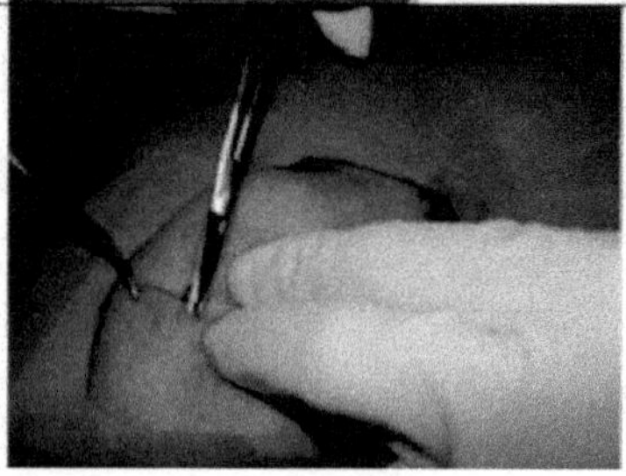

Source: own elaboration using pictures of personal archive

Scheme 1. Lower Face Lift Technique with Barbed Threads

2.1.1.1.3. Results

Barbed threads have two ways of acting. The first is the lifting effect given by the cogs. It is immediate. This effect is poor. The other action is delayed, due to the inflammatory reaction when the thread is placed, producing vas dilatation, increased capillary permeability, inflammatory exude that will be represented by leukocytes, erythrocytes, plasmatic proteins and fibrin which take us to the epitelization; that is: fibroblasts are generating collagen and elastine fibers.

So we can say that the barbed thread face lift has good results that change the angles of the face with an aesthetic expression, giving contour as well as improving the skin. Patients like this technique and ask for more threads. It is long lasting. Experienced doctors can insert more threads several times.

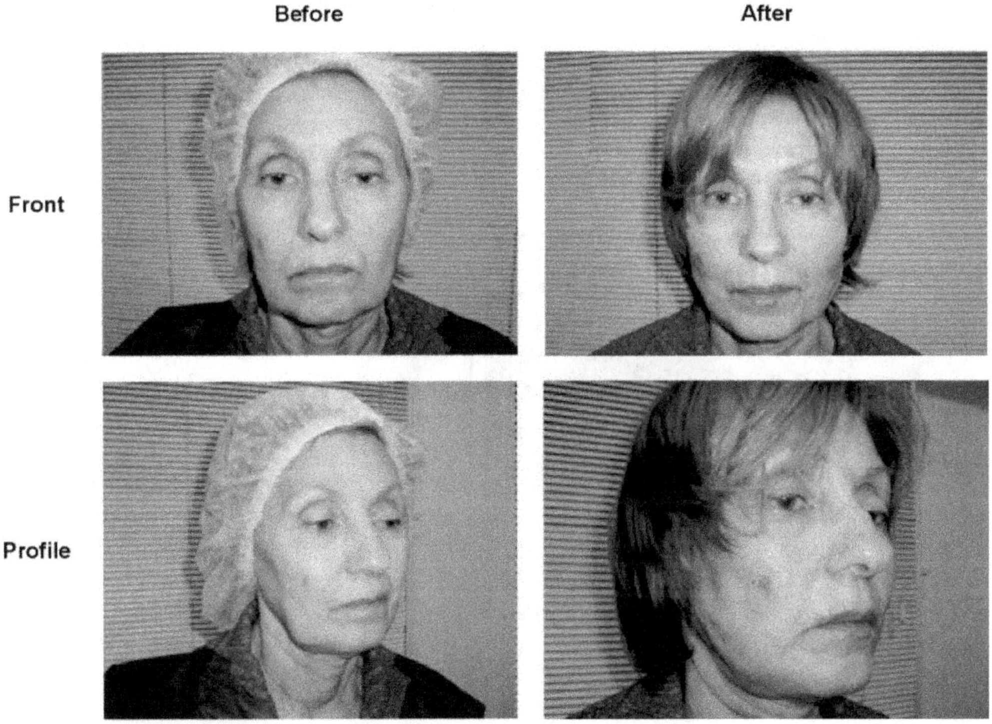

Source: own elaboration based on pictures from personal archive

Figure 8. Lower Face Lift Results

2.1.1.1.4. Complications

This technique has few complications, one of them is cutting a long thread producing it to prick from within. This is the most common complication. Another one is the migration of the thread. We have had a 3% rate in migrations. Extrusion is unusual (1% of the cases). Another authors have found thread visibility, migration, and exposure; linear bleeding along the needle course; skin dimpling; hypocorrection and hypercorrection; transient paresthesias; and a small number of cases of injury to major vessels, nerve branches, and parotid capsule/duct [5] mild asymmetry, ecchymosis, erythema, bleeding, swelling, and discomfort were the only minor. [6]

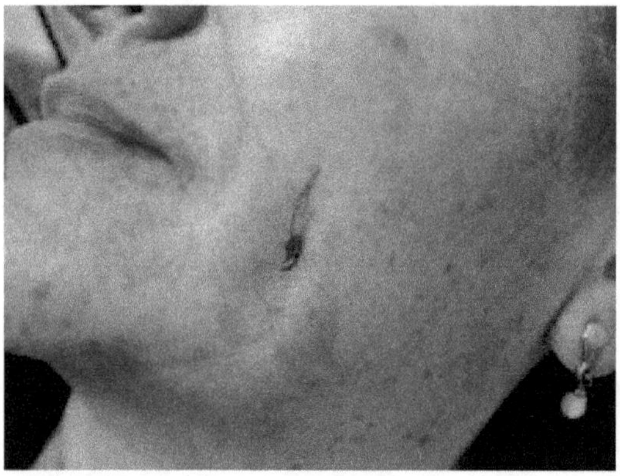

The most common complication is the thread cut long, so it pricks and we have to explore it. If the thread is anchored, we can keep it in the same place but if it is loose we have to remove and replace it.

Source: Personal archive

Figure 9. Thread cut long

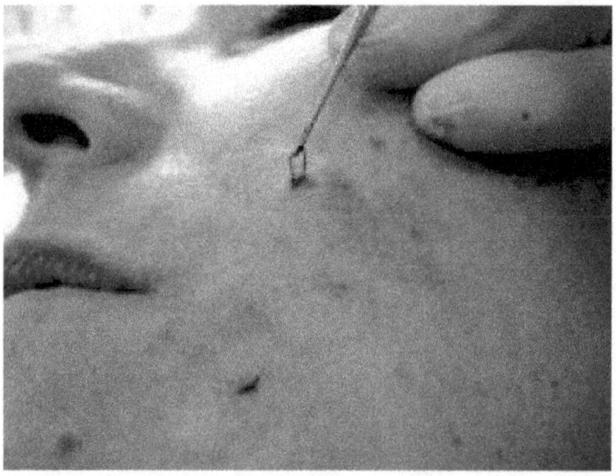

A different way to remove a migrated thread. In this case with a crochet needle

Source: Personal archive

Figure 10. Removing a thread

2.1.1.2. Medial third

The aim of this technique is to lift the cheek bone zone and indirectly also to improve the jawline and smoothing the folds. We insert one or two barbed multifixing thread of 12 cm. long, added to the above procedure in vertical form.

2.1.1.2.1. Materials

FIBERLIFT® MULTIFIX THREADS: Polypropylene 2.0 barbed threads with multidirectional cogs.

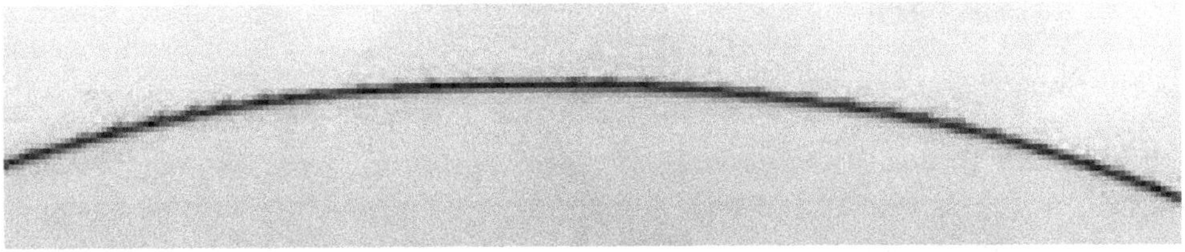

Source: Proesteticamed, 2006

Figure 11. Multifix thread

This procedure allows us to lift the soft tissue and reshape the cheek bone too as well as smoothing the folds and commissures.

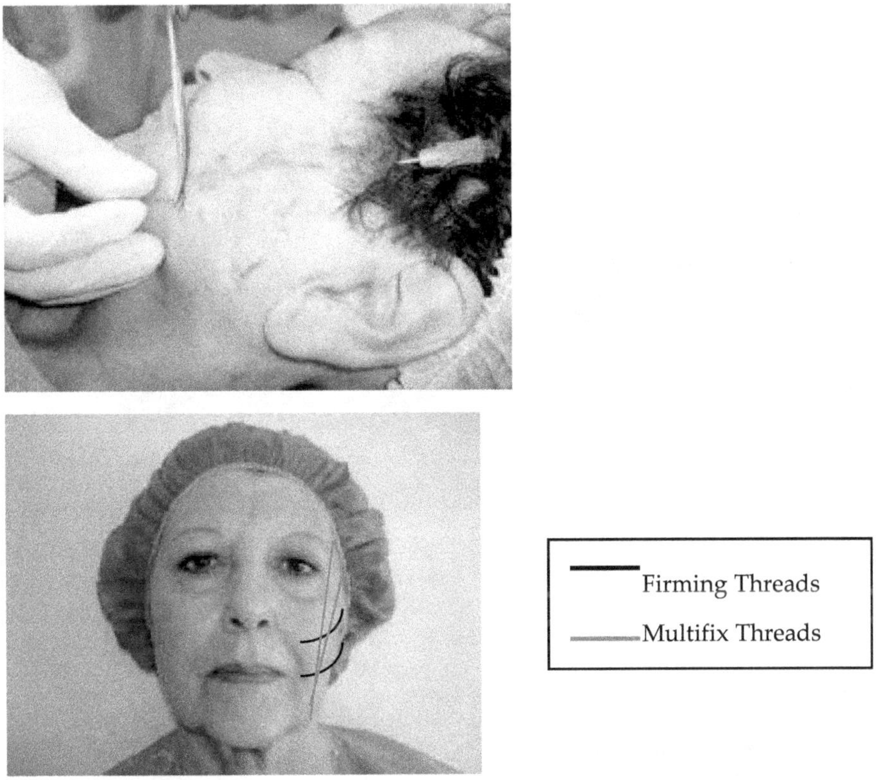

Source: Personal archive

Figure 12. Multifix thread located in vertical form with 21 Gx3 spinal needle

2.1.1.2.2. Procedure

One or two FIBERLIFT® MULTIFIX THREADS are placed in vertical form from the jawline to temporal zone with a 21 G x3 spinal needle, following the same procedure as in the case of Firming Threads.[7]

2.1.1.2.3. Comparative study

Between November 2006 and July 2007 we performed an 8-month study on 32 healthy patients of both sexes, ages ranging between 38 and 66 years old. On 16 of them, we had applied firming threads or anchorage threads as the only treatment. The other half of the patients was treated in the same form except for the extra plus combination of multifix threads. The following was observed:

The patients treated with multifix threads combined with firming threads or anchorage threads presented better results, longer lasting time span, a more important lift effect and a lower number of migrations and extrusions compared to those treated with only one technique. We think due to the multi-directional cogs because they do a more important anchorage surface.[5]

2.1.1.2.4. Results

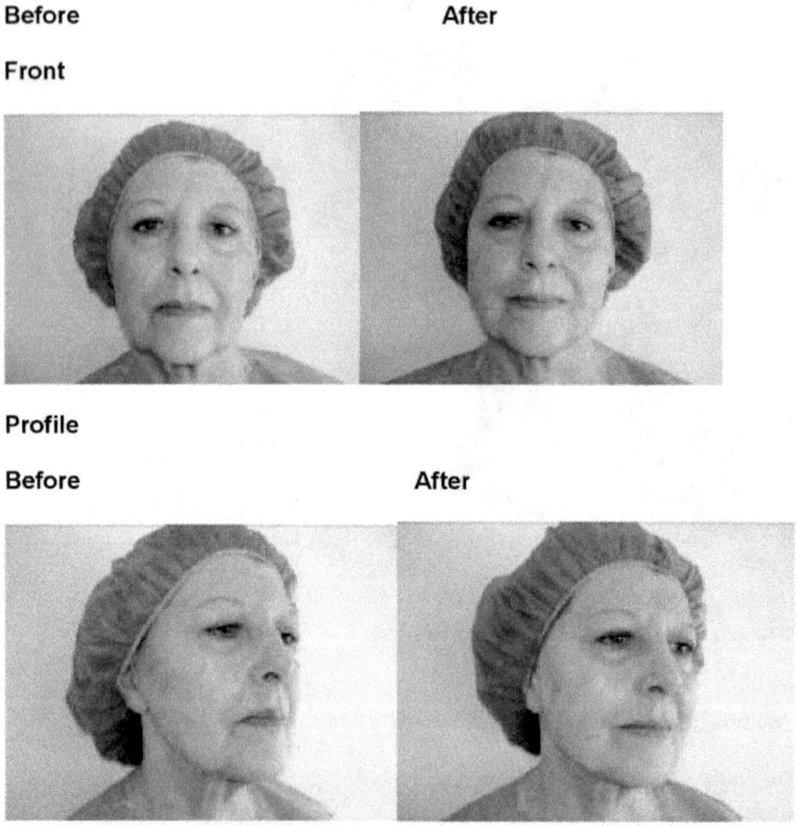

Source: own elaboration based on pictures from personal archive

Figure 13. Multifix threads plus Firming threads. Results

2.1.1.3. Neck lift and double chin

2.1.1.3.1. With firming threads

We can improve the aging neck by using 2 or 3 barbed Firming Threads 10cm's long on both sides of neck. We prefer to place them 2cm away from the midline because we have seen a lot of extruded threads when placed from the midline to the sides. This treatment is good for the neck and double chin. It is simple and only local anesthesia is used, therefore improving 35% of the contour. It is ideal for those patients who elude operations and for those who are knowledgeable on the results attained by this technique. Firming threads are inserted with a 21 Gx2 needle. Entering at point two fingers below the edge of the mandible and below the earlobe, above the sternocleidomastoid muscle to a point located in the same line, 1 or 2cm outside the outer border of the central band of platysma.

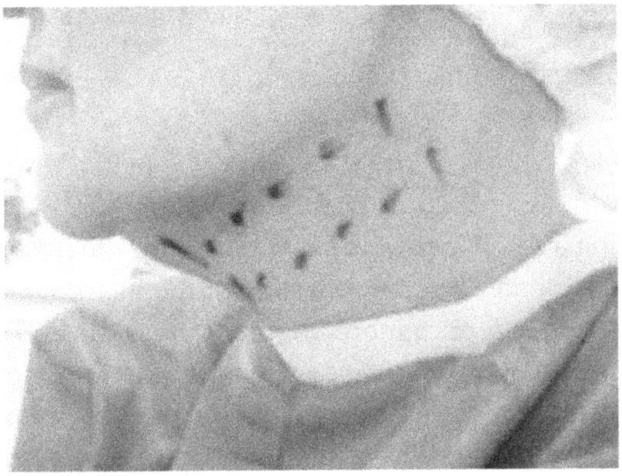

Source: Personal archive

Figure 14. Marcation on the patient's neck

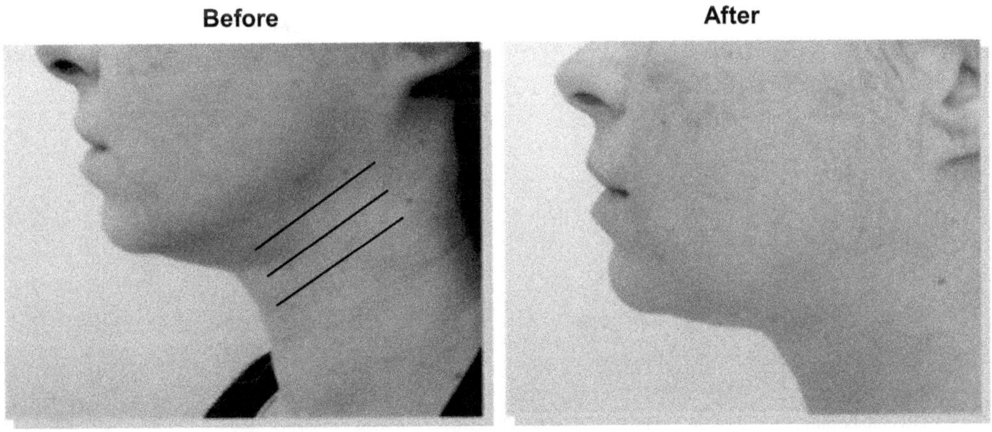

Source: Own elaboration based on pictures from personal archive

Figure 15. Neck Lift and Double Chin with barbed threads Results

2.1.1.3.2. With fiberlift®

FIBERLIFT THREAD (By Fiberlift®) is a barbed polypropylene 3.0, with divergent cogs. It is not an autosustentation thread but an anchorage one, 30cm long, with two parts each consisting of 3cm with divergent cogs separated by a smooth area and two smooth ends.

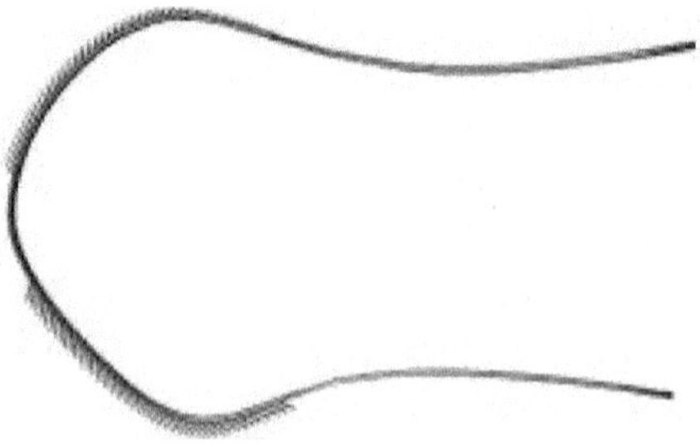

Source: Proesteticamed, 2004

Figure 16. Fiberlift® thread

This method is simple and allows us to lift the neck in a better way than in the FIRMING LIFT. The procedure is done with local anesthesia, using the 21 Gx2 needle, by entering the mastoid zone making a small incision of 1cm. The aim is to introduce the thread in the shape of a "V." Firstly, we enter through one side of the incision and exit on the internal point out of the platysma band, once more holding the needle and entering again on the other side of the incision, secondly, exiting at the same anterior point and out through the platysma band. The results are very good, on the other hand some complications have arisen such as persistent folds and pain. Only one case has been registered of a torn thread.

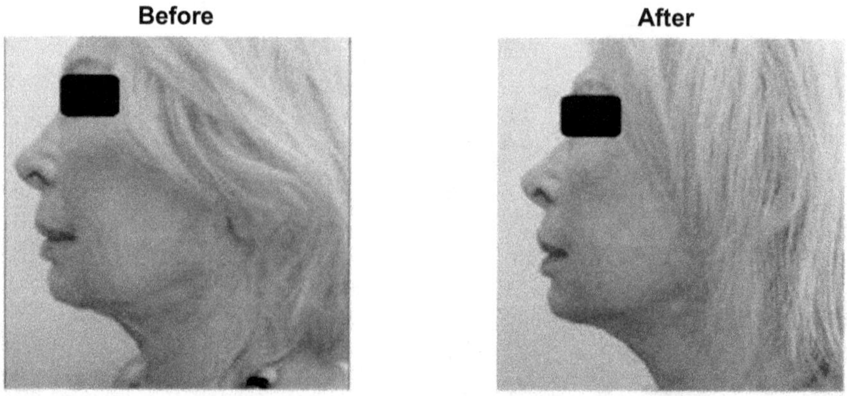

Source: Own elaboration based on pictures from personal archive

Figure 17. Neck Lift and Double Chin with Fiberlift® Results (The patient also has Firming Threads at the lower and medium third)

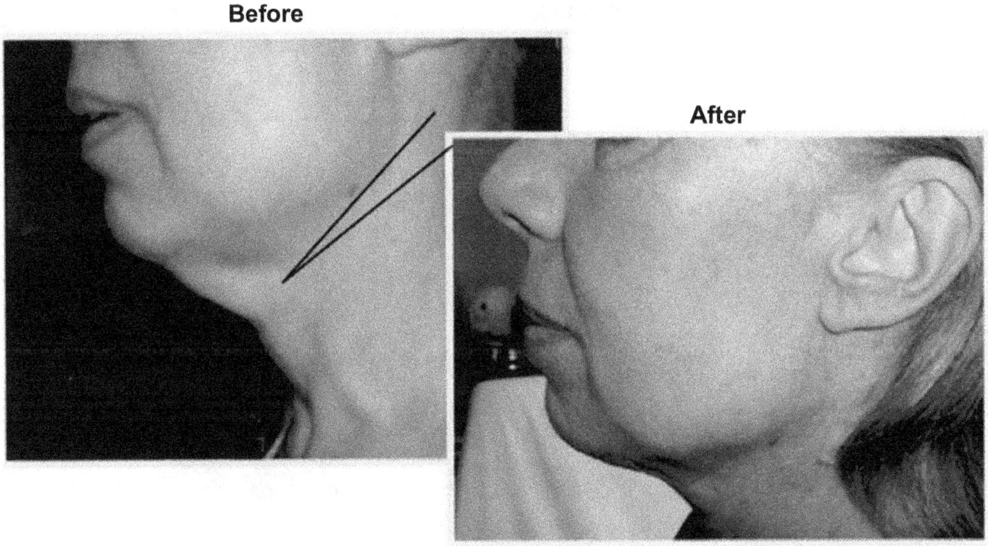

Source: Own elaboration based on pictures from personal archive

Figure 18. Neck Lift and Double Chin with Fiberlift® Results

2.1.1.4. Upper third

2.1.1.4.1. With firming threads

Brow lift may be done with one or two 6cm convergent barbed threads being very careful with the blood vessels. Work on frontal zone is made easier with a curved needle. This is a very good procedure with highly satisfied patients, who do not want an invasive technique and this one is performed in a few minutes.

COMPLICATIONS: only hematomas.

RESULTS are good and long lasting. Patients are very happy.

2.1.1.4.2. With fiberlift®

Fiberlift® is a triple anchorage polypropylene 3.0 30cm divergent barbed thread that is used to lift the eye brow tail. The technique is very simple with only a small incision of 0.5 to 1 cm. at the coronal line. Fiberlift is a procedure of double entrance and triple anchorage. We use a 21 G x2 needle and enter twice. The first entrance of the needle is AC and the second is BC. We put the divergent barbed thread from C to A in the first step and from C to B in the second step. In this way the thread has the first anchorage in C point. The divergent cogs picture the second anchorage and the last one is given by a sub-galea knot in the temporal zone. This method is very good to lift the eye brow, opening the eyes and smoothing the periorbital lines. Patients like it very much. Initially, we have seen few complications. Pain and persistent folds are improving with practice.

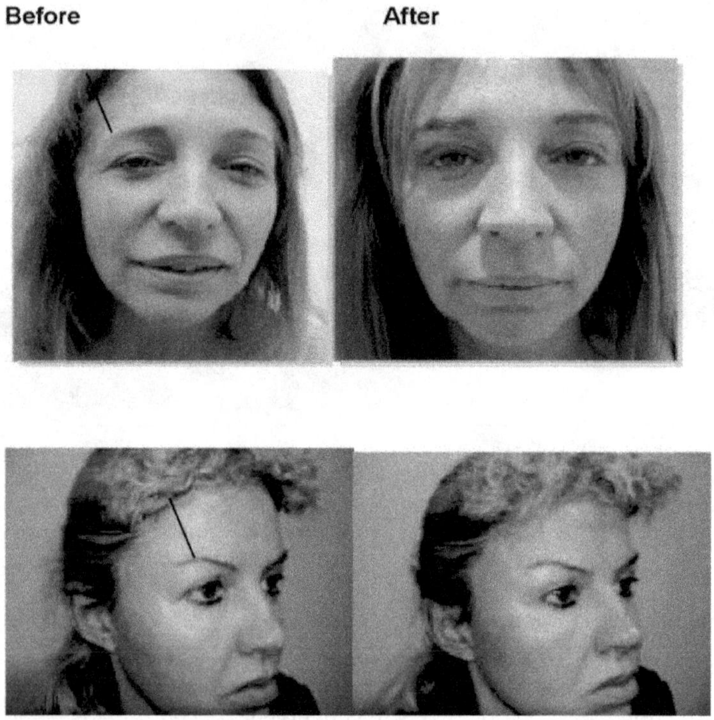

Source: Own elaboration based on pictures from personal archive

Figure 19. Direction of the Firming thread to lift the eye brow. Results

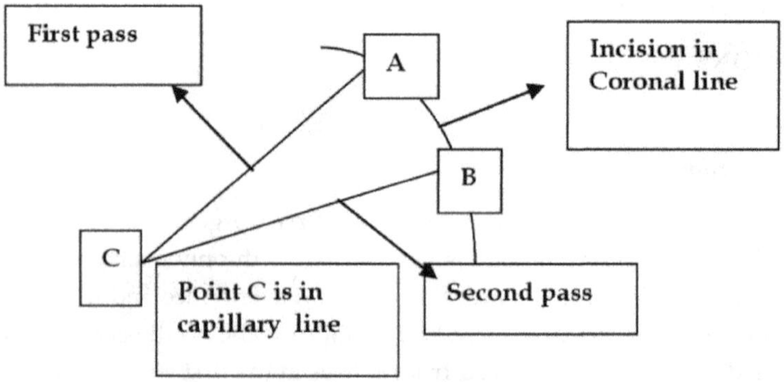

Source: Own elaboration

Scheme 2. Placement of Fiberlift®

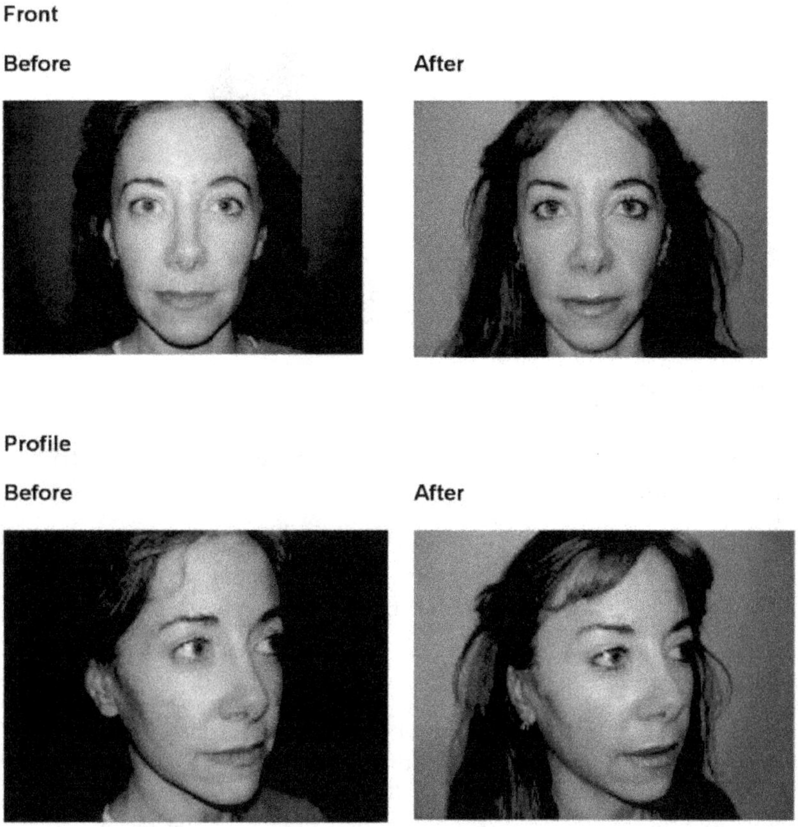

Source: Own elaboration based on pictures from personal archive

Figure 20. Upper Face Lift with Fiberlift® Results

2.1.1.4.3. Complications

In two cases we found a decubitus ulcer that needed surgical treatment.

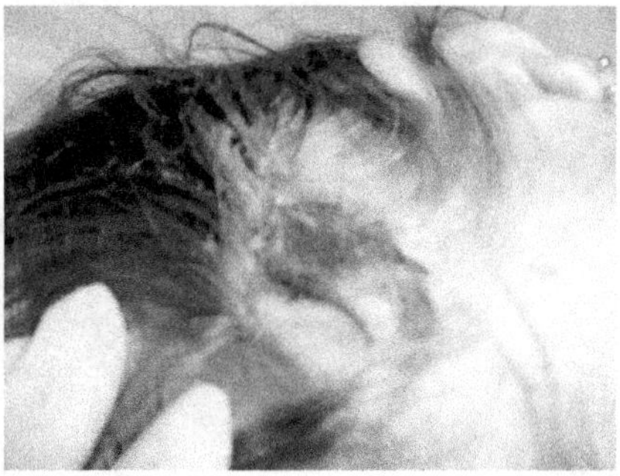

Source: Personal archive

Figure 21. Decubitus ulcer

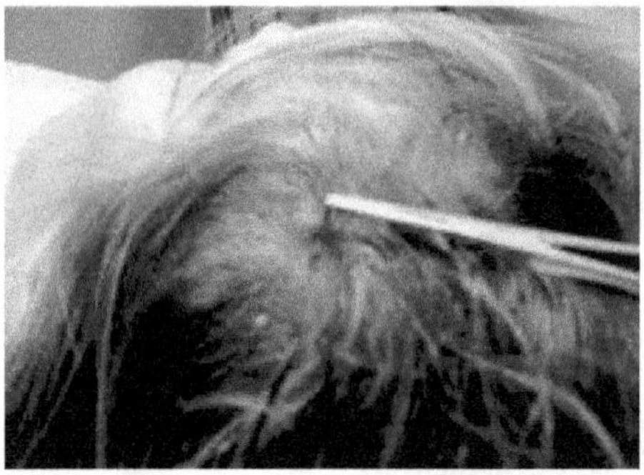

Source: Personal archive

Figure 22. Extrusion of Fiberlift® thread

2.2. Serdev sutures – Serdev methods: Temporal face lift, eye brow lift, medial face lift and chin enhancement

These techniques, created by Nikolay Serdev use semi-elastic polycaproamide, long term absorbable (2-3 years), braided, antimicrobial, Bulgarian materials, called Serdev Sutures. With Serdev's methods we can lift one mobile tissue and carry it to a non movable point.

2.2.1. Temporal face lift without incisions

The Temporal face lift with Serdev sutures not only lifts the soft tissue of the upper face and the zygomatic zone but it also reflects a lifting of the lower face. The results cover in a complete way 'lifting' without an incision. It is significant to know the location of the temporal zone to prevent damage to the temporal branch of the facial nerve. It is very important for us to outline the temporal zone.[8]

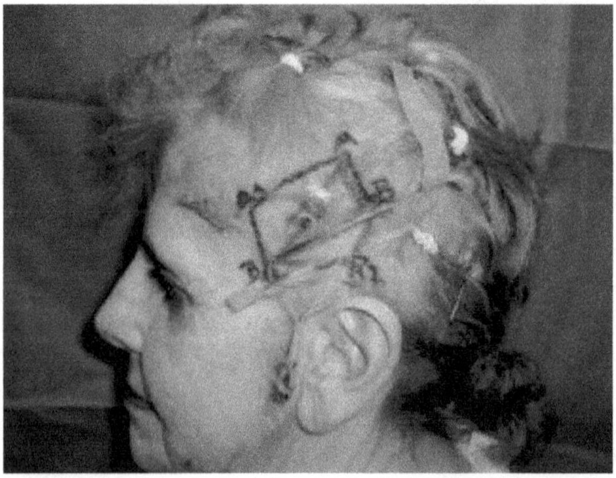

Source: Personal archive

Figure 23. Marcation for temporal face lift

In this outline we have marked with green a second lift treatment, in the same temporal zone to optimize the result. In this case there were another four passes (AB1, B1B2, B2B and B2B)

2.2.1.1. Technique

Insert the suture with a special, curved, semielastic, small or mini Serdev's needle with a tip hole. The passes are A-A1, thread the suture and leave. Go B1A1, thread the suture and leave, then BB1 thread the suture and leave and finally AB, thread the suture, knot it and cut. The passes AA1 and BB1 are sub-galea, the pass A1B1 is sub-dermic, and the last AB is sub-fascia. In this way the SMAS is lifted and fixed to the temporalis fascia.

2.2.1.2. Results

We can see an improvement in the aspect of the face: the eye brows, the skin and the eyes with a change in the tired expression of the face with no traces of an operation. The results of this technique are immediate and the patient's satisfaction is high.

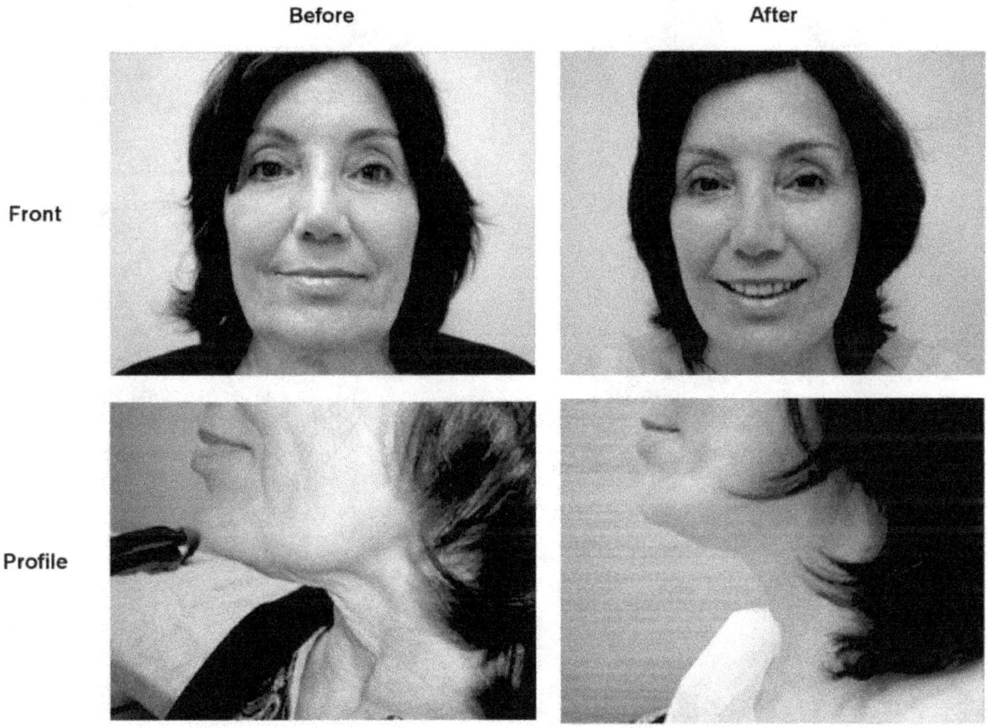

Source: Own elaboration based on pictures from personal archive

Figure 24. Temporal Face Lift with Serdev Sutures Results

2.2.1.3. Complications

Initially, we have seen skin dimpling, pain, edema of the upper face, hematoma below the eye. Skin dimpling is treated with one branch of the "mosquito" claw (Serdev). Pain is tolerable and patients can take analgesics. The edema and hematomas were produced by mistake in the surgical plane of needle puncture and suture insertion. Today, with the experience of 6 years of daily practice with this technique, complications are not significant.

2.2.2. Eye brow lift with Serdev sutures and Serdev method

This method is very simple and fast. It was described by Nikolay Serdev in 1994, [9] without incisions, only a needle perforation between the eye brow hairs. Thus, it is possible to carry

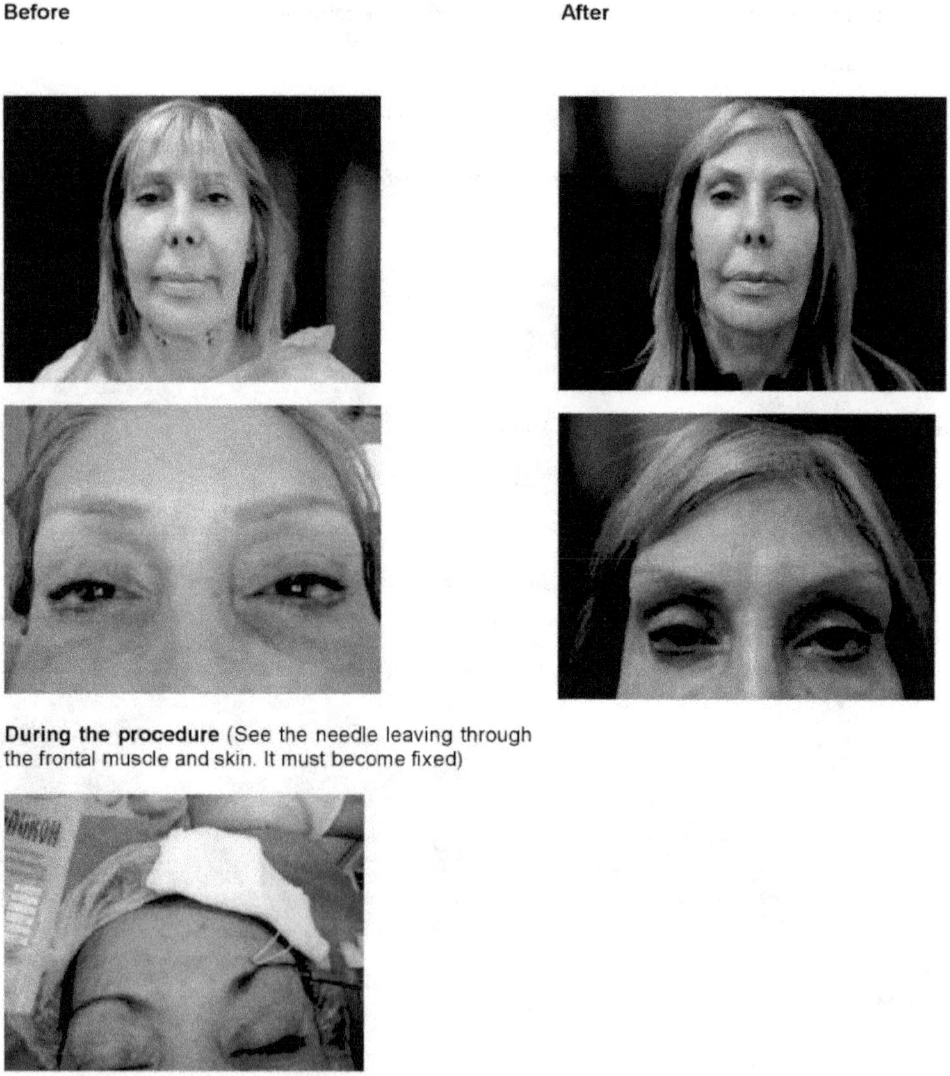

Source: own elaboration based on pictures from personal archive

Figure 25. Eye brow lift with Serdev Sutures and Serdev Method Results the subdermal tissue to the bone periosteum and fix it, using a Serdev suture and a special semi elastic small (mini-mini) needle with a tip hole. The secret for success is not to be afraid of being aggressive in fixing the subdermal tissue to the bone periosteum (Serdev's 2007 Course in Sophia on Serdev Techniques.)

The procedure consists of two steps; using lidocaine 2% with epinephrine in each of the two points that we'll use (positioning previously 1cm above of the orbital rim).

2.2.2.1. First step

Enter in point A with semi elastic, mini Serdev needle. The incision is made with the tip of a Nº 11 scalpel. Get the bone periosteum with the needle tip down and leave through the frontal muscle and skin with the tip up; needle must become fixed, if it is not fixed it could be improperly located in a wrong plane. Thread the suture and remove the needle.

2.2.2.2. Second step

The 2nd needle pass is superficial, it goes through the lower dermis from point A to point B. Then a knot is made with medium tension. The dimpling is removed with a branch of the mosquito claw.

It is a very interesting method with very good and long lasting results. Initially I didn't have good results due to the incorrect position of the needle. It is very important to take the periosteum with the tip down and then turn the needle with the tip up. In 5 years I have only had one complication with a knot extrusion. In that case the suture used was a Nº2 instead of a Nº0. It was removed and replaced by the correct one.

2.2.3. Medial face lift with Serdev sutures

I use only one of the several alternatives that Serdev describes for this method. It is to lift loose medial SMAS and to fix it to the stable zygomatic periosteum. Point A (entrance and fixation) is located in the zygoma 1 cm below the lateral cantus of the eye so the zygomatic periosteum is caught. In this method a Serdev semi elastic, curved needle size small and Serdev elastic braided antimicrobial polycaproamide are used.[10]

2.2.3.1. First step

The needle enters in point A through the bone periosteum and exits in a parallel line beside the nasolabial fold in one of three points that Serdev describes according to the age of the patient.

2.2.3.2. Second step

The needle enters in point A and passes superficially through the soft tissue and exits in point B describing a circle around the zygoma and zygomatic SMAS extension. Then, a knot is made with medium tension. In this way it gives new volume to the cheek bone. It is a good ambulatory method, with good results but at first patients sometimes don't accept it due to the formation of dimples. I haven't seen complications except for some dimples that patients didn't like and there has been only one case of asymmetry. The dimples disapeared in two weeks and the asymmetry, caused by exaggerated tension, was corrected by removing and replacing the suture.

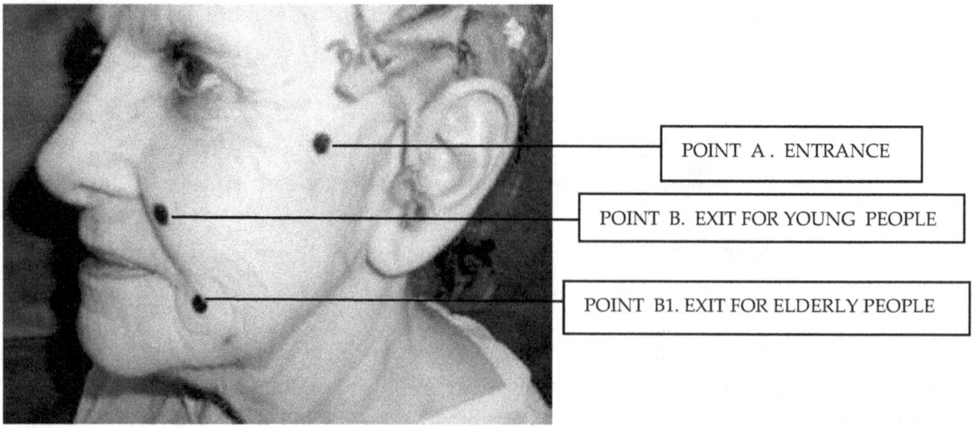

Source: Personal archive

Figure 26. Medial Face Lift Technique with Serdev Sutures

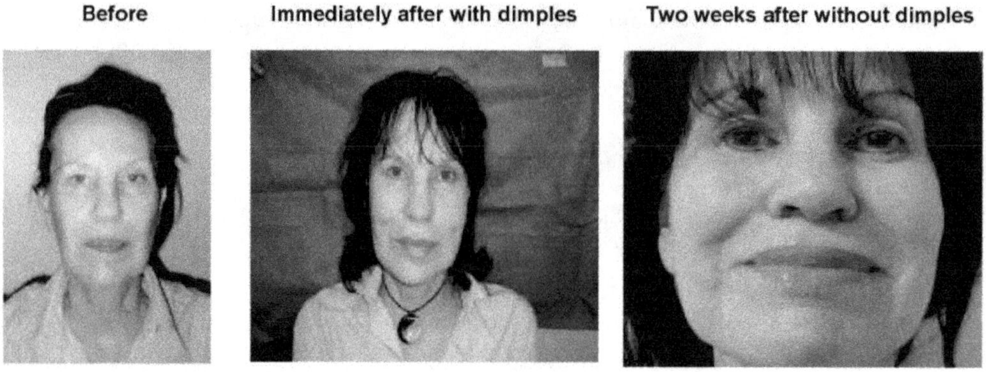

Source: Own elaboration based on pictures from personal archive

Figure 27. Medial Face Lift with Serdev Sutures Results

2.2.4. Chin augmentation using Serdev sutures

The form and position of the chin is very important in the correct and harmonic face proportions and beauty features. It is common to see chin disproportions such as micrognathia aging, asymmetries, etc. Nikolay Serdev proposes a simple technique using non barbed suture to correct these chin disharmonies. The procedure is simple using a small semi-elastic, curve needle with a tip hole and a thin Serdev suture. The entrance may be in point A or B and the exit in the other.

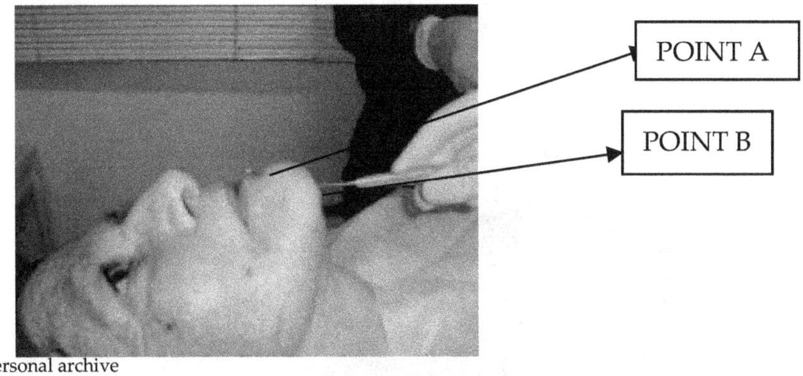

Source: Personal archive

Figure 28. Chin augmentation technique with Serdev Sutures

The aim is to create a circle around the chin's soft tissue, there are two steps to follow. The first pass is depth, entering in point A, going along the mandibular line, exiting in point B, threading the suture and removing the needle.[11] The second pass is done by entering point A but in a more superficial way by going under the skin and leaving through point B in the skin. The knot is done here. If there is dimpling in the skin, it is corrected with the mosquito branch (Serdev). The results are excellent and fast. The patients are satisfied. No complications.

2.3. Threads and sutures in body lift

2.3.1. Barbed threads in body lift

The objective of these techniques are to give a lift effect to the soft tissue of the arms, inner thigh, abdominal zone and outer thigh when there have been sequelae with liposuction effects. They are good for treating flaccid or aging areas. All methods are performed without incisions and without scars. They are simple and fast, obtaining good results, with medium and long term duration due to the new collagen fibers that are generated around each thread and each cog of them.

2.3.1.1. Arm lift

2.3.1.1.1. Materials

We use MULTIFIX THREADS, multifix 12 cm nonabsorbable 2.0 polypropylene with multidirectional cogs. We insert them under the skin in the fat tissue. 4 threads or more can be inserted depending on the size of the arm.

2.3.1.1.2. Procedure

Begin with the marcation three fingers below the axilla. Prior to procedure inject lidocaine 2% with epinephrine in the skin, just 0.5cc in each point is enough.

Do the insertion with a 21 Gx3 needle (spinal needle) beginning from the external point to the internal one, repeating the same procedure many times as necessary. The thread is

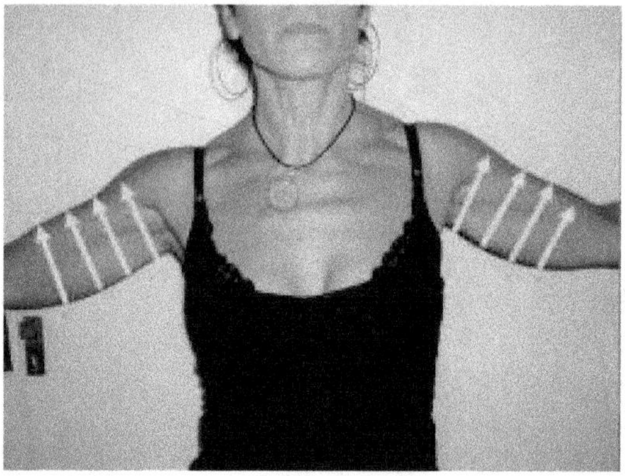

Source: Personal archive

Figure 29. Arms lift

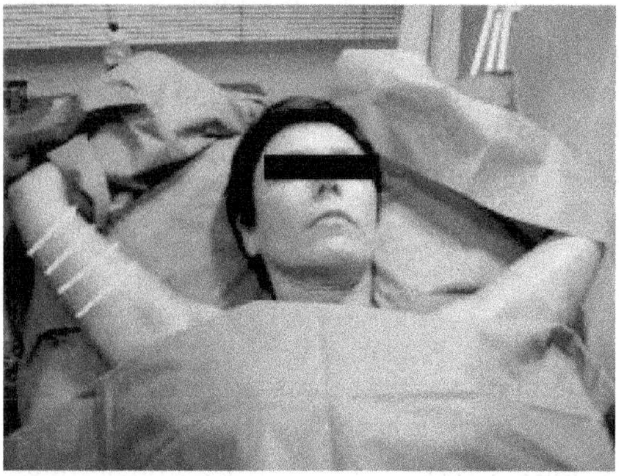

Beware of the humeral artery

Source: Personal archive

Figure 30. Arms lift – Procedure

positioned and anchoraged with a simple and delicate movement with the hand using a Halsted claw and pulling gently in both directions. Then we cut the ends of the thread by pushing the skin down to uncover the thread's end, avoiding a long thread. We use bandages or tight sleeves for 10 days. Nsaids and analgesics are indicated for three days.

RESULTS are good, it is a fast and long lasting procedure.

2.3.1.1.3. Complications

Pain and edema, have been seen. Sometimes a bump under the skin because of the length of the thread. We have had some extrusions in three patients. Bumps under the skin are the most common complications and are corrected by cutting the end of the thread. If it is in the correct position (fix and anchorage), it's not necessary to remove it, if that is the case only cut the end. If the thread is loose it would be convenient to remove it.

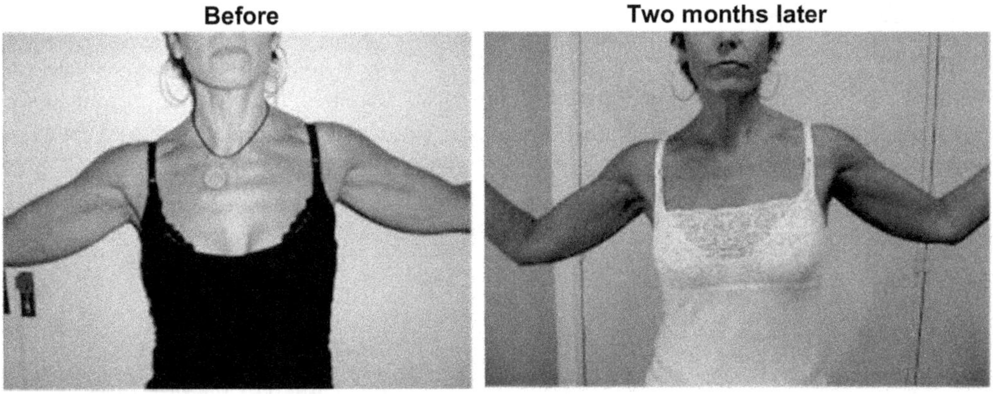

Source: Own elaboration based on pictures from personal archive

Figure 31. Arm Lift with Barbed Threads Results

2.3.1.2. Inner thigh

The inner thigh is a flaccid and aging area that may be improved with 2.0 polypropylene multifix barbed threads with multidirectional cogs. It is a simple application done with a long 21Gx3.5 needle in the fat tissue thickness. We must be careful with the femoral artery and vein as well as with the saphen intern vein. The femoral artery can often be palpated through the skin in the inner thigh at the mid-inguinal-point, halfway between the pubic symphysis and anterior superior iliac spine. [12]

2.3.1.2.1. Procedure

Application of at least 4 threads for each side, from external (A) to internal (B) point using a 21Gx3.5 needle (spinal), being careful when cutting the ends and using an elastic compression for a week.

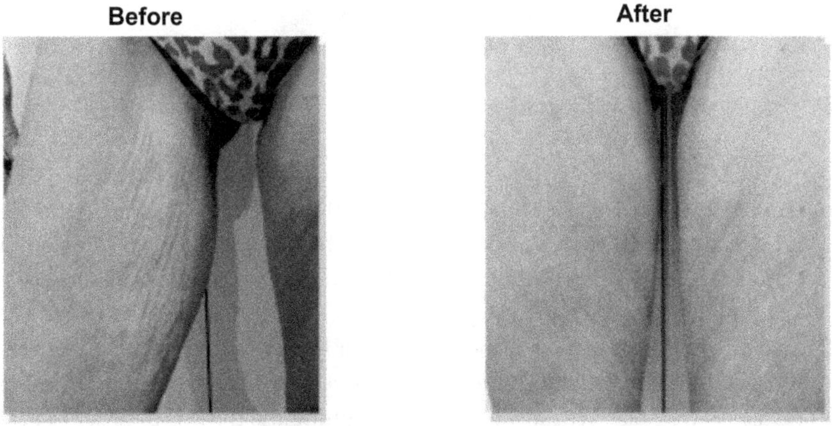

Source: Own elaboration based on pictures from personal archive

Figure 32. Inner Thigh Lift with Barbed Threads Results

2.3.1.2.2. Results

Results are very interesting, patients accept this technique. It allows them to see themselves better as well as returning immediately to their social activities. It is very important to see the changes in the general physiognomy of the skin, produced by the stimulation of collagen formation. This method is easy, fast and with a long lasting time span. In accordance with my experience, I believe the inner thigh is the best place to insert barbed multifix threads in body lift treatment.

2.3.1.3. Front and upper face of the knee

2.3.1.3.1. Materials

The upper and anterior face of the knee share with the inner thigh as the best places to lift with barbed threads. I usually use 2.0 polypropylene antimicrobial multifix barbed threads with multidirectional cogs, 12 cm length and 2.0 polypropylene antimicrobial Firming barbed threads with bidirectional cogs, 8 or 10 cm length. Multifix are inserted in a vertical form and Firming (bidirectional cogs) is used on a horizontal line.

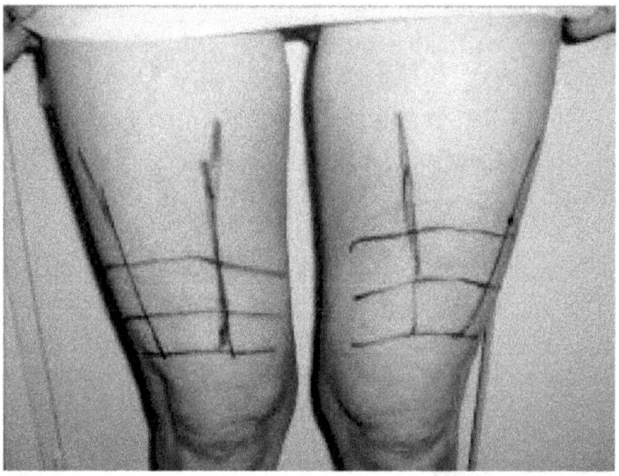

Source: Personal archive

Figure 33. Marcation for front and upper face of the knee lift

2.3.1.3.2. Procedure

It's a simple procedure, using only local anesthesia (lidocaine 2%with epinephrine) at the entrance and exit points; 0.5cc in each one. The insertion is carried out with two kinds of needles a 21 Gx2 is used to insert Firming threads and a 21 Gx3.5 is used to insert Multifix threads. This technique consists of two steps. In the first step insert Firming threads in parallel lines and in a horizontal position place the fat tissue of the anterior thigh 3 or 4 fingers above the knee. In the second step Multifix threads are inserted in diagonal form crossing over the Firming threads. As we finish we have to be careful cutting the threads in order to avoid long threads pricking from within. The use of an elastic compression or tight panties is suggested for a week.

RESULTS are very good. Patients are satisfied with the change in the skin and the improvement of irregularities in the tissue caused by flaccidity.

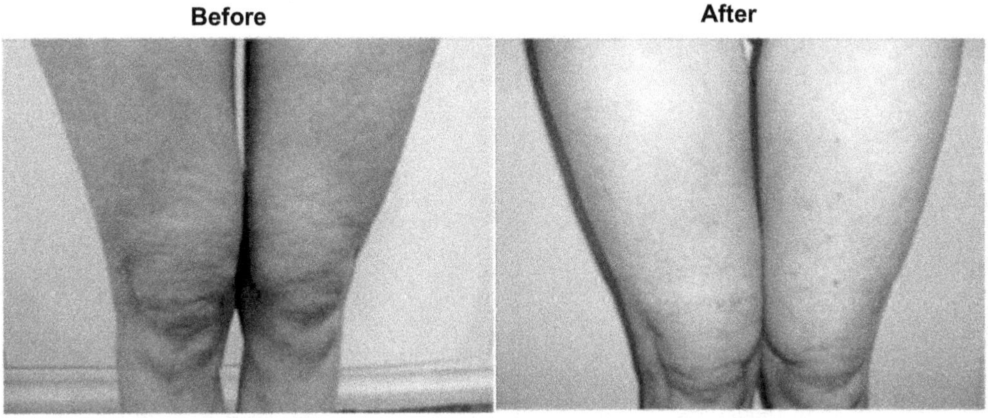

Source: Own elaboration based on pictures from personal archive

Figure 34. Front and upper face of the knee lift with Barbed Threads and Multifix Results

2.3.2. Serdev sutures in body lift

2.3.2.1. Buttock lift

I have experience in buttock lift with Serdev sutures and Serdev's technique. It is a very interesting method to lift buttocks that are flaccid. This is a mini invasive procedure without scars and with a short postoperative. A description of the subject was made by Nikolay Serdev in 2003, in Sophia, Bulgaria. It is an ambulatory procedure and it achieves the reposition of the buttock's subdermal fat tissue by lifting it and increasing its volume and anteroposterior diameter using only a suture that grasps the deep fibrous tissue and fixes it to the upper zone in the gluteus maximus fascia in its sacrum insertion. [13]

We prefer to use the Argentine modified Serdev technique (J. Ferreira, Buenos Aires 2004) due to the gluteus shape of Argentine women. [14] This technique has 3 steps as in the original Serdev's method:

First step: with the patient in a sitting position I mark the lower limit.

Second step: with the patient in ventral decubitus I draw the internal and lower points some centimeters above the inferior limit and 2 or 3 cm from the anus. There is another lateral point, the same as in liposuction. The higher point or sacrum point is in the middle line at the begining of the gluteal fold.

Third step: we then proceed to measure and to check the symmetries, drawing a print line between the three points to give the rounded desired form. It's important for me to draw the inferior limit so as to avoid a long term post-operative pain.

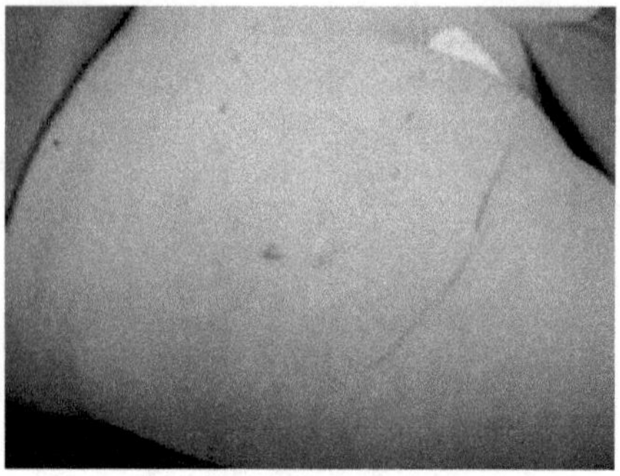

Source: Personal archive

Figure 35. Buttock lift. Marcation

2.3.2.1.1. Procedure

Antisepsis is done, the perianal zone is covered by a sterile gauze. Anesthesia with lidocaine 2% with epinephrine in each point where small incisions between 3 to 4mm will be perfomed with a number 11 scalpel blade. Klein solution is injected with a 2mm cannula into the deep fat tissue which lies on the superficial surface from the maximus gluteus fascia. A way is marked where the path of the Serdev needle will proceed.

We work with a hollow protector in lateral and inferior incision points to avoid taking superficial skin with the needle thus producing a "dimple" on the surface.

The procedure is carried out with a special needle developed by Nikolay Serdev. It is 20 cm, flexible and semi-curved with a top orifice, it is also a polycaproamide, elastic, antimicrobial Bulgarian suture. A liposuction is previously performed on the outer thigh to reduce the volume and weight of the gluteus.

First pass: from external incision to medial or a sacrum one in the shape of an arch with a Serdev needle. We thread the suture and remove the needle leaving out the ends of the suture. Second pass: from inferior perianal incision to the lateral one. Thread the suture and remove the needle.

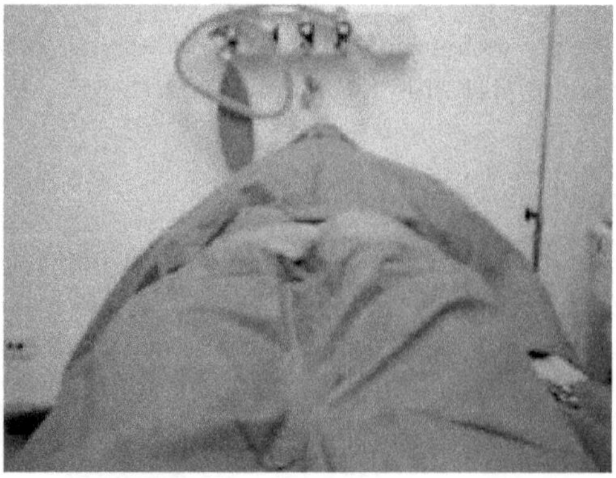

Buttock lift of only one side done

Source: Personal archive

Figure 36. Buttock lift only one side done

Finally we go from the sacrum incision to the inferior internal point and thread the suture, then we remove the needle and we can observe both ends of the suture in the sacrum incision. Adjust the suture to give it the desired form and height and make some surgical knots. Finish by closing the skin with a nylon 5.0 and a micropore.

2.3.2.1.2. Results

The results are very interesting and patients are satisfied. I have performed 104 procedures; 103 were women and only 1 man. The patients were between 20 and 65 years old. A 40% of these were combined with liposuction of the outer thigh. All patients were satisfied with the results.

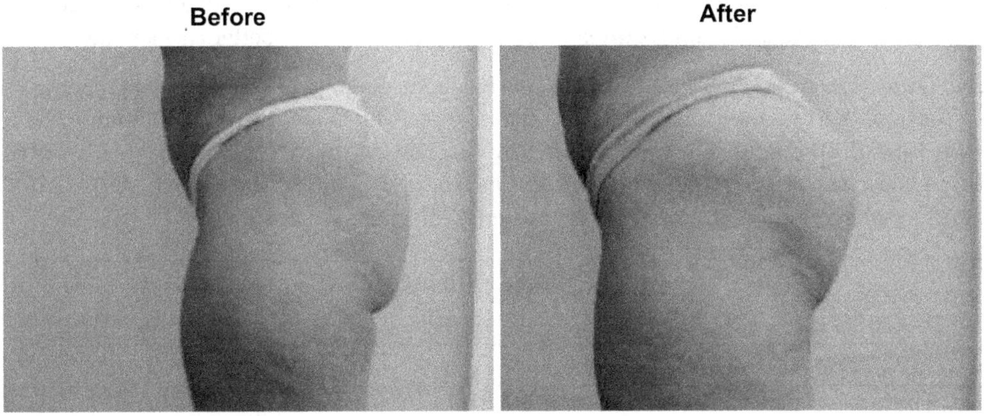

Source: Own elaboration based on pictures from personal archive

Figure 37. Buttock Lift Results

2.3.2.1.3. Complications

There are few complications; such as skin dimples or assimetries due to different tensions found in both gluteus. Pain was the most frequent undesired effect. It had a duration of 15 days and it was treated with Nsaids and analgesics. Every patient had been prescribed with antibiotics. There were neither infections nor hematomas.

2.3.2.1.4. Comparison of both methods, barbed threads and non barbed Serdev sutures

Both methods, barbed threads and non barbed Serdev sutures, are excellent for mini invasive techniques. Patients are satisfied with both of them. Complications are rare and the lifting effect range from good to excellent.

We have found –after 10 years of barbed thread experience and 6 years of Serdev sutures–, that lifting effect is higher with Serdev sutures, patients recover forms, angles and the tissue is repositioned without "operated look." They also improve adding a higher volume and contour. The collagen and elastic fibers generation are very important with barbed threads, improving the skin of the face, giving it light and a glow.

In an experimental study of the morphological changes in tissue with barbed threads carried out by Sulamanidze and co-writers (2002) in order to clarify the mechanism of tissue ptosis correction, it was seen in rats when polyprpopylene barbed threads were inserted subdermally and were compared with non barbed polypropylene in control rats with serial skin biopsies. It was noted that the barbed threads had elicited an earlier inflammatory response followed by a vascular proliferation and fibroblastic reaction thus creating a new collagen generation along the threads and along each barbs. In the case of non-barbed threads in rats it was found (Truswell 2008)[15] that there was neither found a collagen generation nor a vascular proliferation nor an inflammatory response nor a fibroblastic reaction.

Volume and contour were seen with Serdev suture and barbed threads in a less degree. "Z" insertion of Firming and Multifix threads has generated a new and better cheek bone.

The improvement in 1 year is important for both methods as well as the patient's satisfaction. Both methods have no post-operative recovery time. Pain is minimum in both procedures. In the field of complications we can mention that with barbed threads we've seen some cases of migration and some extrusions of the end of the thread. With Serdev sutures we have sometimes seen pain in the temporal zone.

	BARBED THREADS	SERDEV SUTURES
LIFTING EFFECT	++	++++
COLLAGEN GENERATION	+++	+
VOLUME	+	+++
CONTOUR	++	+++
IMPROVE IN ONE YEAR	+++	+++
PATIENT SATISFACTION	+++	+++
POSTOPERATIVE RECOVERY TIME	___	___
PAIN	+	+
COMPLICATIONS	+	+

Source: Own elaboration

Table 1. Comparative chart Barbed Threads vs. Serdev Sutures

2.3.2.1.5. Combined techniques

It is very interesting to combine both methods using barbed threads in the lower third and temporal face lift with Serdev sutures. With this combination we can get fantastic results of the lifting effect and collagen generation. To optimize the contour with temporal face lift with sutures and barbed threads in the neck zone, improving the smoothing effect too. In my daily practice I usually perform a combined formula with temporal face lift and barbed threads insertion in the medium and in the lower third and neck. I can also add one barbed thread in each eyebrow tail.

2.3.2.1.6. Complementary methods

The combination of these methods is very important, with the use of barbed threads and non barbed sutures, and other rejuvenation and beautification techniques as BOTOX, Fillers, IPL, Peelings, Laser, Oxygenesis and Mesotherapy. It's specially interesting Botox application treatment in the lower third as complement of threads. We inject the botulinum toxin in both platysm bands and jawline. Also may be injected into the orbicularis angle depressor muscle to elevate the commisures [16].

3. Discussion

Since the beginning of mankind men and women have always seeked ways to preserve beauty and the fountain of youth. Beauty has always been portrayed through art where you will find the most beautiful features which are in harmony with perfect proportions. In such natural and beautiful forms, why should harmony be altered? There are numerous methods to treat the aging face. Surgical techniques with cuts, pain, edema, scars, long postoperative time, often are used as a matter of surgeons satisfaction who do not even consider the genuine needs of their patients. Already in 1970 R Guillemain published on Curl Lift [17] but at the time the lift with cuts was well regarded by the patients who happily wore their scars. Today the patient ask for mini invasive procedures without scars nor pain and they want to return immediately to their activities. Aging treatments with threads and sutures are chosen for our patients, because they provide a natural effect.

4. Conclusion

In spite of having seen some extrusions, some migrations, some cases of pain or edema, whereas the simplicity of these procedures, the good and natural results that may be seen, the long lasting, the no post-operative time, the few complications and the high satisfaction of the patients we think that threads and sutures are a great answer to our patient's modern life exigencies and their wish: "don't cut". Patient's understanding of these techniques is very important. We are convinced that these procedures are a very good way path in the current cosmetic surgery and the most requested among our patients.

Author details

Vilma L. Padín
CEMEC (Center of Aesthetic Medicine and Surgery), Buenos Aires, Argentine Republic
AIMERA (International Association of Aesthetic Medicine), Argentine Republic

Acknowledgement

I would very much like to thank Professor Nikolay Serdev for allowing me to write this chapter. Dr. Serdev introduced me and opened the way to the fascinating field of the mini-invasive techniques of facial and body lifting.

5. References

[1] Sulamanidze, M. et al., "Removal of facial tissue ptosis with special threads", *Dermatological Surgery* 28 (2002):367-371.

[2] Bacci, P., *Cirugía Estética Mínimamente Invasiva con Hilos Tensores* (Caracas; Amolca, 2008).

[3] SERDEV, N., "Scarless 'APTOS' & 'SERDEV SUTURE' Lifting Methods", *International Journal of Cosmetic Surgery* 4 (2004); 1-10.

[4] Sulamanidze M., Sulamanidze G.,"Avoiding Complications with Aptos Sutures" Aesthetic Surgery,…,2011

[5] Lycka B. et al., "The emerging technique of the antiptosis subdermal suspension thread", *Dermatological Surgery* 30 (2004): 41-44.

[6] Padin, V., "Tratamiento de la Flaccidez Facial con Aplicación de Hilos", *Revista Argentina de Rinología y Cirugía Facial* 1 (2005): 35-44.

[7] Serdev, N., "Ambulatory Temporal SMAS Lift by Sutures with or without Incisions", *International Journal of Cosmetic Surgery* 1 (2001); 97-106.

[8] Serdev, N., "A Suture Method for Scarless Brow Lift", *International Journal of Cosmetic Surgery* 1 (2001); 1-15.

[9] Serdev, N., "Serdev Suture Method for Ambulatory Medial SMAS Face Lift", *International Journal of Cosmetic Surgery* 2 (2002); 1-13.

[10] Serdev, N., "Chin enhancement and form correction using a suture of the soft tissue", *International Journal of Cosmetic Surgery* 2 (2002);16-25.

[11] Padin, V.," Dermosustentación con hilos en miembros inferiores" (presented at the II International Simposium of mini invasive procedures in Flebology, Buenos Aires, Argentina, October 2009,Medicine Faculty, Buenos Aires University).

[12] Serdev, N., "Buttock Lifts. Part I: Ambulatory Buttock Lift Using a Suture Without Incision Scars", *International Journal of Cosmetic Surgery* 2 (2002); 1-7.

[13] Ferreira, J. and Padin, V., "Lifting Glúteo con Tensores Naturales. Hilos Reafirmantes: La Gran Solución No Quirúrgica", *Portal Medestética,* 2005, accessed April 16th 2012 http://www.medestetica.com.ar/informes/informehilos.pdf

[14] Truswell, W. Surgical facial Rejuvenation: A Roadmap to Safe and Reliable Outcomes, October 25, 2008 I ISBN-10: 1588904911 I ISBN-13: 978-1588904911 I Edition: 1

[15] Padin, V. and Lopez Mecle, V., "Mejores Prácticas mínimamente invasivas para el tratamiento del tercio medio e inferior del rostro y el cuello", in Mejores Prácticas en Rejuvenecimiento Facial, ed. Allergan Academy (Buenos Aires: Allergan Press, 2011), 88-113.

[16] Guillemain, R. Le "Curl Lift" :, le Profession Medical,chirr. Plast.E Recon ;Mars 1970

CPSIA information can be obtained
at www.ICGtesting.com
Printed in the USA
BVHW012113190622
640150BV00003B/56

9 789535 111962